D0907116

The Investigative Enterprise

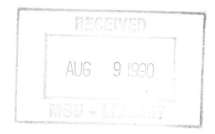

The Investigative Enterprise

Experimental
Physiology in
Nineteenth-Century
Medicine

Edited by
William Coleman
and
Frederic L. Holmes

UNIVERSITY OF CALIFORNIA PRESS
Berkeley • *Los Angeles* • *London*

In Memoriam

William Coleman, 1934–1988

For his scholarship, his buoyant spirit, and courageous example he set for all who knew him and worked with him.

*QP
21
.I58
1988*

University of California Press
Berkeley and Los Angeles, California

University of California Press, Ltd.
London, England

LIBRARY OF CONGRESS CATALOGING IN PUBLICATION DATA

The Investigative enterprise.

  Includes bibliographical references and index.
  1. Physiology, Experimental—History—19th century.
I. Coleman, William, 1934–   II. Holmes,
Frederic Lawrence.
QP21.I58   1988   612'.0-072'4   87-19207
ISBN 0-520-06048-2 (alk. paper)

1 2 3 4 5 6 7 8 9

16578354

*10-15-90
Ac*

Contents

Introduction

William Coleman and Frederic L. Holmes

At the core of the activity we call science is the systematic investigation of delimited aspects of the natural world. Despite the transformations that have altered scientific thought, changed the modes of scientific practice, and called forth new forms of scientific organization, investigation has always been the pivot around which scientific life revolves. Defined narrowly, scientific investigation may seem to consist of reasoning, observation, and experimentation directed at particular problems. Investigative activity, however, inevitably involves much more. Investigators must have access to workplaces, whether these be sea or sky, field or forest, desk and library, laboratory or museum. For all but the simplest or most theoretical of investigations, material resources—at a minimum, instruments, apparatus, and supplies—are a prerequisite. Investigations are not carried out by isolated individuals and never have been, for in one way or another every investigator has been linked to others with similar interests through some form of social organization. Sustained investigative activity has always included an educational function; otherwise one generation of investigators would have no successors. From its start the investigation of nature has suggested applications of the knowledge gained, usually for the welfare of other persons, and has therefore formed connections with social structures beyond the immediate community of scientific investigators.

Historians of science have made sharp distinctions between scientific activity defined in its narrowest sense and its broader dimensions. Pairs of contrasting terms such as "internal and external factors," "science and its context," "science and its institutional framework," or "cognitive processes and social processes" have been used to draw lines of demarcation between perceived inner and outer aspects of the totality of science. The title of the present volume suggests a different approach, one that avoids the artificial boundaries that might be assumed to exist within what is in reality a nexus of overlapping, interlocking thoughts, actions, and conditions. "The investigative enterprise" may, of course, be traced along the fine scale of the single scientist engaged in his or her day-by-day thoughts and operations; yet it extends, too, throughout the network of cognitive, operational, organizational, social, and cultural strands stretching from each investigator to larger or smaller groups of individuals active in or beyond the domain of study in which he or she works. Designing each day's research plan is obviously intrinsic to the investigative enterprise, and it is often a collective act. So, too, is obtaining the support of those agencies that provide the material resources necessary to carry out such plans. For analytical purposes the network, or set of networks, may be dissected into sectors, as is done in the essays contained in this volume. Nonetheless we emphasize that the distinctions so easily drawn between, for example, research and pedagogy, professional and state interests, and scientific activity and institutional frameworks should be recognized as only heuristically useful categories. In the investigative enterprise these boundaries are commonly indistinct and frequently unreal.

The essays that follow explore aspects of the investigative enterprise within a domain loosely bounded by physiology and its connections with medicine during the nineteenth century. The facets of nature encompassed by this field—the structure and functions of the human or animal body and their implications for health and disease—are among the oldest subjects of systematic investigation within the Western cultural tradition. In the fourth century B.C. the Hippocratic treatise *On Ancient Medicine* asserted that studies of human nutrition, carried on over a long prior period, had cumulatively added to knowledge of the diets most suitable for healthy and sick individuals. Aristotle's biological writings reveal a wealth of anatomical knowledge about many types of animals which could have been gathered only through extensive observation and description. In Hellenistic Alexandria human anatomy and physiology were evidently the objects of systematic investigation, most of the details of which have since been lost.

Despite the common characterization of ancient science as aimed at the contemplation of nature rather than at practical control, it is evident that within the anatomical-physiological domain the knowledge gained was medically and in turn socially important. The dietary rules reached by the Hippocratic physicians affected the lives of all who came within their medical orbit. The detailed, accurate knowledge of anatomy acquired through the investigations culminating in the second century A.D. in the work of Galen was deemed crucial to competent surgery.

Anatomy and physiology within a medical context played a prominent part also in the revival of the systematic investigation of nature during the Renaissance. The example of Vesalius and his successors during the sixteenth century is sufficiently compelling. From the seventeenth and eighteenth centuries we can point to a series of brilliant physiological investigations, ranging from William Harvey's discovery of the circulation of the blood, the studies of respiration by his followers, and Marcello Malpighi's microscopic investigations of the organs of the animal body, to Reaumur's and Spallanzani's experiments on digestion, Stephen Hales's measurements of the pressure of the blood, and Antoine Lavoisier's prolonged investigation of respiration. These investigations cannot be understood within the confines of reason and experiment alone, or as pursuits of isolated investigators. They were much broader enterprises and were conducted by scientists who interacted with one another through communication networks shaped by where they lived and worked, where they had studied, and how they published.

Physiological investigation in the nineteenth century continued these earlier traditions. What differentiated the new century from what had gone before is to be found less in modes of reasoning, observation, and experiment than in the scale of scientific activity. The memorable investigations of preceding centuries had been scattered and intermittent. Some were carried out within the framework of organized institutions, as in the case of the professors of anatomy in the sixteenth-century Italian university or in the Academy of Science in eighteenth-century France. Other researches were carried out by gifted amateurs, such as the Reverend Stephen Hales. Some of these investigations involved significant collaboration, but those who collaborated tended to come together in informal association.

During the nineteenth century experimental physiological investigation became intense and continuous, and it came to be pursued characteristically within institutional settings structured in whole or in part for that purpose. The material resources required to carry on physiological research became substantial and the need to work in groups pressing. The potential impact of physiological knowledge on health and disease had become powerful enough to attract the interest of the political world.

Along with many other areas of scientific endeavor, physiology emerged during the nineteenth century as a clearly demarcated discipline, a special field within the arena of natural science (in the German-speaking lands, of *Wissenschaft* or, more specifically, the *Naturwissenschaften*). To establish such a discipline required specialized research facilities. To sustain it required specialized pedagogical activity: the novice now had to be introduced systematically into the regularized practice of investigation. To support it required the argument (demonstration was a much more difficult affair) that physiological investigation would result in improved medical care, better nutrition, or other social benefits.

By means of a small set of selected examples of nodal events occurring in localized settings, the following essays explore major aspects of the development of nineteenth-century experimental physiology. The authors do not attempt a general survey of the period; rather, they examine at close range the intricate interplay among research programs, professional careers, institutional forms, pedagogical objectives, medical practice and training, and state or social interests.

William Coleman discusses the formation of the physiological institute in Breslau, generally viewed as the first of its kind in Germany. He focuses on the close bonds between the research program that Jan Purkyně initiated there and the pedagogical principles that he adapted from the educational reforms of Johann Pestalozzi. The Breslau Institute is central to an understanding of the spread of physiological research centers in Germany because it set precedents emulated later at other universities.

Arleen Tuchman describes reforms at the University of Heidelberg during the 1840s which established both a research institute for anatomy and physiology and a training program that introduced laboratory exercises into the education of all medical students. Jacob Henle, the central figure in these reforms, claimed that he was the first person to turn the microscope into a pedagogical tool used by the students themselves. Tuchman elucidates the way in which the interest of the state of Baden in modernization and in educational reform converged with Henle's plans, brought him to Heidelberg, and enabled him to implement such a program. A similar nexus of interests, according to Timothy Lenoir's essay, brought Carl Ludwig and a physiological institute to Leipzig in the 1860s. The Leipzig example is particularly important because Ludwig's institute became the leading center for research and training in physiology during the era when physiology became the prototypical experimental science associated with medicine. Again it served as a model for other institutes and, above all, became one of the greatest of all training centers for research physiologists.

Moving from Germany to France, the other leading center for experimental physiology in the nineteenth century, John Lesch corrects the widespread historical misperception that the Parisian medical establishment was indifferent to that activity. From its foundation in the 1820s, Lesch shows, the Academy of Medicine not only supported but sometimes participated in physiological experimentation intended to clarify problems relevant to medical practice.

Returning to Germany, Frederic L. Holmes portrays the formation of a distinctive school of physiology eventually housed within the Physiological Institute in Munich. Holmes attributes the shape of the investigative program that matured there to the scientific ideas and objectives of Justus Liebig, Theodor Bischoff, and Carl Voit. He notes, however, that this success was facilitated by a good fit between their plans and the ambition of the Bavarian monarch, Maximilian II, to make his capital a major center for learning.

Robert Frank focuses not on a local setting but on a long line of investigations of recording devices capable of representing graphically the beat of the heart. Frank is particularly concerned with the complex process by which an experimentally successful method may or may not turn out to be employed in clinical practice. The locus for these investigations shifted from place to place and from country to country, yet Frank shows that the local disciplinary interests of each investigator and the institutional arrangements within which each worked conditioned the nature of the investigation pursued.

Just as the particular research programs carried out in the institutions described in this volume were linked to investigative activities pursued elsewhere, so the institutions themselves were particular manifestations of organizational forms repeated in other centers of activity. From country to country, however, the institutional arrangements were more dissimilar than the investigative enterprises. The remainder of our introduction summarizes the general development of the German physiological institute and compares the situation in the German states to that in France.

The scientific institute belonged to the university, and in the nineteenth century the latter both expanded in number and enrollment and changed dramatically in character; the institute, not least the physiological institute, followed these changes. Over a span of three generations institutes were created in German universities to encourage the development of virtually all scientific, medical, and humanistic disciplines.[1] These institutes supported an often numerous staff. They usually possessed their own physical premises and gathered and maintained diverse and expensive equipment, including scientific apparatus and extensive library collections. Their budgets were often quite large. The university institute, and not least the physiological institute, was clearly a great engine of science. But what machinery did it drive? How was it conceived and how brought into being? What was done within its walls? What, in short, was its mission and what its product?

The fundamental fact regarding the physiological institute and one sometimes overlooked is its institutional place. It was an integral component of the medical faculty or its equivalent and not a constituent of the philosophical or arts faculty. In the philosophical faculty the institute served both to encourage the Humboldtian ideal of individual cultural formation (*Bildung*) and to prepare skilled professionals, the latter for the most part destined to offer instruction in the classical and modern languages and in mathematics in the rapidly expanding German secondary-school system. The institutes of the medical faculty prepared other professionals but did so in a manner not radically different from that of the leading humanistic institutes. A second, more familiar point is the physical setting that the scientific institute offered for research and instruction. A third feature, and one that will receive special emphasis in this volume, is the value system of the institute and the relation of these values to diverse medical, administrative, and pedagogical needs, a relation that set the physiological institute squarely within the framework of national political and economic ambitions and expectations. Like virtually all other scientific institutes, the physiological institute rep-

resented itself to the world as an essential foundation for free inquiry into the most complex scientific problems. This surely it was;
but the institute, like the entire university system, was also a public
institution and therefore served state as well as scientific interests.

With few exceptions the German university of the eighteenth century had been little more than the schoolroom raised to a somewhat
higher level. Latin stood at the core of the curriculum, and modern
subjects—vernacular languages and natural science—played a minor
role in comparison to study of the classics. Instruction was composed
principally of lectures and routine drill. Faculties were small and were
organized on the collegiate basis, exercising various degrees of self-
selection and self-regulation. Original research was not essential for
appointment to the professoriate, and most academics neither conducted such research nor wrote for a scholarly audience. Student
numbers were also small, and studies were pursued with an eye to a
relatively stable range of employment possibilities: service in public
administration, school teaching, law, medicine, and the clergy—
careers that in turn offered only a limited number of positions. Perhaps only those who could afford such a luxury, sons of the nobility
and of the more prosperous or influential members of the middle
classes, could contemplate university studies as an end in themselves, a pleasant enough way to acquire the finish of a gentleman
and perhaps some learning as well.

The exceptions to this rule, however, were important. The Prussian university at Halle was founded in 1694 to ensure a reliable
supply of skilled civil servants and to restore and maintain a sense of
devotion and responsibility in the Protestant clergy. Four decades
later the Hanoverian government created in Göttingen a radically
new kind of institution. Göttingen, too, emphasized classical studies, but it did so in a new way. Philological and historical seminars
were created and were guided by professors who had been selected
not because they were particularly distinguished as lecturers or worthy taskmasters in classroom exercise but because they had conducted and were expected to continue to conduct original research
in their areas of interest and expertise. The work of the seminar itself
formed an integral part of this research, the better-qualified student
sharing directly in the inquiry and often preparing a doctoral dissertation based on his studies. The humanistic seminar at Göttingen
(and also that at Halle) has been rightly looked upon as the forerunner of the scientific institute. The subjects studied were very differ-

ent, and research needs and physical facilities were no less different, but there was in common what proved to be the stimulus to and ultimate justification of the later scientific and medical institute— namely, a dedication on the part of both professor and student to original inquiry, a break from the traditional practices of schooling, and the idea that this inquiry was itself a new form of schooling. From the beginning seminar and institute were devoted to eliciting new knowledge and expanding the reach of that knowledge.

With the founding of the University of Berlin in 1810 and the wave of other foundings, refoundings, and university reforms that followed, the research ideal began to spread through the German university system. Institutes appeared in increasing numbers in the philosophical faculties and also in medical faculties. They met resistance from entrenched older members of these faculties, and sometimes they also met resistance from ministerial officials responsible for university affairs. The former were loath to lose the prerogatives of the old collegial system and were alarmed by the openly competitive character that the institute, its research function, and claims on the curriculum represented. The latter often encouraged university expansion and development of the specialized institutes; university officials worried, however, about the costs that the new programs entailed. Some institutes may have begun with small expenditures, but repeated demands for greater support soon revealed that the new university was going to require an unprecedented amount of money.

In physiology the ideal of experimental laboratory investigation was widely announced but only slowly realized. Experimental physiological inquiry was ancient and, as noted earlier, active in the seventeenth and eighteenth centuries. But it was in the nineteenth century that it rose to true prominence, becoming the very emblem of modernity and the aspiration of scientists and administrators throughout Germany and across Europe. Rudolf Virchow spoke for all medical specialties when, in 1847, he wrote of his own specialty: "Experiment is the final and highest court of pathological physiology, for experiment alone is equally accessible to the entire world of medicine, and experiment alone shows the specific phenomenon in its dependency on specific conditions, for these conditions are arranged by choice."[2] Relatively autonomous investigators, exemplified by such figures as François Magendie and Claude Bernard in France, John Hunter and Charles Bell in Britain, and Johannes

Müller and Jan Evangelista Purkyně in Prussia were gradually replaced in Germany at large after 1850 by research institutes in which
a group of researchers worked together, sometimes on a common
problem or set of problems and other times on a diversity of subjects. The institute phenomenon took root primarily in the German
university but appeared also in those universities that built on the
German example. By century's end the institute had become an
essential component of Scandinavian, Russian, eastern European,
Swiss, and Dutch universities. Late in the period the institute idea
crossed the ocean and stimulated major changes in university research and instruction in the United States.

The German physiological institute should be looked upon as the
tangible manifestation of a more active mode in the pursuit of physiological knowledge. As Virchow suggested, by establishing and then
varying the conditions under which specific vital functions are performed, the experimentalist exerts previously unattainable control
over these conditions and thereby gains access to phenomena previously beyond the reach of rigorous inquiry. Much physiological information could be and has been learned by means of deductions drawn
from anatomy and especially comparative anatomy. The 1830s added
to these inquiries microscopical examination of physiologically interesting questions—for example, the specific actions of ciliary tissues or
the structural-functional relations of the secretory capsules in the
kidney.

The physiological institute became the center for these studies.
Experimental work itself was highly varied, ranging from manipulation (for example, neural stimulation, leading to identification of the
action of the different spinal nerves) and organ extirpation (thus
exploitation of the "spinal frog," head removed and body prepared
for analysis of reflex behavior) to simple chemical analysis of body
ingesta and excreta or study of the metabolic activity of whole organs and organ systems. Much of this work was intrusive, involving
vivisection, organ isolation, and the application of a great variety of
chemical and physical stimuli. Repeatability and precision were supreme values in this work, and both were enhanced by the use of
increasingly elaborate apparatus. Indeed, most physiological activities take place rapidly, occur in all and often obscure parts of the
body, and involve numerous interrelated hierarchies of usually subtle changes. Access to these phenomena posed a formidable methodological problem. The conceptual and instrumental power of the

experimental approach offered assurance that one could, in fact, begin to seize the intimate detail of cellular life and related chemical processes.

The institute offered more than the staff and equipment needed for such work. It sustained an ethos for research, awarding discovery high honors and ensuring the discoverer, through the university appointment system, the prospect of advancement and ultimate independence—namely, appointment as director of his own institute and master of its research agenda. Working under the supervision of the director, usually also a professor of physiology in the medical faculty, would be one or more assistants, each with advanced scientific training and now just entering the regular academic succession. The institute also enjoyed the services of a technical staff in whose hands were placed animal preparation, chemical procedures, and the care of specialized equipment. The institute might house a few or occasionally many doctoral candidates whose research would be closely related to or an integral component of the director's own research. Guest researchers were also welcomed. They might stay for only a few weeks, gaining a sense of the institute's research program and learning new techniques, or they might remain for a longer period, carrying out work of their own. The institute was thus a complex social institution serving the needs of a diverse and sizable group of relatively advanced investigators.

None of these several groups or all taken together, however, equaled in numbers the primary clients of the institute: the medical students. Pure research was no doubt valued more highly by faculty and postdoctoral researchers than straightforward instruction. At the same time, these men realized—and their realization received strong reinforcement from administrators in the various educational ministries—that physiology was a subject of fundamental importance for the study of medicine and that every medical student must be introduced to the science in a systematic manner. Ordinarily the professor-director assumed responsibility for a basic course of lectures designed for beginning or intermediate medical students. These lectures were not offered casually: they were the institute's principal public expression of its mission. They also provided a current view of the status of the science, its discoveries, conclusions, and outstanding problems. Lecture responsibilities were heavy but could be immensely rewarding for all concerned. Leaders of the profession understood this point well. They recognized that instruction in the modern university must move beyond encyclopedic learning, repetition, and drill. The student must be brought to engage the phenomena himself (and, late in the century, herself). Thus the lecture might inform and stimulate, but only individual inquiry by the student could truly teach.

The student laboratory, still with us today, is a product of this conclusion, and the institute was the means by which the teaching laboratory attained its original form and its place in the curriculum. Located in the institute and making available an ever more opulent set of basic instruments, the physiological laboratory became a center for indoctrination and instruction. The student learned how to use this apparatus; he learned to ask questions on his own and to find that answers were not at all easy to come by; he learned to doubt the seeming assurance of everyday wisdom and of received knowledge.

At first glance this might seem a strange pedagogical program, especially for a professional faculty most of whose graduates would never turn to original research or participate in the teaching tasks of academic medicine. The program served the personal and research interests of the faculty, of course; without the enrollment of numerous medical students, the institute as we know it would not have received the generous public support that came its way. Disciplinary and professional ambitions thus played a large and expected role. But there was more. In Baden, for example, it is clear that the central medical and educational authorities agreed that exposure to the environment and instruments of research was beneficial to even the least creative of students. The experience produced—or it was hoped that it would produce—a healthy respect for exactitude and for sound reasoning on well-established facts. This lesson presumably would then be carried over into medical practice. One important reward was to be a more reliable diagnosis of disease. "Scientific" medicine thus made its first appearance in the world of medical practice on the diagnostic front, not in the realm of etiology or therapeutics.

Clinical thermometry, chemical tests, microscopical pathology— all had been introduced by midcentury and each reflected a new direction in medicine and made new demands on the skills and understanding of the practitioner. The development of these procedures was as much a concern of the physiologist as it was of the clinician. Furthermore the new practitioner faced the difficult task of remaining abreast with the times. If he was to conduct his practice in the most effective manner, he would need to be able to appreciate, even evaluate in the light of his own experience, the results obtained by investigators who employed sophisticated instrumentation, and he could also be expected to adopt certain new scientific aids in his own practice. These changes and expectations all demanded that the aspiring physician receive a thorough introduction to the tools and reasoning of scientific medicine. The physiological institute was envisaged as a primary point for imparting such knowledge to the student.[3]

The students and teachers associated with a physiological institute worked within a wider world. The hospital and above all the hospital clinic were also open to the inquiring physician. Clinical research and instruction shared the ideals of the institute: investigation of disease moved hand in hand with the task of introducing the beginner to the practice of medicine. The bond between theory and practice was rarely overlooked in the nineteenth-century German medical faculty, and here was the basis for many discoveries and the encouragement of the ideals of scientific medicine.

And in France? In what ways did the rising German or institute model diverge from French scientific institutional practices? At the beginning of the century France stood preeminent among the sciences and in medicine. The Paris medical faculty for a long generation not only dominated the French medical scene but exerted an extraordinary international influence. To the hospitals and dissection rooms of Paris came students from the world over, and the senior staff in the French capital gave direction to medicine for some forty years. But by the 1840s this dominance was being challenged. The medical faculty in Vienna and the London teaching hospitals had long been serious rivals and all maintained their vigor as the century advanced. It was the new challengers, however, those in the many medical faculties supported by the still-divided German states, that evoked greatest interest and concern.

In the French as in the German scientific and medical faculties it was the individual professorial appointment that dominated a particular sphere of knowledge. Gradually at first and only with much difficulty, the German professoriate by the 1840s was attaching its chairs to—or, better, placing its personal appointments in—a commanding position within a new instrument for research, the scientific and humanistic institute. The French professoriate lacked this advantage. Despite no shortage of talent, the French professor possessed at best a small laboratory attached to his chair. He could and did pursue original research, although means for doing so were always limited. He usually lacked supporting staff—above all regular, paid technical assistants—and the scale of his inquiries was severely limited by the equally limited physical facilities at his disposal and by a shortage of funds for the purchase of equipment. Perhaps only in matters directly related to the hospital was this problem readily overcome: material for clinical and pathological investigation was available in abundance in Paris.

While established scientists and research-minded physicians did find ways to conduct and collectively criticize original investigations (Lesch's discussion of the Paris Academy of Medicine makes this clear), France long continued to suffer from an absence of facilities for introducing new students to scientific inquiry. The German institute was a training ground as well as a research center. Here neophytes, postdoctoral students, and advanced professionals found a common home, the special needs of each being provided for and the perennial tension between teaching and research attaining, in most cases, a viable balance. France lacked a comparable institutional foundation for recruiting and training its new generations of scientists and academic physicians. Among the French professors (one need cite only Claude Bernard and Louis Pasteur) there were exceptionally innovative researchers. But until the 1860s and especially the 1870s, they had great difficulty in attracting and then assuring support for the younger men who would provide the creative force of the future. This matter of recruitment and assistance during the crucial early years of a scientific or medical career was greatly facilitated by the German university-institute form of organization. To these bodies were attached junior professorships and assistantships, not to mention the affiliation of *Privatdozenten* whose livelihood depended strictly upon individual teaching skills but who owed their access to the student marketplace to a university or institute connection.

To many observers the German system appeared to work too well. By the late 1880s a glut of highly skilled scientific and medical manpower was visible. Germany, it appeared, had trained too many men prepared for the kind of research career that the university alone was capable of sustaining and who now faced a university system that had completed its expansive phase. French expansion after 1870, modest and always tentative, also had created new opportunities, but the scale of this endeavor never equaled that experienced across the Rhine.

Although clustered within the area of experimental physiology and its connections with medicine, the essays in this volume raise issues concerning investigation and teaching, intellectual vision and institutional setting, that extend beyond these confines. The transitions discussed here were analogous to contemporary changes occurring in other sciences and in humanistic studies. We have invited Kathryn M. Olesko, who has been investigating similar questions in the context of physics in Germany, to write a commentary to conclude the volume. Drawing on her study of the origins of the institution of the teaching-research seminar in German universities, Olesko points out parallels between the developments described in the main essays and those occurring elsewhere within the German educational system during the period. She also points toward some of the subtler aspects of the interplay between pedagogy and the investigative enterprise that should come into consideration as the topics treated in this volume are subjected to continuing scholarly scrutiny.

NOTES

1. On the development of the German university, see Charles E. McClelland, *State, Society and University in Germany 1700–1914* (Cambridge: Cambridge University Press, 1980).

2. Rudolf Virchow, "Standpoints in Scientific Medicine," in *Disease, Life and Man: Selected Essays by Rudolf Virchow*, ed. and trans. Dr. L. J. Rather (Stanford: Stanford University Press, 1958), p. 37.

3. The new "scientific" medicine did not find ready acceptance by all physicians or in all nations. See in this regard the sobering account by Christopher Lawrence, "Incommunicable Knowledge: Science, Technology and the Clinical Art in Britain 1850–1914," *Journal of Contemporary History*, 20 (1985): 503–520.

CHAPTER ONE

Prussian Pedagogy: Purkyně at Breslau, 1823–1839

William Coleman

The claim has often been made that the school of physiology created by Jan Evangelista Purkyně at Breslau constituted the first physiological institute within the German university system. This claim is probably true, but in itself it affords little insight into the character of what proved a decisive innovation in medical pedagogy. "Pedagogy" is the key word, for Purkyně envisaged that learning at every level was a process of discovery. One started in one's youngest years with self-discovery and continued along this course until the line between learning what was already known and discovering the unknown disappeared. A genuine investigator was thus created. His appropriate home was, of course, at the apex of the educational system—namely, the university and its faculties.

At this level the physician and physiologist found in the physiological institute, a component of the medical faculty, the specialized environment needed for original inquiry. The bond between instruction and investigation was assured by the active involvement of the student-investigator in his own education. Training was to be training for discovery; the student was compelled to learn by doing. This was Purkyně's credo. It reflects his own educational experience and also his commitment to pedagogical objectives firmly established by the reform movement of the late eighteenth century and especially by Johann Heinrich Pestalozzi. It provides, too, the essential basis for understanding Purkyně's activities in Breslau after 1823.

The physiological institute attached to the Breslau medical faculty was formally created by ministerial order in 1839. Well before that date, however, and upon Purkyně's personal initiative, supported by occasional curatorial and ministerial assistance, there appeared at the Silesian university a functional unit consisting of professor, occasional assistants, and a number of able medical students, who together pursued a singular program of original research. Most of these students went on to enter the practice of medicine; a few, however, remained in academic medicine and became leading figures in the further development of physiology. For both groups, Purkyně prescribed a program of instruction with a strong practical orientation. The framework within which this program was pursued constituted what Purkyně himself called a "school of physiology," and it is this school that offered the essential outline for others that soon followed.[1]

The origins of the Breslau institute are a complex matter, and dispute might arise at the outset on definitional grounds alone. Essential elements of the "institute" phenomenon are dedicated physical premises and personnel plus equipment, the whole constitutively placed within the university curriculum. Between 1823 and 1839 Purkyně and his associates composed the needed personnel, and they invented and constructed much of their own equipment. Their investigations were an integral part of the university's operations. Purkyně's group had, however, to await the pleasure of a hesitant ministry before obtaining suitable premises. Therefore 1839 is a misleading date: it refers to an accepted administrative entity, together with an independent physical structure and a modest operating budget. But the real life of an institute, or any comparable institution, embraces the work of relevant personnel in both research and instruction, and in Breslau this work had begun much earlier, soon after Purkyně's arrival in the city for the summer semester of 1823.

PURKYNĚ AT BRESLAU

The University of Breslau was itself a new foundation. Much of Silesia had passed under Prussian control in 1742. Already a center of the textile trades, the region was to become during the nineteenth century one of the leading industrial areas of central Europe, a major coal producer and a locus for the production of iron and manufactured goods. Breslau was the vital control center for Prussian authority in Silesia and the seat of ecclesiastical, administrative, and other authorities. As was typical of the German east, the population of Silesia was predominantly non-German, Polish being the language of the larger community. Germans, however, principally Prussians, dominated the military and civil bureaucracies and held vast tracts of land.

In the great era of reform and national reconstruction that followed the disaster of Jena in 1806, Prussia had looked to its schools and universities for guidance. There were only three universities of significance. Halle reflected an earlier reform movement, that of the 1690s, and its role in supplying the state and Church with trained personnel was resumed after a brief interruption. Königsberg also continued with little change. The small university at Frankfurt an der Oder, however, was obviously moribund, and Berlin authorities assured it a rapid death. A decade of reform that brought into being the powerful University of Berlin (1810) and refounded the University of Bonn (1818), Prussia's crucial outpost on the Rhine, also created another, if less celebrated university, that at Breslau (1811).[2] Purkyně's university, the second of these Friedrich-Wilhelms Universitäten, was the most singularly placed, being—and being well understood to be—an agent of *Deutschtum* almost lost in a sea of Slavic-speaking peoples and placed in a region the population of which was generally very poor.

Breslau's university was formed by amalgamation of the faculty of the old Protestant university of Frankfurt an der Oder, the Jesuit philosophical and theological faculty located in Breslau since 1702, and an assortment of independent Breslau medical institutions. Like Berlin and Bonn, Breslau was created as a *Volluniversität*—that is, it provided a complete range of studies and possessed the usual professional faculties as well as the central philosophical faculty.[3] The latter, at Breslau as elsewhere, concentrated upon philological and historical study, utilized the seminar method, and attempted to set a neo-humanist tone of pure scholarly inquiry untainted by the claims of practical applications. *Brotstudien* nevertheless remained strong at Breslau, and Purkyně, appointed to the medical faculty, had a keen appreciation for practical matters. His views often stood in sharp contrast to those of more extreme advocates of German neohumanism.

Purkyně was, in fact, a singular appointee in the Prussian university system. At the time of his appointment as professor of physiology in Breslau he was an assistant in the anatomy department at the University of Prague and had received his medical degree only four years earlier. He had never held a permanent teaching position and had published only two (albeit significant) scientific works. He was, in addition, a Bohemian and had acquired German only as a third language (he was fluent in Latin and, of course, Czech from his early school years). All in all, he appears an odd choice to represent an important medical subject in a flagship Prussian university.[4]

Purkyně (1787–1869) owed his good fortune to personal connections and to a correct scientific disposition. Perhaps even his Czech origins and Roman Catholic background (Purkyně's religious commitment was never feverish and, after his youth, little in evidence) acted in his favor; during his thirty years in Breslau his household became an important meeting point between German and Polish intellectuals.[5] He was, in fact, a great supporter of the latter. The Breslau appointment was decided, of course, in Berlin, and there Purkyně had powerful friends.[6] Foremost among these supporters was Johann Nepomuk Rust, who had moved from service in the Austrian and then Prussian military corps to director of medical affairs within the Prussian ministry of cultural affairs (Kultusministerium). Rust had met Purkyně in Prague, encouraged Purkyně when he despaired of finding a regular university appointment, and urged him to apply for the vacant Breslau position. Above all, Rust introduced Purkyně to Carl Asimund Rudolphi. Rudolphi held the foundation chair of anatomy and physiology at the University of Berlin and was personally acquainted with Karl Freiherr von Altenstein, in 1822–1823 the all-important minister for religious, cultural, and medical affairs. Purkyně was also an immediate and obvious success in the Rudolphi household; on the very day of royal approval of his appointment in Breslau he married Rudolphi's daughter, Julia.

A well-placed and outspoken critic of all speculative tendencies in physiology, whether the product of the *Naturphilosophen* or the then ascendant Berlin mesmerists, Rudolphi surely could not approve of Purkyně's youthful fascination with such congenial indulgences.[7] Nonetheless he obviously favored Purkyně's approach to investigation of the physiological events that seemed to lie close to the heart of such speculative systems—namely, experimental study of sensations and of the operation of the human sensory apparatus. This perspective leads directly to the basic principles of Purkyně's physiological outlook and to the relation of the latter to his program for a physiological institute.

In his initial researches Purkyně had sought to establish the objectivity of the subject, meaning thereby scrupulous experimental analysis of sensory function. He conducted this analysis on his own person, seeking to establish an association (or, when indicated, lack of association) between mental images and specific measurable sensory stimuli. This was self-experimentation in seemingly classic *naturphilosophische* manner. The goal, however, was significantly different. Purkyně sought to establish by means of the phenomena alone, and the latter evoked as far as possible in controlled manner, the regularity and necessity of quite singular and unexpected sensory impressions. Hence, although Purkyně's reports on these curious experiments are marked by patent enthusiasm and delight in the richness of experiences evoked, they also display restraint and sobriety.

These studies paralleled those of another, somewhat younger physiologist, Johannes Müller (1800–1858). In 1826 Müller published two volumes dealing with a multitude of themes in sensory (visual) physiology, each filled with original observations and important conclusions (including the so-called law of specific nerve energies).[8] In 1823, the year following his completion of medical studies and at the same time that Purkyně was beginning his career in Breslau, Müller was in Berlin. He soon became another protégé of Rudolphi and received the warmest encouragement from his life-long protector, Johannes Schultze, perhaps the most influential figure in Altenstein's Kultusministerium. The latter, in fact, acted in an extraordinary manner; he called on the still unknown Müller to provide a professional estimate of Purkyně's *Habilitationsschrift*, a work of long gestation but now rapidly completed and published so that its author could rightfully assume an instructional position in Breslau.

Müller's assessment of Purkyně's dissertation is highly revealing not only of the methods favored by the two investigators but of the latitude of ministerial opinion and also, no doubt, of the decisive role of personal relationships in academic appointment and advancement.[9] Müller applauded Purkyně's many important discoveries but disapproved of his approach: the Czech was too objective in his inquiries. Müller himself at this time was still bemused by the speculative approach to scientific inquiry that he had acquired through his medical studies in Bonn, a veritable hotbed of *Naturphilosophie*. Purkyně had approached the subject of common regard, vision and visual impressions, by assaying the organ of vision, the eye. For this purpose he employed varied experimental apparatus, including what is probably the original form of the ophthalmoscope. Müller disliked these physicalist, intrusive measures. He favored ingeniously contrived observation, a position that he maintained throughout his career and that distanced him increasingly from the physiological community, not least from those among his own students who conducted after 1840 a vigorous campaign to bring experiment, both conceptually and in terms of physical and chemical apparatus, to the center of physiological inquiry.

Purkyně was adept at all forms of experimentation and did not hesitate to use, and to create, physical apparatus for probing the nature of vital processes; experimental work was intrinsic to his hands-on conception of scientific training and investigation. Müller, save for an early and productive period of vivisectional work, greatly preferred systematic observation to intervention; his was the comparative anatomical and zoological approach. This approach is fully exhibited in his essays of 1826.[10] From the ministerial perspective, however, it is evident that, although Müller stood in highest favor, receiving Rudolphi's chair in Berlin in 1833, Purkyně's program was also to receive official recognition: his demands for a physiological institute, an institute in which "objective" inquiry was to be the rule of the house, were heard and then met. Müller's gently critical remarks obviously influenced Altenstein little if at all, and furthermore they were never published, although it is a fact that in his publications Müller made no reference to Purkyně's *Habilitationsschrift*. Nonetheless behind these methodological disagreements and this professional competition can be seen the primary feature of Purkyně's entire scientific and pedagogical career—namely, the conviction that only through immediate contact with the object under scrutiny, even so fleeting an object as a visual impression, can genuine knowledge be obtained. This conviction had been formed early in his life and later found concrete institutional form in the Breslau physiological institute.

Medicine diverted Purkyně from becoming a model schoolmaster, yet the prospect of pedagogical reform that he conceived in his youth he never lost from view. Carried over from Purkyně's dreams of reformed primary and secondary instruction, particularly in the natural sciences, was a view of how best to develop the abilities of the university student. This view occupies the center of the following discussion. First I shall describe the Breslau physiological institute and its activities and its creator's perception of the undertaking. I then turn to Purkyně's pedagogical philosophy, its roots in the Pestalozzian reform tradition, and the relevance of this outlook to the institutionalization of the ideals of experimental science. The discussion concludes with comment on the much-discussed notion of neohumanism and the asserted preeminence of the *Geisteswissenschaften* in the reformed German university. My purpose here is to indicate that our focus on these issues, and thus inevitably on the affairs of the philosophical faculty, is needlessly narrow and may obscure understanding of the origins and nature of the scientific institute, an integral component in the creation of that remarkable machine for scientific inquiry, the German research university and its worldwide offspring.

THE INSTITUTE AND ITS PROGRAM

Purkyně's institute was formally inaugurated on 8 November 1839. It was the product of a decade's insistent solicitation of the Prussian educational authorities—in fact, of action and demands that reached back almost to his arrival in Breslau. In his second year at the university (1824) he had introduced regular experimental demonstrations as an integral component of the general lecture course on physiology. By 1828 he was conducting "experimental courses." These might have included student participation in the demonstrations but more probably continued the traditional practice in which the professor or his assistant conducted a so-called experiment before an audience of students. The latter's role was limited to observing the demonstration.[11] But by the early 1830s at the latest Purkyně was introducing a number of qualified students to the use of available scientific apparatus. Indeed, he had succeeded in launching a collective research project with these same students, a project devoted to study of human histology and related functional questions and which helped lay the foundations of the cell theory.

There was nothing inadvertent in these initiatives. Purkyně knew very well the kind of institutional basis he needed to advance physiology, and from 1831 on he laid virtual siege to Berlin to obtain the physical premises, equipment, supplies, and assistance needed to satisfy his ambitions. He submitted his first formal appeal in 1831 and sent the second, a veritable program for the new world of experimental physiology and a capital document in the history of the science, to Berlin in 1836. The latter proved successful, although bureaucratic wheels turned slowly, and its product, further refined by yet another request, was the institute of 1839. The 1831 appeal never moved beyond the university curator in Breslau, who observed that no German university as yet possessed a physiological institute and that Breslau was obviously not the place to begin. The full text of this document has apparently disappeared, but Rudolf Heidenhain, the second great figure in Breslau physiology, published a brief and revealing extract therefrom in a biographical notice of his predecessor. Here Purkyně observed that

> physiology has today moved beyond the idle speculation of earlier decades and has turned to the empirical sciences. She finds here not only bibliographical assistance and factual material but actively joins these sciences [in their work]. The physiologist qua physiologist must be able to do work in physics, chemistry and biology (*Organik*) if, [as is to be expected], physiologically interesting results are to be obtained in these areas of the natural sciences. If, in order to assure its tangible existence, physiology, which is an independent science just like any other, has to go begging before the precarious liberality of other institutes which tradition has given a well-fortified position, it can prosper only in most limited fashion and in the end even the most courageous physiologist will weaken. If it is appropriate to assign physiology a standing equal to that of anatomy, zoology and other specialties in the university, then it follows, and also reflects intelligent scientific administrative practice, that physiology should be given autonomous status and fitted out with all that is needed for productive activity.[12]

Purkyně thereupon requested, Heidenhain reported, separate physical facilities, his own assistant, and an annual appropriation for research purposes. These requests, fruitless in 1831, formed the core of the renewed and successful 1836 appeal.

Much was at stake that cannot be explored here. Purkyně did not base his plea for independence, for example, on general principles alone but invoked also the exasperating local factors, above all his dependence for space and equipment upon the tempered generosity of the director of the well-established anatomical institute, A. W. Otto. The latter, whose primary ambition was to expand his already enormous collection of pathological specimens, had no interest in experimental work, much less in Purkyně's newfangled notions of mingling physics and chemistry with physiology, and was also among the many in Breslau who had opposed Purkyně's appointment.[13]

A continuing theme in Purkyně's programmatic statements and in his daily approach to instruction was his castigation of those who teach by the book. Worst of all was instruction that never reached beyond repetition of what was contained within a textbook. Purkyně himself did not hesitate to use textbooks as part of his course on physiology, but he understood well their limitations. Physiology was not to be communicated by words alone: science deals above all with sensory perceptions, not simply with words or combinations of words. To be sure, language was crucially important. It constituted an essential element in the Pestalozzian notion of learning and it was the indispensable coin of all scientific exchange. But language was only a part of science, the more familiar and perhaps the easier part; Nature herself posed the fundamental challenge. The nascent scientist-physician must therefore be brought into intimate contact with the phenomena themselves. The lecture-demonstration was a first step along this road and, as will be seen, one widely available in German universities during the 1820s. In this setting, however, the student remained only a passive observer of the phenomena produced by the lecturer-demonstrator. The distinguishing feature of Purkyně's pedagogical reform was to replace the professor by the student, to assure the direct engagement of the latter with these same phenomena. To do this an appropriate setting was required, a setting that virtually defined the character of the scientific institute.

The physiologist, Purkyně declared, must deal with both man's "mental and bodily activities."[14] In this his views were one with the prevailing interpretation of the unity or, at very least, constant and intimate interaction of the moral and physical attributes of man. This position was most clearly formulated by the French ideologue and physician, P. J. G. Cabanis and was shared by many in Germany, including those moved by the macro-microcosmic analogy restored to favor by the *Naturphilosophen*. Experimentation—namely, self-experimentation—when addressed to a first domain, to visual imagery and the many other sensory perceptions, appeared to deal with this "moral" realm in a manner that assured unanticipated rigor. In fact, the work of Purkyně, Müller, and contemporary Leipzig physiologists offers the beginning of a deliberately experimental psychology. Purkyně cited no specific material needs for prosecuting this part of the inquiry, although his remarks do tend to bring the subject close to mechanics, with the body-soul/physical-moral interaction seemingly understood in terms of vital materialism.[15]

For the demonstration and study of another domain, however, the patently physical phenomena of life, diverse and often expensive apparatus was required; provision for its care, use, and elaboration was needed, and assistants had to be trained and paid. Of course equipment, supplies, and assistants had to be housed and suitable space provided for the use of students, visitors, and staff. Here, obviously, one meets the tangible needs of a scientific institute as a social institution, and regarding these needs Purkyně displayed no reticence.[16] Well before formal creation of his institute, he was granted funds to purchase a major research tool, the Plössel microscope, and further funds were allowed to hire a part-time assistant. At the outset Purkyně spent his own money for research but was soon granted a small annual sum for this purpose. With these funds, some of which had to be used for expendable supplies, he and his associates devised and constructed a wide range of physiological apparatus, including an early form of the microtome and, in the early 1840s, means for photomicrography and photographic methods for recording bodily motions.

The Plössel microscope, a powerful new achromatic instrument, was probably the single most important piece of equipment in Purkyně's laboratory (by 1846 he had managed to purchase three of these instruments). The regular manufacture and sale of achromatic microscopes was begun by Charles Chevalier in Paris in 1825; soon thereafter Giovan Battista Amici in Modena and Pistor and Schiek in Berlin offered their improved versions of this instrument. In 1828 Simon Plössel of Vienna joined this group, producing a microscope that, despite its optical limitations and awkwardness in use, stood for twenty years as a standard of excellence and power.[17] The arrival of a Plössel microscope in Breslau in 1832 was the stimulus for a dramatic advance in knowledge of human histology and related aspects of general physiology. Purkyně, who had begun his microscopical researches in the 1820s (plant structures; early chick embryogenesis) with a simple lens and then progressed to using the most sophisticated available apparatus, exhibited singular enthusiasm for the instrument and its applications. The Plössel microscope was particularly well suited to histological inquiries. The numerical aperture of Purkyně's early instruments probably did not exceed 0.2–0.3, but their lenses offered suitable resolution (about 1 micron) for exact observation of whole cells, gave a magnification of about 200 to 300 diameters, and provided the great depth of field needed for study of tissues.[18]

The achromatic microscope, particularly as it was improved after 1840, provided the foundation for an extraordinarily exciting new area of inquiry—histophysiology and histopathology—and thus appeared to move the study of animal functions definitively from the organ to the cellular level. During the 1830s Purkyně's group in Breslau stood at the forefront of these developments, and the discoveries made by these men, for the most part accomplished before formal creation of a physiological institute in 1839, gave notice to the scientific world that the combination of new apparatus *and* a stimulating pedagogical-research situation could be expected to yield rich rewards. Of course to instructor and to student, and especially to the observant Kultusministerium in Berlin, all of this activity, while encouraging the expansion of scientific and medical knowledge, was also producing or could be expected to produce useful knowledge. Medicine was beginning to enter the era of physical and chemical diagnosis (Purkyně's microscopes were available to and used by local pathologists in their own work), and this entailed not only the invention and improvement of medical instruments but the systematic training of students in the use of these tools. Obviously the scientific institute played a major role in this work, matched only by direct instruction, when available, conducted in the hospital ward or other clinical settings. In the early 1840s instruction at the new Breslau institute offered a model for emulation.

The microscope was by no means the whole either of Purkyně's program for physiology or of the outfitting of the institute. Ample chemical reagents and apparatus were provided and were used by all; the same was true for physical apparatus. Acquiring this equipment preoccupied Purkyně and his staff throughout the former's ten-year leadership of the institute. His definitive request for creation of an institute (July 1839) contained a detailed itemization—including projected costs—of the required apparatus, supplies, and salaries. Two additional microscopes were requested, along with an air pump, a galvanometer and other electrical apparatus, a fine balance, gasometers, anatomical and surgical instruments, and glassware. Salaries were requested for a full-time and qualified scientific assistant and a janitor, and other funds were needed to pay for the

preparation of drawings. Still further requests were made for ex-
penses directly associated with anatomicophysiological researches
(cadavers, experimental animals, injection materials, preservative
spirits) and for the routine operations of the building.[19]

Surprisingly most of these demands were satisfied. The Breslau
institute grew gradually but healthily through the 1840s.[20] Purkyně,
however, was fifty-two years old when the institute was created and
for the next several years was wholly preoccupied with its organization and routine operations. This was for him, therefore, a period of
much-reduced scientific productivity, although advanced students
continued to be active at the institute. The decade ended not with
his return to vigorous physiological research but his departure for
Prague, where another organizational effort was required. Only
slowly did Purkyně there renew his physiological investigations,
and these were no longer his principal objective: a second career,
bringing modern science into the mainstream of Czech life and bol-
stering the cause of Czech nationalism, had begun.[21]

Fifteen students completed medical dissertations in Breslau under
Purkyně's supervision between 1824 and 1838, and another eleven
did so between 1839 and his departure for Prague in 1850. The
majority of these publications presented original observations and
dealt with the microscopic examination of various human tissues.
This was primarily descriptive work, contributing to the creation of
the subject of human histology. Purkyně was, as is well known, an
early spokesman for the cell theory, but he ventured no general
statement of such a theory and did not participate in the often divi-
sive theoretical disputes that rent microscopical anatomy during the
1840s.[22] A leading figure in the Breslau institute was G. G. Valentin,
one of Purkyně's early students and soon to become a major physiologist in his own right: Valentin and Purkyně published jointly
(1834) their epoch-making discovery of ciliary motion in vertebrates,
a model instance of the microanatomical elucidation of physiological
activity. Analogous work was accomplished by Samuel Pappenheim, who examined the microscopic structure of the stomach lining
and its secretory cells as part of an experimental analysis of digestion. Pappenheim also joined Purkyně in close examination of the
muscle fibers of the heart and the application of microscopical findings to understanding the physiological properties of the eye.[23]

All of this work took place in buildings that were not truly suited to such a role. Between 1823 and 1825 Purkyně worked in a single small room in the crowded anatomy institute; from this he was ousted by Otto, who needed more space for his pathological collections. Physiology moved to the attics of the main university building and remained in this cramped location until November 1839, when a separate building was provided. Purkyně found the latter quarters unsuited to physiological work: the building was exposed to the dirt and vibrations of heavy nearby traffic and had few windows that received direct light, a crucial matter in early microscopical investigation, and he hesitated to move in. The interior arrangements were, however, if not ideal, a great improvement over previous facilities. Purkyně now had a small room for his personal researches plus two larger rooms for microscopical and chemical investigations and a small cabinet for physical experiments. The institute also possessed a lecture hall and quarters for the service staff.[24]

The effectiveness and renown of the Breslau institute obviously could not be attributed to the unimpressive physical locale available to professor and students. It was, instead, a matter of personnel and guiding ideas that made Breslau a model for others to emulate. Pedagogy was important in its own right, but it was all the more important with regard to physiology, for Purkyně had no small vision of his chosen science. "Just as the human individual," he told Altenstein, "may be called the little world, so is physiology, which takes man as its principal subject, the synthesis of all the natural sciences. And so, too, [must] an institute dedicated to physiology unite in itself and in suitable manner the leading aspects of all the other sciences."[25] Purkyně understood well the potential for useful knowledge offered by physiology and understood even better the appeal of scientific utility to the popular as well as to the ministerial mind.[26] But these convictions, no less than Purkyně's fascinating personal style and unfailing ingenuity, were perhaps not the decisive point. Under the watchful but supportive eye of Altenstein and Berlin, Purkyně found himself free in Breslau to give reality to what he deemed the proper principles of pedagogy. He thereby moved the training of physiologists from an era of lectures and reading drawn from an assigned text and from theoretical discussion undisturbed by close association with firsthand observation to another world, to the world of the classic scientific institute, in which he who learns, the student, becomes the principal agent of his own instruction. If, as Purkyně fervently believed, learning is doing, scientific education must both adopt a hands-on attitude and educate the senses; in reality, it would do the latter by means of the former.

PEDAGOGICAL REFORM

These were and remain powerful pedagogical principles, and they have transformed the character of schooling in Western society. Purkyně belonged to a reform movement that began with Jean Jacques Rousseau, Johann Bernhard Basedow, and Johann Heinrich Pestalozzi and which has continued with only changing emphases into the twentieth century. Born of the Enlightenment's hope to create new men and women, independent, self-aware, and productive citizens, the reformers began with the premise that it is the cultivation of the individual person, and not religious catechization, rote learning, or iron discipline, that best forms the personality and renders the unformed boy or girl a responsible, happy, useful man or woman. These sentiments were developed and systematized by Rousseau in his philosophical romance, *Emile,* and the movement quickly thereafter acquired social identity with a singular group of vigorous Swiss reformers, of whom Pestalozzi was a leading figure.[27]

But what was Purkyně's connection with this world? And what bearing, if any, did it have on his selection for a position on a medical faculty in far-off Silesia? The orphaned son of a Bohemian estate manager, Purkyně received an altogether extraordinary education and proved capable of drawing great benefit from it.[28] After primary schooling near his home, he traveled to the Piarist Gymnasium in Mikulov, in Moravia on the Austrian border. The Piarist order (Pauline Congregation of the Mother of God), founded in Rome in the early seventeenth century, had grown into a great teaching order, in central Europe always a formidable rival of the Jesuits. Upon finishing his studies at Mikulov Purkyně entered the order; his religious commitment was not great, however, for he soon returned to the secular world. Nonetheless from the Piarists he received intensive training for the scholastic calling and was sent to teach in the order's colleges in Straznice and Litomysl.

Purkyně obviously learned much from these two years in the classroom. Straznice was, moreover, sacred ground to teachers. Here, on the very site of the Piarist college, had stood the school of the Bohemian Brethren and here Comenius, foremost among pedagogical reformers, had been educated. The Piarists as a group had no favorable view of their heretical forerunners and looked upon the earlier institution as "that Godless school; that seat of pestilence; the Devil's synagogue."[29] Purkyně, however, had no taste for such religious disputes and held Comenius in highest regard, a model for the teacher's calling. Later in life he tracked down and rescued in Poland the surviving manuscripts of his predecessor.

After this Piarist youth, dominated by language instruction and including mathematics and natural science, together with extensive reading in the new German idealistic philosophy, Purkyně pursued varied self-instruction and university studies. He first studied philosophical subjects (1807–1810) and then turned to preparation at the Charles University in Prague for a medical career (M.D., 1819). A crucial interlude in these studies (1810–1812) was passed on the estate of Baron Hildprandt at Blatna, a few miles south of Prague. Here Purkyně served as tutor to the baron's son. Warmly supported by his employer, he was able to act independently as a teacher and to develop his own understanding by constant and wide-ranging reading. From this experience and from continued contact with friends in Prague he conceived the notion of founding for the Czech nation a model school in the natural sciences. The Swiss pedagogical reformers, Pestalozzi and Emmanuel Fellenberg in the front rank, and German philosophical and pedagogical principles and polemics, the latter also inspired by Swiss writers, were the acknowledged source of his inspiration.[30]

War, however, intervened. The Napoleonic conflicts were coming to a head in 1812–1813. Austrian and Czech affairs were in turmoil; military mobilization was the order of the day; and Prussia, not yet a part of Purkyně's plans, was about to recapture its national pride by force of arms at Leipzig. These confusions launched Purkyně upon a medical career. Young Hildprandt, Purkyně's pupil, went off to war, and Baron Hildprandt provided his employee and friend means for study in Prague, insisting that his protégé carry his work to completion. Obviously the opportunity to create a new school for molding both the student and a sense of Czech national identity had, for the moment, passed.

But what is of importance is that the essential notion behind this plan—that instruction must be based on practice, that learning is the product of the direct interaction between student and object—was not lost. Its effect marked all of Purkyně's subsequent dealings with educational matters, not least those at the university and institute levels. If not an out-and-out zealot, as was many a pedagogical reformer, Purkyně was at very least an enthusiastic advocate of change and of systematic modernization. He lived in dramatically changing times. The French invasions had shattered traditional German social and economic forms and had reduced proud Prussia to seeming impotence. There were many lessons to be learned from these events and from this defeat, and the agenda of the great age of Prussian reform that followed the catastrophe of 1806 included rebuilding the nation from the ground up, a program that entailed thoroughgoing reconstruction of the entire Prussian educational establishment.

Prussian reform mixed ambiguously—indeed, it joined in contradictory manner—allegiance to Enlightenment ideals of self-development and the priority of the individual and a demand for better-trained and obedient civil servants.[31] Neohumanism pressed the former ideal to its extreme; more practical minds, intent on efficient administration, modernization, and rapid economic expansion, had the latter goals most in mind. Although himself a person of startlingly wide learning, Purkyně had no sympathy for the extreme neohumanist position. His eye turned always to practical matters. The Pestalozzian program—one shared, verbally at least, by practical men and by neohumanists such as Wilhelm von Humboldt alike—was pragmatic to the core. But as will be seen, Purkyně believed that individual development could, and emphatically should, follow upon close engagement with the natural world and with the realia of daily life and should not be confined to or even emphasize the cultural ideals of ancient Greece. There was a commonality in pedagogical methods on the university level between the classical or historical seminar and the nascent scientific institute, but there was also a clear division in their subject matter and in their understanding of the social mission of such training.

"There are times," Purkyně observed, "when men appear who try to make it possible, by improving methods of instruction, to reach the infinite potential of the mind. Pestalozzi may be named first among these men. He built his method upon the most correct insight into the mechanisms of mental activity." These remarks were published in 1847 and within the frame of yet another assault on the cultural exclusivities of the neohumanists, yet they represent the abiding conviction of Purkyně's entire pedagogical career. The only shortcoming in Pestalozzi's outlook, the physiologist noted, was that he had confined his attention to "elementary matters," when in reality the approach was equally fitted to preparing students for work in the "higher sciences."[32] Purkyně himself had set about to bring Pestalozzian learning-by-doing into the university.

Pestalozzi (1746–1827) was born in Zurich and sought to make a career in the church.[33] His political outlook and activist stance soon made this impossible, and he moved, inadvertently it seemed, into charitable work with small children. This experience inevitably led him to educational questions. He drew further inspiration from Rousseau, other reformers, and the widespread humanitarian sentiment of the epoch. Demands for pedagogical reform in the German-speaking lands considerably antedated both Pestalozzi's proposals and the programs of the Prussian reformers. The ever-robust enemy was mindless learning, be it the Protestant catechism or Roman Catholic latinity, and the new goal was formation of an informed populace capable of independent (but not socially disruptive) judgment and amenable to effective employment in an increasingly complex economy.

Pestalozzi not only formulated in systematic and popularly accessible terms a definite philosophy of education but attempted on several celebrated occasions to put his principles into practice. He created a series of model schools in Switzerland and enjoyed a dual success. His schools created useful citizens from seemingly unpromising material—namely, orphans and children of the poor, the principal focus of all of his concerns—and also served as magnets attracting interested observers from across Europe. That interest was perhaps strongest in Germany at large and in Prussia in particular. A key figure in the Berlin educational bureaucracy was Johannes Wilhelm Süvern. A product of the classic training ground of the neohumanist and the philological seminar, and who became the leading advocate of the neohumanist ideal within the Kultusministerium, Süvern was a crucial stimulus to introducing Pestalozzian practices into the Prussian primary school.[34] With missionary zeal and governmental encouragement, Germans and others visited the Pestalozzian establishments in the Swiss cantons and returned home prepared to create new schools and new citizens. Purkyně himself, in the decisive year 1812, had completed plans to journey to Switzerland in order to gather impressions and guidance for the school that he and Baron Hildprandt expected to open at Blatna.

Pestalozzi built upon Rousseau's central notion of the "natural" child. First of all, the Swiss pedagogue announced, one must know the character or nature of one's raw material: the uninstructed child. How does it learn? At what pace should instruction move and in what sequence should the subjects be presented? What is the best environment for teaching? To Pestalozzi, whose focus was on the young child or what has come to be called primary education, the fundamental issue was not *what* a child learns but *how* it is learned. Primacy thus went to the pedagogical process, and to this was added, a truism of eighteenth-century epistemology, the assertion that sensory experience is an intrinsic element in training the mind. Children learn in a definite and ascertainable order, a natural order that must be discovered and exploited. The child must be guided toward knowledge, particularly self-knowledge, by assured presentation of concrete experiences. The child is to work with its own hands, involve its own senses in the phenomena of daily life; the teacher is to organize instruction to meet this goal, assist at difficult moments, and offer aid in generalization. Central, therefore, to the Pestalozzian method were such practices as manipulation of lettered, numbered, or colored blocks, repeated exercise of lessons, and carefully articulated sequential building upon previously acquired knowledge. Ideally such learning would proceed in a group setting, the varied interaction of individuals offering stimulus to all and intense social contact establishing common values.[35]

All of this means, of course, that genuine education is self-instruction, activity that permits (even compels) the child to build his or her own view of the world, and this a world the form of which is not given by ancient authority or the written word. Pestalozzi presented his views in literary form. His extraordinarily popular sentimental fictional narratives, *Leonard und Gertrud* and *Wie Gertrud ihre Kinder lehrt*, like Rousseau's *Emile*, spread the good word to readers who might never touch a philosophical treatise on education. Herself an attentive and loving mother, Gertrud realized that a child's only meaningful activity is self-activity. She knew that what I, the child, am to become is what I make myself to be. Knowledge is a product, to be sure, but what matters is that it is a self-generated product. Not least because we have so created our own place in the world and have done so by forming our own fund and view of knowledge, as well as begun to come to grips with what is transmitted by cultural tradition (an important fact not overlooked by the reformers), our knowledge is intrinsically our own. It gives us freedom and independence and also confidence.

All of the foregoing is to say that learning—real learning—necessarily ensues upon individual activity. "Man!" cried Pestalozzi, "needing much and desiring all, thou must to satisfy thy wants and wishes *know* and *think*, but for this thou must also (and *can*) *do*. And knowing and doing are so closely connected that if one ceases the other ceases with it." The teacher, whether this be a child's mother, *primus inter pares* to Pestalozzi, or a teacher in the schools, had therefore a limited but crucial role to play. She or he must act

> in a *continual benevolent superintendence,* with the object of calling forth all the faculties which Providence has implanted; and [education's] province, thus enlarged, will yet be with less difficulty surveyed from one point of view, and will have more of a systematic and truly philosophical character, than an incoherent mass of "lessons"—arranged without unity of principle, and gone through without interest—which too often usurps its name.[36]

For Pestalozzi a teacher's responsibility was to lead, to put the student on the path to veritable *e-ducatio*—not telling the child what but above all how, thus setting that child upon a pleasant but probably arduous course of self-discovery of his or her faculties. Training of these faculties assured that the student in maturity would be able to know his or her own capabilities and make a useful contribution to society.

Curiously the Pestalozzian pedagogical ideal stands, at best, in ambivalent relation to the study of natural phenomena. Pestalozzi's purpose was to train the young mind, to create an *Anschauung* and perfect the basics of (the vernacular) language; these were to be the essential tools for life. But Pestalozzi did not stress close, continued, and critical consideration of sensory impressions received from natural phenomena; that is, his agenda urged awareness and classification, not doubt and analysis. With regard to translation of his program to elementary and secondary instruction in the natural sciences, the results appear to have been few and dismal; it seemed that one had found only a new theoretical basis for pedantry.[37]

But this sobering conclusion ignores the larger possibilities of Pestalozzianism. The heart of his doctrine was, in fact, not directed toward imparting any one or another body of knowledge. It was, instead, an assertion of the power of the human mind, if only that power were properly cultivated. Purkyně fully understood this mission, but he realized as well that knowledge was also a matter of content and that education was meant not only to train the mind but to train the senses such that sensory impressions aided mental training. Perhaps this goal could not be reached at the elementary level; perhaps it was too remote even for the secondary schools. Purkyně accepted neither of these limitations, but save for a brief period in the classroom in Straznice, long before he turned to medicine and probably prior to his study of the writings of the pedagogical reformers, he had no opportunity or cause to introduce his views into the first years of study. Once launched in natural science, however—this being the real product of his philosophical and then medical training in Prague, and thoroughly immersed in these pedagogical writings, the result of the years in Blatna—a fertile combination was produced. It was Purkyně's ambition to launch training at the university level based upon direct contact with natural phenomena.

Strictly pedagogical writings from Purkyně's Breslau years (1823–1850) are rare. His detailed annual reports during the 1840s to the Prussian Kultusministerium do offer sustained comment on the operation and accomplishments of the new institute and ample announcement of his plans and expectations for the dual program of instruction-as-research (the reverse, research-as-instruction, might better fit the situation). In all of this, exercise, practice, the repeated use of one's senses and bodily machinery offered a leading theme. It may be noted, too, that Purkyně not only had his own teaching and tutorial experience to guide him and the writings and examples of the Swiss reformers to provide further inspiration and guidance but had had, from an unexpected quarter, a course of learning that surely confirmed both thought and action. From earliest childhood he had shown himself an accomplished vocalist and supported his studies in Mikulov from the stipend received as a choirboy. To him singing was a realm of acquired and perfected expertise. It entailed sure coordination of the senses and the organs of voice. Purkyně understood well that such coordination was not a given, however apt one's potential, but was to be developed through use. One must hone one's tools, perhaps the foremost lesson in all pedagogy, and this Purkyně did.

Purkyně began his professional career by calling for a "natural history" of the senses. "Each of our senses can be captured and de-

scribed by means of observation and experiment. We can thus appre-
hend the peculiar character of each sense as well as its characteristic
reaction with the external world."[38] Thirty years later, in announcing
his program for the new Prague institute of physiology, he reempha-
sized this psychological theme, giving his auditors a brief formal review of the five senses and the need for the development of each if a
student is to make progress in the science.[39] Such thoughts and this
emphasis were anything but new, having occupied a privileged position in pedagogical discourse since at least the time of John Locke.
What is striking and original in Purkyně's use of the argument is his
conviction that one must build an institutionalized program for physiological research and instruction at the university level upon an effective epistemological basis—namely, sensationalism mediated by the
master-pupil—really the craftsman-apprentice—relationship. Purkyně's program and his experience in Prussia exhibit the priority of
method in the creation of the scientific institute and they also exemplify the essentially guild structure of advanced scientific work in the
German university that has been emphasized by Charles E. Mc-
Clelland.[40]

Pedagogical discussion in the early (and late) nineteenth century in
the end often reduced to consideration of the place of language in
instruction. For the secondary schools and above, this meant consideration of the classical languages, the respective merits of Latin and
Greek. An associated question was the role, if any, of the vernacular
in these schools. On the elementary level the only issue was the
legitimacy of classical training at all. Purkyně took the hard line on
this question, and his views return us once again to the absolute
priority of individual sensory experience in gaining knowledge. The
classical languages, he believed, and in fact all foreign languages,
must be withheld from the child.[41] These several tongues denied that
immediacy of contact, contact with objects as well as persons, that
only one's mother tongue could assure. It may be noted that Purkyně's remarks were published in German and utilized the neutral
expression "mother tongue"; the tone of his remarks indicates, however, that other and definite national languages, notably Czech, were
also intended. The problem with a foreign language was that it was
"unnatural" to the child. It divorced the child from living reality, from
the commonalities of daily experience and discourse, and created the
harmful illusion that in and through words alone might one gain

access to true knowledge. Foreign words were only sounds; they lacked the concrete reference and repeated connection with real things that came naturally with one's mother tongue.

Let it be noted that Purkyně did not slight the advantages of having a solid command of both ancient and modern languages. He himself was a formidable linguist, knowing well four to five Western European and Slavic languages as well as having a good knowledge of classical Greek and Latin. He made several translations of poetry between Polish, Czech, and German. The important question was, for what purpose does one learn these languages, especially Greek? What has a classical curriculum, built upon Latin and Greek and the literary culture conveyed in these languages, to do with training scholars and students for life in the nineteenth century? Purkyně spoke out vigorously on this crucial matter: it bore directly upon the training offered students in the German Gymnasium, which had now become the unavoidable preliminary to university study and thus the machine that molded the product whose abilities and shortcomings he repeatedly met in the university laboratory and classroom.

To Purkyně both the classical Gymnasium and the *Realschule,* which mixed Latin with modern subjects, including the natural sciences, were false creations. They both denied the essential fact of humanity that all experience is the proper province of man. Pushed to its extreme, as the Gymnasium was doing in the 1840s by building its pedagogical program on extensive training in Greek and using this as the basis for general moral and cultural formation (*Bildung*), these schools put before the young student a false "separation of knowledge and life."[42] Of course, the sin of the Gymnasium was the more serious, for it divorced the student more extensively from the real world and thus deprived him of that greatest of teachers: experience. While not overlooking the high ideals that were often expressed and perhaps more rarely pursued by its advocates, Purkyně had little patience with the pieties and pretensions of the *Bildungsbürgertum.* The educational program of classical *Bildung,* he observed, fitted no man for life in this world:

> One studies grammar, logic and philosophy for their own sake, and not because one wants to learn [to use other] languages or learn to think or to comprehend thoughts expressed in the real world. In this way [the classical student] elevates himself to a most distinguished level indeed and one which has nothing at all to do with the common

realities of life. Here you have the school of the intellect and not that of real things.[43]

Nothing, of course, was unusual in these remarks. Purkyně's was but another voice in the continuing battle in nineteenth-century Germany that had as its public focus the character, development, and preservation of the Gymnasium and often as its private purpose the role of classical training in the establishment of cultural values and the cultural control of social mobility. Purkyně opposed the exclusivity of this philological-historical program. He saw, again, all experience as part of a unitary field, and he insisted that this fact guide instruction at every level, from first schooling to the completion of university studies. This was the essential message he had received from the pedagogical reformers, although, in Pestalozzi's case, that message was both socially and politically very conservative. Purkyně's view was only reinforced by repeated frustration in the Breslau institute with evidently intelligent medical students, Gymnasium graduates yet students who knew little or nothing of the facts of natural science and who had not been trained to cope with natural phenomena in a confident and informed, much less an original manner. These students had never learned to make thought and experience work together.

In short, to Purkyně *Bildung* based upon immersion in the classics was out of step with the times and the Gymnasium a flawed institution. The times required training in the natural sciences and an awareness of the languages spoken today—that is, those used by such improving nations as England, France, and even Germany. Admittedly, specialist training should come at the end of one's education, yet it was vain to attempt to guide the aspiring economist or physician, lawyer or engineer to the forefront of his subject if he had spent his school days assiduously ignoring essential foundations of his intended subject matter. Purkyně therefore demanded the implementation of a sequential pedagogical program reaching from the elementary school through the Gymnasium/Realschule to the university.

His scheme, surely, could expect little success. It boldly contradicted the curricular plans and social expectations inherent in the new Gymnasium; it seemed to its confident critics more fit for the creation of technical narrow-mindedness than for gentlemanly ideals; and at the university level it could be read as a threat to the student's cherished *Lernfreiheit*. But in fairness to Purkyně, his fundamental pedagogical ambition was to promote the development of a fully formed human being. His reservations regarding the Gymnasium were based less on the presence there of study of the classical languages and culture than on the fact that these studies preempted other subjects, and, the crucial matter, these studies removed the student from regular interaction with the world in which he lived. The gymnasialist was thus urged to reflect anew on the root meaning of his proud title—*Übung*: exercise, practice, use.[44] There was far more here than repeated grammatical drill and textual exegesis; genuine exercise demanded directed contact with the real world, with contemporary society and its economy; it required mastery of modern languages and, not least, familiarity with natural phenomena and with the basic natural sciences.

THE INSTITUTE PHENOMENON

We have seen that in the routine activities of the Breslau physiological Institute, Purkyně and his associates practiced what the master preached. The Breslau school had constructed or acquired considerable physiological apparatus well before an institute was formally created, and with this apparatus numerous important discoveries were made. After 1839 the institute was better equipped and original work continued. The outfitting of the Breslau' Institute is clearly portrayed by Samuel Pappenheim, and the continuing research life of Purkyně's school can be easily read from the detailed bibliography of its publications prepared by Vladislav Kruta.[45]

What was distinctive about this institute was the direct involvement of the student in the research process. The involvement may be taken as a major and perhaps the essential characteristic of the institute phenomenon. The institute was, it must not be forgotten, an integral element of the university, and the latter had as its mission the training of students. Education remained its unchanging goal, but the nature of that education changed dramatically. New subject matter was introduced, new organizational forms devised, and, what is significant for present purposes, a new conception of the student's own role in his or her training made its appearance.[46] The Breslau Institute illustrates well the form being assumed by the new organization of scientific instruction. Purkyně realized, of course, that he was an innovator and took pride in his creation; this can be seen in the annual *Berichte* he directed to the Kultusministerium and is evident, too, in the description of his work that he sent to Rudolph Wagner (to be noted later). Purkyně did not compare his endeavor in detail with that of others who also might be considered to have introduced an institute form of organization into the natural sciences, particularly physiology. Such comparisons, however, have been ventured or at least implied by later scholars, usually with the intent of settling the ever-renewed question of the origin of the first such institute.

In 1821, for example, Carl August Sigmund Schultze introduced an "experimental" course in physiology at Baden's university in Freiburg.[47] This course continued until Schultze's departure for Greifswald in 1831, where apparently he did not repeat his effort. The course received financial support from university authorities and in 1828 was provided with a "physiological *Assistant*." Schultze was a harsh critic of *naturphilosophische* speculation and believed that his course, which was based upon direct experience with the experimental animal itself, provided the necessary antidote to this not uncommon mental poison.

Himself an experimenter of considerable ingenuity and great dexterity, Schultze developed a highly successful course of instruction in experimental physiology. Lectures were based on Friedrich Hildebrandt's *Lehrbuch der Physiologie*; the demonstrations offered Freiburg students a view of vivisection, microscopical preparation, and chemical analysis. For the period this was a sophisticated approach to physiological instruction but not a unique one. Purkyně offered similar demonstrations to his students in Breslau, and comparable "experimental" courses were available in several other German universities.[48]

Schultze regarded the experimental approach as one ideally suited to the needs of medical students. The course is important to us, however, not for what was done but for what was omitted. At Freiburg Schultze provided experimental demonstrations only as an accompaniment to his physiological lectures. At Breslau, in contrast, perhaps in the mid- to late 1820s and certainly after 1830, Purkyně moved beyond the lecture-demonstration and sought to involve his students directly in the "demonstration"—that is, he placed them in the position of making their own observations and conducting their own experiments.

The entire class did not join in these exercises; only a few students did so. Perhaps these few were self-selected, or perhaps Purkyně himself made a selection from among his more promising students, as Johannes Müller was notoriously doing during the 1830s in his rudimentary laboratory in Berlin.[49] Purkyně's innovation was thus a limited one, but it was nonetheless a point of profound importance in the creation of the scientific institute, in exposing the student to a research environment, and in asserting the research ethic within the German university. The self-involvement of the student and the creation of an institutional basis for such involvement opened the way to the possibility that a student might make an original discovery and to the prospect that the student might elect to follow a career in medical or scientific research. The realization of Purkyně's pedagogical plan meant that an investigator was being trained by doing, and it also meant that he had transcended the passivity of the auditor, an inherent feature of the lecture-demonstration. Of course, this step was also a supremely Pestalozzian gesture, now brought to bear at the summit of the educational system, the university and its specialized institutes.

From this point of view, it deserves renewed emphasis that Purkyně's innovation constituted but one and a still quite tentative step along the path leading to the general functions of the nineteenth-century scientific institute. In her essay in this volume, Arleen Tuchman demonstrates that, in physiology at least, it was Jacob Henle at the University of Heidelberg who, during the early 1840s, began to make bench experience in the physiological laboratory a necessary part of the education of all medical students rather than the undertaking of a select few.[50] This extension of a pedagogical scheme, she shows, was welcomed by the Baden public authorities, and it also expanded the reach of the research ethic. Purkyně's "school" of physiology was in full vigor throughout the 1830s and attained permanent institutional status in 1839. But it was always a small affair and never seemed to realize its full potential, especially in bringing modern instruction to all levels of the (medical) curriculum. Henle's work in Heidelberg and that of others during the 1840s were indispensable in translating this ideal from modest realization to broad acceptance and widespread implementation.

A small affair, yes, but one that nonetheless was noticed. In this domain many questions remain open and I can deal briefly with only two. First, what was the later history of the Breslau institute? It was recognized, not least by Purkyně himself, that his own original investigations declined rapidly over the 1840s. He reported that the principal reason was the urgent need to organize and outfit the new institute and to perfect its instructional program. There are indications, however, that he was already thinking of returning to Bohemia, and he was also becoming increasingly active during this politically agitated decade in the question of Czech nationhood and the creation of an indigenous Czech scientific culture.[51] After his appointment (1850) to the chair of physiology in Prague and departure from Prussia, the Breslau institute changed character.[52] Purkyně's replacement was Carl Theodor Ernst von Siebold, a zoologist whose researches focused on parasitic worms.

In 1853 Carl Bogislaus Reichert, a microscopical anatomist working in the Müllerian tradition, assumed responsibility for the institute. Reichert was not an experimentalist. He nevertheless completed the plan of organization as laid down originally by Purkyně. Scientific work in the institute was to be pursued in three separate but interrelated units, each with its assistant: microscopical anatomy, physiological chemistry, and experimental physiology, the latter including vivisection and physical inquiries. This organizational pattern offered a model for other physiological institutes, most notably the famous Leipzig Institute built for Carl Ludwig and opened in 1869. Reichert went to Berlin in 1858 and received there the professorship of anatomy created when Müller's combined chair of anatomy and physiology was divided after his death. Breslau physiology then lay dormant for a year, but in the spring of 1859 a new life began.

Under Rudolf Heidenhain's vigorous direction and with the assistance of Lothar Meyer, the Breslau institute rose rapidly to a commanding position in European physiology and remained there throughout Heidenhain's long career.[53] Breslau became a center for the study of metabolism, animal energetics, and all aspects of glandular secretion. The institute was a prosperous division of one of the best-attended German universities and it performed well its dual function of instruction and research, preparing many physiologists of the next generation. Only in 1898, however, the year following Heidenhain's death, did a new and specially designed building for the institute finally become available.

All in all, there is no doubt that the Heidenhain years brought to rich fruition the plans laid by Purkyně in the 1820s and 1830s. These early years had been especially difficult not only because of frequent doubts regarding the utility and even propriety of such an institute but because public funds in general were limited and seemed to be, for academic purposes, even more constrained. After 1859 and especially after 1866–1871, when Prussia gained hegemony in Germany and the Kaiserreich was created, explosive economic development began. A more favorable political situation for the universities also emerged and university funding became both more secure and more generous. Heidenhain obviously knew how to make the most of these opportunities.

Purkyně's efforts in Breslau were quickly noticed by other physiologists. In the absence of a detailed comparative history of the physiological institute it is impossible to deal satisfactorily with the question of the possible influence of the Breslau Institute on similar foundations in other universities. Purkyně was, in fact, consulted by physiologists who sought to create comparable institutes at their own universities, and a portion of this widespread conversation was recorded. In 1846 Purkyně proudly reported to Altenstein that "interest in creating physiological institutes is beginning to catch on everywhere."[54] He also reported at this time the receipt of inquiries from Bonn and Prague. A few years earlier Rudolph Wagner had solicited his advice regarding the creation of a new center for physiological training in Göttingen. Wagner was Johann Friedrich Blumenbach's successor, the latter in the closing decades of his life an increasingly minor figure in his science, a sad end to what had been a very influential career. Wagner thus was called upon to reestablish the great tradition of physiological study that had been inaugurated a century earlier by Albrecht von Haller. From Purkyně he received a detailed account of the plan and activities of the Breslau Institute, a document that provides the best description of Purkyně's school before and on the eve of the creation of his institute. Wagner did in fact persuade the Hanoverian authorities to establish an institute at Göttingen and himself provided a detailed public apologia for it.[55]

Finally, to conclude with a suggestively dubious possibility, in 1838 Friedrich Hermann Stannius brought into being in the small university at Rostock an institute for "comparative and general pathology as well as physiology." Stannius had received most of his medical training under Müller in Berlin but took his M.D. degree in 1831 in Breslau (not, however, with Purkyně). He had written Wagner regarding the Rostock Institute, and the latter informed Purkyně vaguely that an "institute of this sort" had arisen in the Baltic city. Stannius's letter to Wagner seems lost, but other sources indicate that Stannius, too, was convinced that "academic instruction . . . can prosper only when the student is assured of gaining his own insight (*Anschauung*) into the objects" under scrutiny. The description of this institute given by Heinz Gunther Wischhusen and Ernst Ehler suggests, however, that instruction in Rostock was based upon preserved anatomical and pathological exhibits and did not involve the students in either the preparation of these materials or in experimental work of any kind.[56] At the moment there is no way to decide this question and no way to know whether Stannius was working under the stimulus of Purkyně's Breslau practices.

A negative reply to the latter inquiry may nonetheless be ventured, and we might perhaps expect this reservation to extend to other institutes that closely combined physiology and anatomy. Increasingly in the nineteenth century, and very much so in the case of Purkyně, physiologists saw themselves placed in opposition to anatomists, the latter being traditionally the accredited students not only of bodily structure but of organic function. A major point dividing the two specialties was methodology. Physiologist and anatomist came to differ on methods applicable to both instruction and inquiry. The physiologist wanted direct access to vital processes and was eager to exploit physical, chemical, microscopical, and vivisectional techniques to gain that access; his institute was to be built around this proposition. The anatomist, in contrast, continued to stress skill in dissection and to offer a comparative view of function by means of preserved materials. Microscopical anatomy might be expected to have belonged to anatomy; but whenever possible it was seized by physiologists (and pathologists). As noted earlier, the microscope and its celebrated creation, the cell theory, promised a new approach not only to structure but to function and dysfunction. In the tradition of the German universities, microscopical anatomy was distinguished, de facto if not always de jure, from gross anatomy. It was made a responsibility of the chair of physiology or of a second, "histological" anatomical appointment and thus came to be represented by students of function and development.[57]

For reasons that I have been unable to establish, anatomy and physiology at Breslau were assigned wholly independent status at the foundation of the university. This was a singular novelty within a German university and one not easily repeated; the separation of the chairs of anatomy and physiology in the medical faculties of these universities came about only gradually, and the process of separation offers a major theme in the story of the arrival of so-called scientific medicine in these faculties. For example, Müller personally never, and Berlin institutionally only in the 1850s, separated physiology and anatomy. In 1855 Emil du Bois-Reymond became *extraordinarius* for physiology and in 1858 he received the new chair in physiology at Berlin created by the division of Müller's combined responsibilities. To compound the confusion, however, Reichert received the new chair of anatomy in Berlin. Reichert came from the physiological institute in Breslau; he was an outstanding microscopical anatomist; and he had a keen interest in functional questions. No doubt it was not part of du Bois-Reymond's concern to appropriate the microscope as the emblem of his craft; his talents and tasks obviously ran in the physicalist direction indicated by electrophysiology. But perhaps in the 1850s and even much later du Bois-Reymond was a conspicuous exception. Heidenhain fought vigorously and successfully throughout his career in Breslau to keep microscopical studies within the bounds of physiology; microscopy constituted a major feature of Ernst von Brücke's work in Vienna and of Carl Ludwig's laboratory in Leipzig.[58]

Questions such as these will remain moot until study of the institute phenomenon moves beyond concern with the nominal designation of one or another chair or institute and explores in a detailed and comparative manner the character of the instruction offered and the research conducted by the occupant of a given chair or chairs: it will be necessary also to explore the actual program of an institute and the instructional activity and research of its varied staff. Physiology often entered the German university under another name. Siebold, for example, whom we have seen as professor of physiology in Breslau, moved to Munich in 1853 as professor of anatomy and physiology. His real interest, however, was zoology, and in the following year he shifted to a chair with that designation. He was immediately replaced as professor of anatomy (and physiology) by Theodor Ludwig Wilhelm Bischoff, a veritable physiologist. In 1856–1857 Emil Harless received a new *ordinarius* (physiology), yet a truly autonomous chair of physiology appears to have come to Munich only in 1863, and this position was filled by Carl Voit.[59]

In such a situation it is as fruitless to attempt to identify the "first" physiological institute as it would be meaningless to succeed in such a task. I intend to leave the impression that Purkyně at Breslau was a leader in the rapidly accelerating movement toward the creation of such institutions, but I hope that I have not suggested that it is the novelty of his endeavor (which seems genuine) or even the modest success that he enjoyed during the 1830s and 1840s that is of major interest. To be sure, we may fairly conclude that the physiological institute had acquired a definite and enduring form by the early 1840s (Breslau, 1839; Göttingen, 1842; Jena, 1846), and many others followed after 1850. The real interest of the Breslau institute is that it reveals with exceptional clarity the meeting point of a new physiology, one changing character after the 1820s and beginning to adopt a much more interventionist methodological stance, one that took its stand on the rapidly growing instrumental or technical culture of science, and public (that is, administrative) recognition of the importance and needs of this new approach. The Breslau program or, if one will, "institute" truly began with Purkyně's appointment in 1823. That appointment was a result of favorable personal connections in Berlin, but even more it came about through recognition by Prussian educational authorities that in this Czech physiologist they had found an individual both determined and able to extend to a promising and important domain the research ethos that was to become the hallmark of the major German universities.

THE RESEARCH IMPERATIVE

The ideal of original investigation conducted by the professoriate acquired great celebrity in the nineteenth-century university. The origins of this research ideal are varied and still problematic, although recent scholars tend to agree that these developments found their earliest home in the German university and, within the university, among the members of its philosophical faculty.[60]

The neohumanist program that pervaded the philosophical faculty stressed the ideal of *Bildung*. *Bildung* or, loosely put, the pursuit, by means of advanced instruction and the directed development of individual skills, of cultural depth and socially favored values, was to be encouraged by study of classical languages and cultures, above all the Greek language and Greek history and thought. The overriding goal of this program was moral in character, and the principal mission of the university's philosophy faculty was to prepare the instructors for the secondary-school system, whose own students were of an age most suited to moral formation. A lesser goal was to prepare professional philologists and historians. A few among those enrolled in a historical or philological seminar would, in fact, go on to a university career, but most could look forward to teaching in the reorganized

Gymnasien of Germany, there to impart to their students the glories that were Greece. Aesthetic sensibility was cultivated and that sensibility by no means had natural phenomena as its principal concern. The neohumanist found himself entering a "second Paradise," that of the "human mind" (*Geist*), a new and happier paradise that transcended the limited "first Paradise" of "human nature."[61]

Historians of science have also examined the possible meaning of the research ideal that apparently emerged from the philological and historical seminars established in Göttingen and Halle in the 1780s and 1790s and which soon thereafter appeared in the reformed universities of Prussia and elsewhere in Germany.[62] A seemingly improbable but nonetheless very important connection has been sought: the link between the early neohumanist-inspired research ideal and the later but powerful research impulse exhibited throughout the natural sciences. The latter, emerging under the stimulus of the neohumanistic example, has been seen to assume recognizable form during the 1830s; the mathematical-physical seminar launched in 1835–1836 by C. C. G. Jacobi and Franz Neumann in Königsberg provided the model for this new form of organized scientific inquiry.[63]

But there are serious problems with this conclusion. First, although special attention has quite properly been directed to the singular conditions surrounding the creation of the philosophical faculty and to its extraordinary brilliance and expansion during the nineteenth century, it is a fact and one too often overlooked that strictly humanistic studies—classical languages, Germanistics, history—did not alone constitute this faculty, nor did humanistic studies alone bear the burden of high research expectations. At Breslau, for example, chemistry formed part of the philosophical faculty, and the chemical institute dedicated itself from the outset to both regular instruction and original research. The same was true for Justus von Liebig's celebrated chemical laboratory in Giessen, begun in 1824, where the hands-on approach for the student was rapidly brought to a high art.

I do not intend these remarks to diminish the novelty and general significance of the revolution that was effected after 1780 in classical studies. I do suggest, however, that we must view the philosophical faculty and, even more, the university in the same manner as did the neohumanist. The neohumanist knew very well that classical studies did not represent the entire faculty and that the latter alone did not compose the university. The neohumanist was pleased, of course, to view his as the most important because morally the most elevated body of studies offered by the university; he made no small contribution to the growing separation of the no longer so liberal arts and the natural sciences, and his scientific colleagues showed themselves prepared to respond in kind.[64] The neohumanist condemned the specialization and fragmentation of knowledge that seemed to accompany scientific advance. He deplored the natural scientist's emphasis on mere practical matters and reacted with apparently genuine horror to the smell of materialism that often accompanied his scientific colleagues.

"Philosophical" studies had come to the fore only with the rise of post-Kantian idealism and the new-found veneration of the Greek world. They enjoyed apparent dominance within the philosophical faculty throughout the nineteenth century, often reaffirmed by the strength of a new economic power and cultural arbiter, north Germany. The appeal to Hellenism was also well received in Protestant circles as a counterforce to the Roman-Latin tradition of Catholicism. By century's end, however, as Fritz Ringer has strikingly demonstrated, the ideal itself was becoming corrupt and its advocates shrill in their defense of what others saw as an outdated, arrogant, and socially destructive set of values.[65] For the historian of science the problem is that although we know the research ideal best through its incarnation in the neohumanist program, this does not mean that the neohumanist program wholly or even best represents that ideal. The appearance of a strong leadership role for neohumanism may, in addition to its well-founded claim to such a position, derive also in part from its own uncommonly effective self-advertisement and our continued ignorance of other possibilities.

One must not overlook the existence in nineteenth-century Europe and not least in Germany of a veritable culture of science.[66] Perhaps all university graduates, because of the need of an *Abitur* from the Gymnasium for matriculation in the university (a firm rule in Prussia after 1834), had received extensive training in the classics during their school days, and perhaps, too, many of the students who elected to pursue a university career in the natural sciences continued to value highly and defend fiercely the stringent classical curriculum and its broader cultural program. Nonetheless, although such a self-reproducing elite may easily set standards and expect many others to follow its example, it is obvious that these standards did not offer a norm for the entire community. Neither did scientific culture, but its reach was wide and its message, although it is still inadequately explored, was unmistakable. Natural science was seen to offer its own distinctive measure of rationality. It appeared to offer positive knowledge and a set of methods by which reliably to increase the fund of such knowledge. It easily set aside (or so it seemed) older authorities, particularly scriptural authority. Especially when appearing in conjunction with the great engineering marvels of the age, science also seemed to furnish a new and exciting aesthetic, one peculiarly suited to the needs of modern man. Again in conjunction with the many applications to which it was bent, science notoriously made its claim to be the true foundation of economic development, general progress, and the construction of, almost indifferently, both the liberal and illiberal state.

Spokesmen for these several values held a respected place in the German university and many presumably found their home within the philosophical faculty. The scientist might or might not share the neohumanist value system, but certainly he did share the research ethos. This matter, however, must here be left unresolved; the presumed origin of the research imperative uniquely within the philosophical faculty, and the question of whether that value was principally represented by its humanistic or scientific members, requires much further investigation. Naturally, such an examination will need to attend closely to appointments, budget, and outfitting and explore the conduct of instruction and research in each of the ever more numerous scholarly and scientific specialties that found themselves within the philosophical faculty.

My discussion is not directed to this question, however, but to an additional doubt regarding the preeminent role of neohumanism in generating the research imperative and assuring for it a respected and effective place within the university. The fact is that the philosophical faculty had to make its way amid or, one could say almost equally well, against well-entrenched rivals: namely, the traditional studies of law, theology, and medicine. In the late eighteenth century these faculties still assured general cultural formation as well as study of the particular professional subject to which each was dedicated. They offered "arts" as well as "sciences." But dramatic changes transformed German university life between 1789 and 1815. The new philosophical faculty claimed for itself the right to provide aspiring men with the cultural trappings befitting their destined place in society.

After 1815 the faculties of law, theology, and medicine were viewed increasingly as training or professional schools, their cultural functions now largely lost. They prepared students for careers with the state or for independent service dedicated, loosely speaking, to the public interest. Naturally these faculties emphasized practical subjects (*Brotstudien* in the harsh polemical coin of the day), and they employed Greek and Latin, the essential arms of the neohumanist, only as tools of the trade. Professional literature in all three areas of study continued to be published in Latin well into the nineteenth century. In medicine, where the ancient Greek physicians had become idealized figures to be emulated even as they remained authors to be read for their seemingly eternal contributions to the healing art, a reading knowledge of Greek still had its place. It offered, however, no entrée into a distant culture the standards of which were to be restored for the modern world.

What is true of the philosophical faculty has also been true of the medical faculty: we lack incisive conceptual and institutional assessment of the creation and evolution of the cognitive demands, specialized facilities, administrative interests, and realized practices that informed the emergence of this faculty and its members as leaders in the strong movement toward original research that was characteristic of the early nineteenth century. Several essays in this volume attempt to deal with this problem, and one can hope that other investigations, focusing on other time periods and other national traditions, will follow.[67] The case of Breslau makes clear (Berlin or Leipzig, Göttingen or Heidelberg would probably serve as well) that the unit of principal interest—the scientific research institute in the medical faculty—came into being contemporaneous with and in some cases earlier than comparable centers of research in the natural sciences located in the philosophical faculty.[68] The question before us is, again, not one of priority but of when and where and above all how and why the institutionalized form of the research ideal made its way into the university community. Certainly motives were many. Purkyně, like others before him, found in medicine the only way to obtain advanced training in the natural sciences, and, again like many others, he saw in medicine the surest hope of securing a "scientific" position within the university. The medical faculty in most German universities was especially favored by responsible authorities, and in the Prussian universities the faculty was at the forefront of institutional modernization. The Berlin Kultusministerium had its own agenda, one embracing the sciences as well as the humanistic disciplines, and pursued its purposes across the university, not simply in the philosophical faculty.

Obvious points, perhaps, but nonetheless insufficiently explored. Less obvious is a second issue, one that calls into question the sharp division so often presumed to have existed between the demands of the neohumanist and the aspirations of the natural scientist. I have respected this distinction, but, like other observers, I am also obliged to examine the possibility that these notorious disciplinary battle lines, however sharply drawn between bodies of knowledge and sociocultural purposes, are less clearly expressed on the methodological level.[69]

Did the classical-neohumanistic ideal exclude the study of natural phenomena or reduce such study to a derisory level? So it would appear in the programmatic literature of many of its late as well as its early proponents. Purkyně's remarks on the proper role of the Gymnasium, for example, were provoked by the demand of Carl Gustav Carus, himself a physician and an artist and leading figure in the administration of medical affairs in Saxony, that the Gymnasium, a "school of the spirit," exclude all scientific studies, these to commence only with entrance into the university (that is, the medical faculty).[70] Carus's views exhibit once again the radical proposition that the natural sciences deal with matters that are not an integral part of all human experience and can be reserved for later study by those few who have declared a professional interest in such concerns. Purkyně, as we have seen, would have none of an argument that steered a youth or university student to a spiritual diet alone and deprived him of direct experience with the natural and social world.

To be sure, it might be claimed that Purkyně was an exception— not the exception that proves the rule but one which, like most exceptions, leads essentially nowhere. I find this charge unwelcome, and I immediately place against it the important fact that however much his views collided with those of some members of the university community, Purkyně's organizational efforts were recognized as meritorious by distinguished members of his own discipline and, the decisive point, by influential figures in the Prussian Kultusministerium. One must shift perspective here, from Purkyně the individual physiologist to the administration's view of Purkyně's endeavor and to the perception within the Kultusministerium that the Breslau Institute constituted a novel and worthy undertaking. Purkyně's affairs, like his objectives, were by no means his alone. Academic appointments and institutional accoutrements in the nineteenth-century German university were closely controlled by governmental authorities and were always subject to the needs of national educational, social, and economic policy. For almost thirty years Purkyně enjoyed the undiminished support of the same cultural authorities who created and supported the philological and historical seminar.

Moreover, the Berlin Kultusministerium did not favor Purkyně and Breslau alone but encouraged the spread of scientific work in other Prussian medical faculties and universities. Schultze, for example, a product of F. A. Wolfe's epoch-making philological seminar at Halle and an experienced Gymnasium teacher, during his long years as Altenstein's deputy in the Kultusministerium provided even-handed support for all innovative and promising young scholars and scientists who sought and found a place in the Prussian university system, whatever their special subject. It is clear that, rhetoric notwithstanding, the neohumanist program qua program did not preclude vigorous efforts to further the study of the natural sciences in the university. This is only to be expected, for public authorities were not blind or opposed to the important role that technical expertise, the essential product of a professional faculty, played in assuring social stability and measured economic development. This is only to restate the essential point made by McClelland: in the state bureaucracies and among many university professors, predominantly those found in the professional faculties, approval and encouragement of practical studies at the university level were always to be met.[71] This was the enduring and ultimately successful counterforce to doctrinaire neohumanism.

Opinions varied as to whether self-development by means of individual experience was appropriate to all stages or only to one or another stage in the educational process. Insofar as local conditions permitted, the Kultusministerium supervised every stage of a student's career, beginning with primary education and continuing through university studies. Süvern had made the Pestalozzian program an integral part of Prussian pedagogical intentions on the primary school level. This was done in the early years of the reform movement and before the arrival of both Altenstein and Schultze at the head of educational affairs. The Gymnasium was another matter entirely. It was claimed by the neohumanists and it became their own very effective instrument for the propagation of the classical ideal. The curriculum of the Gymnasium included much Latin, ample Greek, German, Hebrew and scriptural studies, and some mathematics. Physics and natural history commanded only a small proportion of the student's time in the early history of the Gymnasium, and even this proportion would decline sharply by the 1840s.[72]

What is in question, however, is not subject matter or the social function of this subject matter but how the university student would best be trained. The representative neohumanist indeed believed that emphasis upon classical studies and mathematics—the latter meant to discipline the intellect, not to become the handmaid to scientific inquiry—served a high cultural purpose: the inculcation of moral standards and social values that would replace the gentlemanly ideal of the eighteenth-century *Gelehrter*. In the minds of the early reformers, at least, and before these high ambitions degenerated into routine, relentless drill and indoctrination, education for the university student was to be an exciting exercise in discovery and self-development. When this is kept clearly in mind, the circle of pedagogical aspiration within which Purkyně moved appears much larger than is suggested by the easily formulated but ambiguous rivalry between classical and scientific studies.

The common ground was pedagogical method, and the method in question, one shared by all reformers, had as its common feature the urgent need to bring the student into active involvement in his own education. The critical addition to this plan was, in Purkyně's case, to arrange that this involvement, now taking place in the university, be applicable to work in the natural sciences. The Gymnasium, to Purkyně's anger and continued frustration, offered slight or no prospect for applying at the secondary level a hands-on approach to scientific study, but the university (that is, the medical faculty) did provide this opportunity. Seconded by the Berlin authorities, Purkyně seized the occasion; his creation was not perfectly formed but it suggested the program that a scientific institute should develop and pursue, exemplified how such an institute might be organized, and, in its scientific work and the students it prepared, demonstrated both the feasibility and value of such an endeavor.

The scientific research imperative in the German university did in fact emerge with shifting or, better expressed, emerging "professional" concerns, these revolving around such sociologically interesting processes as specialization, the cultivation of technical expertise, modernization, and intense methodological dispute. The creation of the Breslau Physiological Institute indicates the capital importance of this last factor and places stress on the methodological continuity between the school and the university. Purkyně's contribution was to implement the Pestalozzian program at a new and higher— indeed, the highest—educational level and to reveal the hidden creative impulse of that program. He showed that proper attention to self-development meant more than merely effective schooling, the point at which Pestalozzi had left the subject. Instead it directed the student's attention to what was as yet unknown. The possibility of preparing a qualified student for original research and discovery followed from this conclusion, and the social realization of Purkyně's program, the physiological institute, followed in its turn.

ACKNOWLEDGMENTS

I am grateful for the suggestions of F. L. Holmes, Timothy Lenoir, K. M. Olesko, and Arleen Tuchman, as well as for comments on a rudimentary version of this essay offered years ago by members of the Johns Hopkins Institute of the History of Medicine. My thanks, too, to helpful staff members at the Zentrum für interdisziplinäre Forschung and at the Universitätsbibliothek, both in Bielefeld.

NOTES

1. J. E. Purkyně, Bericht H: 1844, *Opera omnia/Sebrané spisy*, ed. Vladislav Kruta and Blanka Eberhardova, 12 vols. (Prague: Czechoslovakian Academy of Sciences, 1918–1973), XII: 287. Between 1839 and 1849 Purkyně sent numerous reports on the activities of his institute to the Prussian Kultusministerium in Berlin. These Berichte carry no titles and have been labeled by the editors of Purkyně's works in an alphabetical series beginning with E (1839) and continuing to N (1849); items A to D are pre-1840 documents pertaining to the foundation of the institute. These reports are preserved in the Deutsches Zentralarchiv, Merseburg, and have been transcribed in full for the aforementioned edition. All of this material is of utmost importance for understanding the institute phenomenon in its earliest years, and my references thereto follow the form just described; that is, Bericht + assigned letter + year for which the report was filed.

2. See C. E. McClelland, *State, Society and University in Germany 1700– 1914* (Cambridge: Cambridge University Press, 1980), pp. 101–149; Thomas Nipperdey, *Deutsche Geschichte 1800–1866* (Munich: C. H. Beck, 1984), pp. 33–69, 454–482; L. Petry, "Die Gründung der drei Friedrich-Wilhelms-Universitäten Berlin, Breslau, Bonn," *Festschrift Hermann Aubin zum 80.*

Geburtstag, ed. O. Brunner et al., 2 vols. (Wiesbaden: Franz Steiner, 1965), I: 687–709.

3. Georg Kaufmann, ed., *Festschrift zur Feier des hundertjährigen Bestehens der Universität Breslau*, 2 vols. (Breslau: Ferdinand Hirt, 1911), I: 1–44.

4. A Prussian appointment was highly regarded in Prague. A friend wrote to Purkyně: "Sie haben das Ziel erreicht! soll ich mich freuen? soll ich trauern? wir verlieren Sie; ein neues Land, neue Verhältnisse, ein neues Leben fesselt Sie weit von hier! Die Gränzgebirge einmal im Rücken, überschreiten Sie solche nicht so bald wieder. Wie Cäser können Sie sagen: ich kam, ich sah und siegte." To another friend Purkyně confided (8 February 1823): "Nun aber, da sichs entschieden hat, so betrachte es mit mir als ein besonderes Lebensglück, welches auch selbst manche kühne Hoffnung mein früheren Jugend übertroffen hat. Ich bin an einer der ansehlichsten Universitäten Deutschlands, in einem Fach das von jeher mein Lieblingsfach war, mit einem mehr als zureichendem Gehalte (800 Thl [Thaler] Fixum und wenigst 400 Th Honorar), in einem wenigstens erträglich geistesfreien Lande, meine bisher begonnene und weiter zu verbreitende wissenschaftliche Existenz auch academisch begründet." *K. Pocatkum Vedecké Drahy J. E. Purkyně/Beginnings of the Scientific Career of J. E. Purkyně*, ed. Vladislav Kruta and Vladimir Zapletal (Brno: Medical Faculty of the J. E. Purkyně University, 1964), pp. 130, 136.

5. See H. J. John, *Jan Evangelista Purkyně. Czech Scientist and Patriot 1787–1869*, Memoirs of the American Philosophical Society, vol. 49 (Philadelphia, 1959). The best overall guides to Purkyně's scientific work are Vladislav Kruta and Mikulas Teich, *Jan Evangelista Purkyně*, trans. Samuel Kostomolatsky and Alice Teichova (Prague: State Medical Publishing House, 1962); Vladislav Kruta, *J. E. Purkyně [1787–1869] Physiologist. A Short Account of His Contributions to the Progress of Physiology, with a Bibliography of His Works* (Prague: Academia, 1969).

6. John, *Purkyně*, pp. 15–17; Erich Witte, "Die Berufung Purkyněs nach Breslau," *Anatomischer Anzeiger* 92 (1941): 68–77.

7. Johannes Müller, "Gedächtnissrede auf Carl Asimund Rudolphi," *Abhandlungen der Akademie der Wissenschaften zu Berlin*, 1835 [1837]: xvii–xxxviii; Walter Artelt, *Der Mesmerismus in Berlin*, Abhandlungen der Akademie der Wissenschaften und der Literatur in Mainz, Geist-und Sozialwissenschaftliche Klasse, no. 6 (1965). Purkyně's vocabulary and general outlook preserved many traces of his earlier philosophical infatuations, but these latter left little mark on his later scientific work or on the conduct of the affairs of his institute. On the former point, see Richard Toellner, "Naturphilosophische Elemente im Denken Purkyněs," in *Jan Evangelista Purkyně 1787–1869. Centenary Symposium*, ed. Vladislav Kruta (Brno: Medical Faculty of the J. E. Purkyně University, 1971), pp. 35–41.

8. *Zur vergleichenden Physiologie des Gesichtssinnes des Menschen und der Thiere* and *Ueber die phantastischen Gesichtserscheinungen*. See Gottfried Koller, *Das Leben des Biologen Johannes Müller* (Stuttgart: Wissenschaftliche Verlagsgesellschaft, 1958), pp. 51–60.

9. J. E. Purkyně, *Commentatio de examine physiologico organi visus et syste-*

matis cutanei (1823), *Opera omnia*, I: 163–194; English translation in John, *Purkyně*, pp. 54–59. Müller's comments remained unpublished until presented by Vladislav Kruta, "Unrecognized Discoveries. Johannes Müller's Report on Purkyně's Treatise 'On the Physiological Examination of the Organ of Vision and of the Cutaneous System' (1823)," *Clio Medica* 2 (1967): 159–177. Purkyně's view of the disputed question of "subjective" and "objective" approaches to sensory phenomena is vigorously stated in "Johannes Müller. De sensibus libre duo," 1827, that is, review of *Physiologie des Gesichtssinnes* and *Phantastische Gesichtserscheinungen: Opera omnia*, V: 27–54.

10. On method, see Johannes Steudel, "Müller, Johannes Peter," *Dictionary of Scientific Biography*, ed. C.C. Gillespie (New York: Charles Scribner's Sons, 1970–1980) IX, esp. pp. 573–574. Müller's move to Berlin in 1833 was not without its difficulties, Friedrich Tiedemann having first received and declined a call. The Berlin medical faculty favored both Tiedemann and Müller, stressing that each represented *both* observation and experiment; the university's rector, the chemist and mineralogist Christian Samuel Weiss, was much more skeptical, noting that several other candidates, including Purkyně, better represented the (desired?) experimental approach than did Müller, who had restricted himself to physiological observation. See the full discussion of this very complicated affair in Manfred Stürzbecher, "Zur Berufung Johannes Müllers an der Berliner Universität," *Jahrbuch für Geschichte Mittel- und Ostdeutschlands* 21 (1972): 184–226, esp. pp. 192–199.

11. The chronology is that stated by Purkyně himself: Vladislav Kruta, "J. E. Purkyně's Account of the Origin and Early History of the Institute of Physiology in Breslau (1841)," *Scripta Medica* 39 (1966): 1–16. Kruta here offers an English translation of Purkyně's description of his work sent to Rudolf Wagner in Göttingen; a transcription of the German original appears as Purkyně, Bericht A: 1841, *Opera omnia*, XII: 213–218. See also Karl Hürthle, "Die Gründung des physiologischen Instituts in Breslau durch Joh. Ev. Purkinje, mit Enthüllung der Büste Purkinjes," *Jahresbericht der Schlesische Gesellschaft für vaterländische Cultur* 86 (1908): 1–12.

12. Quoted by Rudolph Heidenhain in "Purkinje, Johannes Evangelista," *Allgemeine Deutsche Biographie*, XXVI: 720; "ohnmöglich" read as "ohnmächtig." Kruta could not locate this document in either the Prussian Kultusministerium archives now in Merseburg or the university archives in Wrocław (Breslau): "Purkyně's Account," p. 5, n. 7.

13. The faculty's candidate was F. P. Gruithuisen, another able sensory physiologist who, however, turned to astronomy in 1826. On Otto and anatomical studies in Breslau, see Paul Dzillas, "Die Geschichte der Anatomie an der Universität Breslau," *Jahrbuch der Schlesische Friedrich-Wilhelms Universität zu Breslau* 18 (1973): 212–241; A. W. Otto, "Ueber die neue Anatomie zu Breslau," *Medizinische Zeitung* 7 (1838): 139–141; idem, *Einige geschichtliche Erinnerungen an das frühere Studium der Anatomie in Schlesien, nebst eine Beschreibung und Abbildung des jetzigen Königlichen Anatomie-Instituts* (Breslau: Grass, Barth, 1823). C. G. Carus, "Adolph Wilhem Otto. Über Sein Leben und Wirken," *Janus* 1 (1846; reprint 1931): 691–698. Purkyně was evidently a

very poor lecturer, and Otto provided the Berlin authorities a private and vicious account of that fact. As stated by Heidenhain, Otto reported: Purkyně "spreche nicht fliessend und deutlich, es fehle ihm oft an den deutschen Ausdrücken, die Vorträge sind zu philosophisch und abstract, die gangbären Ansichten nicht genügend hervorgehoben. Otto bezweifelt, dass P[urkyně] je ein guter Lehrer werde, vielleicht könne er trotzdem ein brauchbarer Docent werden, wenn er Lateinische vortrage, denn die lateinische Sprache ewinge zu präciser Ausdrucksweise, und nicht nach eigenen Heften, sondern nach einem gangbaren Compendium, wozu sich etwa Lenhossek empfehle, da Rudolphi's Lehrbuch für P[urkyně] zu gelehrt sei." Heidenhain, "Purkinje," in *Allgemeine Deutsche Biographie*, p. 719. This amazing outburst tells much not only of the personal relationship between Otto and his new colleague but of the great divide between the old university conceived as a training school (especially in its professional faculties) and the rising research ideal. Purkyně taught from his own knowledge and that which he had received from others but worked over after receipt; he had no use for teaching by the book. "Lenhossek" is probably the *Institutiones physiologicae* (Vienna, 1822) of Michael von Lenossék; see Erna Lesky, *The Vienna Medical School of the 19th Century*, trans. L. Williams and I. S. Levij (Baltimore: Johns Hopkins University Press, 1976), pp. 72–73. The ministerial influence was indeed strong at Breslau. Chemistry in association with botany had received virtual "institute" status upon university foundation in 1811; the active hand belonged to Johannes Wilhelm Süvern in the Berlin Kultusministerium, who, like many a later statesman pursuing a personal as well as public agenda, saw in chemistry a new foundation for industrial development. See Julius Schiff, "Das erste chemische Institut der Universität Breslau," *Archiv für Geschichte der Mathematik, der Naturwissenschaften und Technik* 9 (1920–1921): 29–38.

14. Purkyně, "Ueber den Begriff der Physiologie, ihre Beziehung zu den übrigen Naturwissenschaften, und zu andern wissenschaftlichen und kunst-Gebieten, die Methode ihre Lehre und über die Bildung zum Physiologen Praxis, über Errichtung physiologischer Institut" (1851), *Opera omnia*, III: 64–79; the quotation is from the incomplete translation by John, *Purkyně*, p. 39.

15. Purkyně, Bericht C: 1836, *Opera omnia*, XII: 227.

16. See his first round of demands in ibid., pp. 231–232.

17. Josef Hölzel et al., "Simon Plössel (1794–1868). Optiker und Mechaniker in Wien (Zur Entwicklungsgeschichte der Plössel-Mikroskope)," *Blätter für Technikgeschichte*, no. 31 (1969): 45–89; Viktor Patzelt, "Die Bedeutung des Wiener Optikers Simon Plössel für die Mikroskopie," *Mikroskope* 2 (1947): 1–12. On related microscopical tools developed in the Breslau institute, see Josef Sajner, "Jan Evangelista Purkyně and Adolph Oschatz," *Nova acta leopoldina* N.F. 24 (1961): 133–139; Rudolph Zaunick, "Adolph Oschatz' Leben und Wirken," ibid., pp. 139–145.

18. Ed. Frison, "De microscopen waarmee Jan Evangelista Purkinje (1787–1869) heeft gewerkt," *Scientiarum historia* 14 (1972): 165–180; idem, "Les microscopes de Simon Plössel examinés et appréciés par les micrographes contemporains," *Mikroskopie* 12 (1957): 289–298. See also Purkyně, "Uber ein für die hiesige Universität gebautes grosses Plössel'sches Mikroskop" (1832),

Opera omnia, II: 81–84. Purkyně's appreciation of the microscope, this marvelous "potentiated eye," as he called it, and his vision of the new world of microscopy is stated in "Mikroskop (Anwendung und Gebrauch bei physiologischen Untersuchungen)," in *Handwörterbuch der Physiologie mit Rücksicht auf physiologische Pathologie*, ed. Rudolf Wagner, 5 vols. (Braunschweig: Friedrich Vieweg, 1842–1853), II: 411–441.

19. Purkyně, Bericht D: 1839, *Opera omnia*, XII: 236–241.

20. My purpose is to offer an assessment of Purkyně's objectives for his institute and not a portrait of its operations. The latter, however, may be traced in some detail through the several reports sent to the Kultusministerium in Berlin (Berichte E–N, *Opera omnia*, XII: 242–309) and in Samuel Pappenheim's complete public declaration of intentions and description of first operations: "Mittheilungen über die Thätigkeit des Königl. physiologischen Institutes zu Breslau, von Ende Januar bis Ende August 1843," *Beiträge zur physiologischen und pathologischen Chemie und Mikroscopie* 1 (1844): 486–512. Of Purkyně's reports, that of 1844 (Bericht H) is especially detailed; it may also represent major elements of an (unpublished) popular statement of the Breslau program promised the reader by his colleague, Pappenheim (ibid., p. 512). No doubt study of the institute's account book, complete from November 1842 until Purkyně's departure in November 1851 and preserved in the university archives in Wrocław, would offer much information regarding day-to-day operations: see Otakar Matousek, "J. E. Purkyně's Leben und Tätigkeit im Lichte der Berliner und Prager Archive," *Nova acta Leopoldina* N.F. 24 (1961): 128 n. 16.

21. See John, *Purkyně*, pp. 35–50. Also Matousek, "Purkyně's Leben und Tätigkeit," pp. 121–126, who points out that by the late 1850s Purkyně, then in his seventies, had become politically suspect to the reactionary and diligent Austrian authorities and found his professional life seriously disturbed. Purkyně's political activities are generally ignored by his biographers; see, however, the anonymous and obviously disapproving Austro-German account: ["Purkyně, Johann Evangelista Ritter von"], *Biographisches Lexikon des Kaiserthums Oesterreich*, 59 vols. (Vienna: K. K. Hof- und Staatsdruckerei, 1856–1890), XXIV: 94–102.

22. This large subject has often been reviewed: F. K. Studnicka, "Joh. E. Purkinjes und seiner Schule Verdienste um die Entdeckung tierischer Zellen und um die Aufstellung der 'Zellen'-Theorie," *Acta societas scientiarum naturaliae Moraviae* 4 (1927): 97–168; "Joh. Ev. Purkinjes histologische Arbeiten," *Anatomischer Anzeiger* 82 (1936): 41–66; Véra Eisnerova, "The Anatomy of Plants and Its Contribution to the Origin of Cellular Theory in the Early 19th Century," *Acta historia rerum naturalium necon technicarum* (Prague), Special Issue no. 5 (1971): 269–333; Vladislav Kruta, "J. E. Purkyně's Contribution to the Cell Theory," *Clio Medica* 6 (1971): 109–120. Purkyně published a number of suggestive short statements regarding the new notion of the living cell, but his only general discussion is the brief review, "Theodor Schwann-Microscop. Untersuchungen üb. die Übereinstimmung in d. Structur u. d. Wachstum der Tiere und Pflanzen" (1840), *Opera omnia*, V: 178–183.

23. Mikulas Teich, "Purkyně and Valentin on Ciliary Motion: An Early

Investigation in Morphological Physiology," *British Journal for the History of Science* 5 (1970): 168–177; Bruno Kisch, "Forgotten Leaders in Modern Medicine: Valentin, Gruby, Remak, Auerbach," *Transactions of the American Philosophical Society* 44 (1954): 137–317, esp. pp. 142–192. Also Brian Bracegirdle, *A History of Microtechnique. The Evolution of the Microtome and the Development of Tissue Preparation* (London: Heinemann, 1978), pp. 309–318; L. S. Jacyna, "The Romantic Programme and the Reception of Cell Theory in Britain," *Journal of the History of Biology* 17 (1984): 13–48.

24. A detailed verbal description is given by Pappenheim, "Über die Tätigkeit des Institutes zu Breslau," pp. 487–490; a sketch of the floor plan (the original was sent to M. J. Schleiden in Jena, who was then planning a new institute) appears in Ilse Jahn, "Diskussions-beiträge," *Nova acta leopoldina* N.F. 24 (1961): 209; a photo of the battered last physical vestige of Purkyně's institute is reproduced by Matousek, "Purkyně's Leben und Tätigkeit," p. 115. Purkyně had found the university's attics so unsuited for physiological work that between 1835, upon the death of his young wife, and 1839 he used his own home as a scientific laboratory.

25. Purkyně, Bericht H: 1844, *Opera omnia*, XII: 281. Such expansive thoughts came easily to Purkyně; see also his concluding comments in a review (1833) of K. F. Burdach's *Physiologie als Erfahrungswissenschaft, Opera omnia*, V: 117–122.

26. See his remarks quoted by John, *Purkyně*, p. 40.

27. H. M. Pollard, *Pioneers of Popular Education, 1760–1850* (Cambridge: Harvard University Press, 1957), pp. 1–131, who states clearly (p. 125) the common theme: the reformers held "that the victims of want would have to be helped if a more reasonable future were to be opened up for Europe, and that it paid better to have intelligent human beings than ignorant beasts of burden." Also see R. H. Quick, *Essays on Educational Reformers* (New York: Appleton, 1907), pp. 239–383.

28. The best account of Purkyně's younger years is given by John, *Purkyně*, pp. 4–17; his medical studies are described by Bozena Matouskova, "Purkyně's Studienjahre an der medizinischen Fakultät der Prager Universität," *Nova acta leopoldina* N.F. 24 (1961): 15–30. On Purkyně's teaching, see J. R. Berg and Josef Sajner, "J. E. Purkyně as a Piarist Monk," *Bulletin of the History of Medicine* 49 (1975): 381–388.

29 John, *Purkyně*, p. 5.

30 Ibid., p. 9. In one of several autobiographical fragments that Purkyně published during his second period in Prague (1850–1869), he recalled at length his early ambition: "Während meines Aufenthaltes in Blatna, wo ich ganz unbeschränkt freie Zeit geniessen durfte, und mich mit Lesen von neueren Philosophen und römerischen Klassikern, besonders aber der pädagogischen Schriften von *Pestalozzi*, befasste, verfolgte mich immerzu das Bild der Schule von Sais, das sich allmählich sozusagen der Wirklichkeit näherte und sich schliesslich in meiner Gedankwelt zu einer wissenschaftlichen Anstalt für Knaben formte . . . Kurz und gut, ich wollte aus freien Stücken die Methode von *Pestalozzi* verwirklichen und ich hoffte, dieselbe bis zu den äussersten Asten der wissenschaftlichen Ausbildung entwickeln

zu können. Deshalb sollte man mit meinen Knaben bis zu den höchsten Stufen der wissenschaftlichen, namentlich der mathematisch-naturwissenschaftlichen lehre fortschreiten, und es sollte überall als letztes Ziel die Virtuosität, die Meisterschaft erreicht werden." Quoted from the translation (of Purkyně's Czech) by Erich Witte, "Beitrag zur Kenntniss der Bildung von Purkinjé," *Sudhoffs Archiv für Geschichte der Medizin und der Naturwissenschaften* 35 (1942): 238–356, passage quoted, pp. 352–353. The "school of Sais" is a reference to the singular unfinished novel by Novalis, *Die Lehrlinge zu Sais*, in which the great mystery is self-knowledge and the uncertain character of natural knowledge is exposed; see John Neubauer, *Bifocal Vision. Novalis' Philosophy of Nature and Disease* (Chapel Hill: University of North Carolina Press, 1971), pp. 113–127.

31. Despite its almost exclusive emphasis upon classical studies, the standard work remains Friedrich Paulsen, *Geschichte des gelehrten Unterrichts auf den deutschen Schulen und Universitäten*, 2 vols. (Leipzig: Veit, 1897), esp. II: 189–403. But see also Peter Lundgreen, *Sozialgeschichte der deutschen Schule in Ueberblick. Teil I: 1770–1918* (Göttingen: Vandenhoeck und Ruprecht, 1980) and the essays by Karl-Ernst Jeismann ("Gymnasium, Staat und Gesellschaft in Preussen") and Lundgreen ("Schulbildung und Frühindustrialisierung in Berlin/Preussen. Eine Einführung in den historischen und systematischen Zusammenhang von Schule und Wirtschaft") in Ulrich Hermann, ed., *Schule und Gesellschaft im 19. Jahrhundert. Sozialgeschichte der Schule im Uebergang zur Industrialgesellschaft* (Weinheim and Basel: Beltz Verlag, 1977), pp.44–61, 62–110. Hermann and Gerd Friederich provide in the same volume (pp. 462–480) a comprehensive bibliography of the large recent literature on the history of German education.

32. Purkyně, "Ueber Reform der Gymnasien, mit Rücksicht auf Naturstudium, nebst kurzer Darlegung eines cyclischen Unterrichtsystems" (1848), *Opera omnia*, II: 112–127, passage cited, p. 117. With this theme, of course, one meets the crucial divide. The neohumanist could and did easily accept a Pestalozzian view of primary education. Pestalozzi attended only to elementary instruction, but the neohumanist knew that his party had to control secondary education, above all, the Gymnasium, and also the university. The latter together assured *Bildung* along classical lines and were open to only a minority of the population; their exclusivity in curriculum and numbers offered selective acculturation and preservation of social lines, a very important consideration for the upper-middle class. Purkyně, on the other hand, saw a need for practical work at every level of the educational system, that need being perhaps greatest at the university. Politically he was no egalitarian but belonged to the convinced liberal camp whose members saw in the modernization of instruction and an increase in student numbers the foundation for economic expansion and the general freeing of nineteenth-century thought. Purkyně, too, as a Czech nationalist only temporarily based in Prussia, probably entertained, despite his high status as university professor, no particular need to support a cultural bias defended by the German elite and shared by the dominant and despised Austrian regime in Prague. In the social domain, these struggles are analyzed by Leonore O'Boyle, "Klas-

sische Bildung and soziale Struktur in Deutschland zwischen 1800 and 1848," *Historische Zeitschrift* 207 (1968): 584–608; at the university level, they are portrayed by R. S. Turner, *The Prussian Universities and the Research Imperative, 1806–1848* (Ph. D. diss., Princeton University, 1973). The great Aristotelian scholar Werner Jaeger almost a century after Purkyně stated the matter radically, succinctly, and plaintively: "Wissenschaft and empiricism [Empirie], the latter word taken in the antique sense of practical experience, are two fundamentally different things, and Wissenschaft has no place where *Empirie* is required, for theory kills the instinct." Quoted in F. K. Ringer, *The Decline of the German Mandarins. The German Academic Community, 1890–1933* (Cambridge: Harvard University Press, 1969), p. 110.

33. See Kate Silber, *Pestalozzi. The Man and His Work* (New York: Schocken, 1965).

34 Wilhelm Dilthey, "Süvern, Johannes Wilhelm," *Allgemeine Deutsche Biographie* 37, pp. 206–245.

35. Pollard, *Pioneers of Popular Education*, pp. 35–39; Quick, *Educational Reformers*, pp. 364–370.

36. Quoted in L. F. Anderson, ed., *Pestalozzi* (New York: McGraw-Hill, 1931), p. 80.

37. Walter Schöler, *Geschichte der naturwissenschaftlichen Unterrichts im 17. bis 19. Jahrhundert. Erziehungstheoretische Grundlegung und schulgeschichtliche Entwicklung* (Berlin: de Gruyter, 1970), pp. 133–138. Was Pestalozzi's program aimed only at assuring competence and confidence but not encouraging creativity? Silber thinks not (*Pestalozzi*, p. 140), but the use made of Pestalozzian principles by the celebrated geographer Carl Ritter at least suggests if it does not prove this claim; see Rudolf Kuenzli, "Teaching Method and Justification of Knowledge: C. Ritter—J. H. Pestalozzi," in *Epistemological and Social Problems of the Sciences in the Early Nineteenth Century*, N. H. Jahnke and M. Otto, ed. (Dordrecht: Reidel, 1981), pp. 159–181, esp. pp. 168–171.

38. Purkyně, *Beiträge zur Kenntniss des Sehens in subjectiver Hinsicht* (1819), *Opera omnia*, I: 4.

39. Purkyně, "Der Begriff der Physiologie" (1851), *Opera omnia*, III: 72–74; these comments are omitted in the translation by John, *Purkyně*, pp. 40–41.

40. McClelland, *State, Society and University*, pp. 180–181.

41. Purkyně, "Ueber die Wichtigkeit der Muttersprache" (1820), *Opera omnia*, II: 3–4.

42. Purkyně, "Ueber Reform der Gymnasien," p. 115.

43. Ibid., p. 114.

44. Ibid., pp. 112–113.

45. See notes 5 and 20.

46. The rapidly changing character of the German university is admirably portrayed by McClelland, *State, Society and University*, pp. 58–149.

47. See K. E. Rothschuh, "Carl August Sigmund Schultze (1795–1877) und seine Vorlesungen über experimentale Physiologie in Freiburg (1830)," *Sudhoffs Archiv* 47 (1963): 347–359. Also E. T. Nauck, "Bemerkungen zur

Geschichte des physiologischen Institutes Freiburg i. Br.," *Bericht der Natur-forschende Gesellschaft, Freiburg i. Br.* 40 (1950): 147–159; Mauritz Dittrich, "Motive und Hintergründe des Greifswalder Anatomie-Baues. Ein Beitrag zur Biographie von C.A.S. Schultze (1795–1877)," *Medizinhistorisches Journal* 4 (1969): 271–286.

48. The shift from experimental demonstration to student participation in experimental work constitutes a decisive turn in the development of the institute and generalization of the research ethic. I am arguing that Purkyně made this shift probably during the late 1820s and certainly after 1830; I am also, again, suggesting his originality in making this move, at least in the physiological domain. Nonetheless, other possibilities exist; see the spirited descriptions in H. F. Kilian, *Die Universitäten Deutschlands in medicinisch-naturwissenschaftlichen Hinsicht betrachtet* (Heidelberg-Leipzig: Groos, 1828, reprint, 1966). Among these possibilities the program of the still unknown Carl Mayer in Bonn stands foremost. Mayer's stated purpose (1821) is particularly suggestive: "Verbunden ist mit demselben [lectures?] eine besondere Anstalt zum Behufe der Experimentalphysiologic. . . . In dem Cursus der Experimentalphysiologie erhielten die Studierenden Gelegenheit, unter Leitung des Direktors, Versuchen an Thieren anzustellen, und eine Reihe merkwürdiger Experimente beizuwohnen." Quoted in H.-H. Eulner, *Die Entwicklung der medizinischen Spezialfächer an den Universitäten des deutschen Sprachgebietes* (Stuttgart: Ferdinand Enke, 1970), p. 50. Mayer clearly did not satisfy the medical faculty in the long run, for the move that brought the experimentalist Hermann von Helmholtz to Bonn's chair of physiology and anatomy (1855) was largely inspired by dissatisfaction with Mayer's cumulation of positions coupled with a disastrous decline in enrollments. See Friedrich von Bezold, *Geschichte der Rheinischen Friedrich-Wilhelms-Universität von der Gründung bis zum Jahr 1870* (Bonn: Marcus und Webers, 1920), p. 476. Purkyně, too, viewed the repetition of previous experiments by students to be an essential part of his institute's program. From Mayer's statement one cannot determine whether all students in a given course were to be involved in the activity or, as was often the case in these first years of organized laboratory instruction, only a select few participated. The experimental demonstration itself has a long history, being well represented by William Harvey's Lumleian Lectures beginning in 1616, Albrecht von Haller's teaching in eighteenth-century Göttingen, and the highly influential practice of Purkyně's great contemporary, François Magendie. See J. E. Lesch, *Science and Medicine in France. The Emergence of Experimental Physiology, 1790–1855* (Cambridge: Harvard University Press, 1984).

49. See Friedrich Bidder, "Vor Hundert Jahren im Laboratorium Johannes Müllers," *Münchener medizinische Wochenschrift* 81 (1934): 60–64. Needless to say, neither Purkyně nor Müller ceased to offer lecture-demonstrations, an effective pedagogical device that continues to the present day.

50. See Arleen Tuchmann, "From the Lecture to the Laboratory: The Institutionalization of Scientific Medicine at the University of Heidelberg," in chapter 2 of this volume.

51. Purkyně's aspirations acquire a particularly poignant quality in light of twentieth-century experience. In reviewing an English anthology of Czech poetry, he observed: "Die älteren Litteraturen Europas, die Italiänische, Spanische und Französische, waren von jeher in England nie ganz fremd gewesen, die Bekanntschaft mit ihnen gehört sogar mit unter die Requisite höherer Bildung. Auch die Deutsche scheint in neuerer Zeit einen gleichen Rang erwerben zu wollen. . . . Die Schlawischen Nationen beginnen erst in neuerer Zeit in diesen geistig-organischen Verband mit bedeutenderem Erfolg einzutreten. . . . wir schliessen unsern Bericht über diese Englische Dollmetschung Böhmischen Volksgeistes, mit der Ueberzeugung, dass auch bei den Deutschen die gelungenern Productionen dieser neustehenden, mehr als nachbarlichen Litteratur erregen werden . . . Möge bei zuerwartendem, sich steigerndem Aufschwung auch dieses Interesse in gleichen Masse zunehmen, und, ungleich früheren brudermörderischen Zeiten, sich zwischen Deutschen und Slawen im geistigen Bereiche immer mehr ein freudliches bruderliches Verhältniss herstellen, wie es der Schöpfer und Herr der Geister nicht anders wollen kann" (1832), *Opera omnia*, V: 100, 110.

52. Karl Hürthle, "Physiologisches Institut," in Kaufmann, *Festschrift der Universität Breslau*, II: 274–281; more generally, see Werner Gottwald, "Beiträge zur Geschichte der Medizin in Schlesien 1850–1914," *Jahrbuch der Schlesische Friedrich-Wilhelms Universität zu Breslau* 21 (1980): 188–221.

53. K. E. Rothschuh, *Geschichte der Physiologie* (Berlin: Springer Verlag, 1953), pp. 137–139.

54. Purkyně, Bericht J: 1846, *Opera omnia*, XII: 301.

55. See note 11. Göttingen in the 1840s still reflected the great tradition of teleomechanical physiology: see Timothy Lenoir, *The Strategy of Life. Teleology and Mechanics in Nineteenth-Century Biology* (Dordrecht: Reidel, 1982), esp. pp. 156–245. In time the Göttingen institute under Wagner's direction also acquired an experimental orientation: Rudolf Wagner, *Ueber das Verhältniss der Physiologie zu den physikalischen Wissenschaften und zur praktischen Medizin, mit besonderer Rücksicht auf den Zweck und die Bedeutung der physiologischen Institut* (Göttingen: Vandenhoeck und Ruprecht, 1842); "Universität. Physiologisches Institut," *Nachrichten von der G.A. Universität und Königl. Gesellschaft der Wissenschaften zu Göttingen* no. 16 (1860): 165–175.

56. H. C. Wischhusen and Ernst Ehler, "Friedrich Hermann Stannius (1808–1883) als Begründer des Instituts für vergleichende und allgemeine pathologische Anatomie so wie für Physiologie in Rostock (1838)," *Wissenschaftliche Zeitschrift der Universität Halle*, Math. Naturw. Reihe, 23, Heft 4 (1974): 112–120.

57. Eulner, *Die medizinische Spezialfächer*, pp. 38–39.

58. Ibid., pp. 49–50. Also Erna Lesky, *The Vienna Medical School*, pp. 228–237, esp. p. 235, where Brücke sneers at "pure observers and chaste microscopists"—that is, those who fail to make their microscopy physiological; Heinz Schröer, *Carl Ludwig. Begründer der messenden Experimentalphysiologie 1816–1895* (Stuttgart: Wissenschaftliche Verlagsgesellschaft, 1967), pp. 76, 142–143.

59. Eulner, *Die medizinische Spezialfächer*, p. 58.

60. See Turner, *The Prussian Universities and the Research Imperative*, pp. 371–391; "The Prussian Professoriate and the Research Imperative," in Jahnke and Otto, eds., *Epistemological and Social Problems of the Sciences*, pp. 109–121.

61. Such was the enthusiastic image of the philosopher-classicist, G. F. W. Hegel, quoted in Paulsen, *Geschichte des gelehrten Unterrichts*, II: 207.

62. Turner, *The Prussian Universities and the Research Imperative*, pp. 200–323; Herbert Butterfield, *Man on His Past. The Study of the History of Historical Scholarship* (Cambridge: Cambridge University Press, 1955), pp. 32–61.

63. Turner, *The Prussian Universities and the Research Imperative*, pp. 405–408. See also K. M. Olesko, "The Emergence of Theoretical Physics in Germany: Franz Neumann and the Königsberg School of Physics, 1830–1890" (Ph.D. diss., Cornell University, 1980).

64. Isaiah Berlin, "The Divorce between the Sciences and the Humanities," *Against the Current. Essays in the History of Ideas* (New York: Viking, 1980), pp. 80–110; the mandarins were highly sensitive on this issue: see Ringer, *The Decline of the German Mandarins*, pp. 295–302.

65. Ringer, *The Decline of the German Mandarins*, pp. 367–434.

66. The subject regrettably lacks synthetic treatment, but see F. M. Turner, *Between Science and Religion. The Reaction to Scientific Naturalism in Late Victorian England* (New Haven: Yale University Press, 1974). Also see Siegfried Gideon, *Mechanization Takes Command. A Contribution to Anonymous History* (New York: Oxford University Press, 1948) and the many suggestive essays in Tilmann Buddensieg and Hennig Rogge, eds., *Die nützlichen Künste. Gestaltende Technik und bildende Kunst seit der industrielle Revolution* (Berlin: Quadriga Verlag, 1981).

67. Both Eulner, *Die medizinische Spezialfächer*, and Lesky, *The Vienna Medical School* provide a large-scale map of the domain requiring additional exploration.

68. The point is reaffirmed by R. S. Turner's silence regarding developments within the medical faculty and his willingness to emphasize Bonn's teacher-training school, the Seminarium für die gesammten Naturwissenschaften (1825), as being "Prussia's first step toward the network of large research institutes which by 1880 had made the German organization of science world famous" (*The Prussian Universities and the Research Imperative*, p. 403).

69. The tide, as Max Weber pointed out long ago, in the last third of the century set strongly in favor of discarding the cultural message of "*Wissenschaft*," whether met in humanistic or natural scientific study. Rhetorical flourish aside, the new reality was largely given by sober, positive study in a supposedly "value-free" scientific world. See Herbert Schnädelbach, *Philosophy in Germany, 1831–1933*, trans. Eric Mathews (Cambridge: Cambridge University Press, 1984), pp. 27–29.

70. Purkyně's views and those of Carus provide a superb view of opposed positions, the one advocating the quickest and most complete possible assimilation of natural science by the aspiring student and the other insisting that medicine remains supremely an art and its practitioner a man

of culture, although a gentleman who did require a major but only late introduction to scientific study. Said Carus, offering in a few lines the position that Purkyně set out to destroy: "Sind wir also jetzt so weit in unsern Betrachtungen gekommen, dass wir erkannt haben, nur der aufgeschlossene Geist könne mit Erfolg die Wissenschaft aufnehmen, so werden wir nun auch noch die Frage entscheiden haben, welche *Vorbereitungen sind es denn eigentlich,* wodurch der Geist in dieser Hinsicht zuerst im Allgemeinen entwickelt werden muss, wenn er fähig genannt sein soll, dem Besondern irgend einer, und so auch der ärtzlichen Wissenschaft mit Erfolg sich zuzuwenden? Wehen wir aber bei der Beantwortung einer so wichtigen Frage mit der grössten Umsicht zu werken, so wird es darauf doch zuletzt nur die eine antwort geben, nämlich: dass diese Mittel der vorbereitenden Entwicklung des jungen Geistes für ein-und allemal sind und bleiben werden: a) die Sprache, b) die Mathesis, c) die Geschichte, d) die Poesie und e) die Philosophie." C. G. Carus, "Von den Forderungen der Zeit an eine Reform des Medicinalwesens," *Janus* 2 (1847; reprint, 1931): 155–192, passage quoted, p. 164.

71. McClelland, *State, Society and University*, pp. 106–111; Ringer, *The Decline of the German Mandarins*, p. 121.

72. See the shifting emphases in subject matter reported by Brita Rang-Dudzik, with mathematics, natural philosophy, and natural history in decline in the period 1820–1848, "Qualitative and Quantitative Aspects of Curricula in Prussian Grammar Schools during the late 18th and early 19th Centuries and Their Relation to the Development of the Sciences," in Jahnke and Otto, eds., *Epistemological and Social Problems of the Sciences*, pp. 207–233.

CHAPTER TWO

From the Lecture to the Laboratory: The Institutionalization of Scientific Medicine at the University of Heidelberg

Arleen M. Tuchman

The growth of scientific research in nineteenth-century Germany and its institutionalization in the state university system have long been topics of interest to both historians of science and sociologists. Attempts to account for this remarkable proliferation in scientific knowledge have included both ideological and institutional factors. Much attention has been paid to the importance of the neohumanist notion of *Wissenschaft* for early nineteenth-century Prussian reformers.[1] To them education was a process in which the personal search for knowledge had precedence over the mere acquisition of information. This led, naturally, to a higher estimation of the value of research, and in the nineteenth century expectations rose that a professor must be not only a good teacher but a renowned scholar as well.

In the early decades of the last century a professor of the natural sciences or medicine usually carried out his research in a few small rooms that were equipped with only the simplest instruments. Perhaps a few advanced students had the privilege of sharing these cramped quarters, but for the majority of students education took place in the lecture hall alone. Not until midcentury, when the construction of scientific institutes began, did this change. As Joseph Ben David and Awraham Zloczower have argued, this transition must be looked at within its institutional context.[2] The decentralized structure of the German university system created a competitive market that permitted professors to set conditions for their acceptance of academic appointments. In the 1840s and 1850s, as adequate laboratory

space became one of the central demands, the local state governments—pressured by the competitive market, concerned with the
reputation of their universities, and interested in attracting the best
scholars—began to finance the construction of these new institutes.
Within a few decades laboratory training and research had become a
fully integrated part of the university curriculum.

Both the neohumanistic ideology and the decentralized university system were essential in fostering the production of scientific
knowledge, but, as I shall argue in this chapter, they do not present the entire picture. A competitive system that placed a high
premium on *Wissenschaft* characterized the German scene by 1815,
yet major laboratories did not appear until decades later. Moreover
an essential tension existed between the holistic, anti-utilitarian emphasis implicit in the neohumanistic definition of *Bildung* and the
kind of laboratory training provided in the latter half of the nineteenth century—training intended not for an elite group alone but
for all students of the sciences and medicine. These discrepancies
can, however, be accounted for by taking into consideration the
parallel between state interest in the natural sciences and the modernization of Germany; that is, by adding a third, socioeconomic
dimension to the aforementioned ideological and institutional factors. The model of competition, which has been applied effectively
to account for macro-level developments, would thus be comple-
mented by a more detailed analysis of the decision-making process
found at the local level of ministerial reports, parliamentary proceedings, and correspondence.

In this essay I focus on the southern German state of Baden to
demonstrate that the institutionalization of scientific medicine at the
University of Heidelberg, and the government's decision to build
new scientific and medical institutes, were part of a broader process
of social and economic change defined by a society responding to
the early pressures of industrialization. Although the real explosion
in construction of research laboratories did not occur until the 1860s
and 1870s, concerted interest in the promotion of science education
dates from an earlier period. I begin, therefore, with a brief description of the sweeping educational reforms in Baden in the 1830s,
focusing specifically on parliament's decision to promote scientific
knowledge in the interests of modernizing the state's economy. In
the second section I introduce Jacob Henle and Karl Pfeufer, two
professors hired by the Baden government in the 1840s to instruct

medical students in the new methods of the natural sciences. Last, I look more closely at the years Henle and Pfeufer spent at Heidelberg (1844–1852), during which time the government began investing significant sums in the construction of the first science and medical institutes intended for student instruction.

I

In the 1830s the Baden government, guided by a liberal lower parliament, began implementing reforms that would promote modernization of the state. The representatives of this Vormärz parliament were only too well aware of the changes in manufacture, trade, and transportation that had been transforming European society since the beginning of the century. In Germany alone, significant improvements in the waterways and canal system had been carried out, not only benefiting agriculture but greatly advancing long-distance travel even before the construction of the railroad in 1834. In addition, modernization of the iron industry had already led to greatly increased production, with major consequences for many other branches of manufacture. The spinning industry, as important to the industrial revolution in Germany as textiles had been in England, changed from hand- to steam-driven mills in the 1830s, increasing the use of raw cotton within the *Zollverein* by a factor of eight within twenty years.[3] It was the dream of the men in parliament that Baden be able to keep pace with these developments, and they believed that lifting restrictions on the economy would encourage a first step in this direction. Consequently they fought for such reforms as abolition of the tithes system, introduction of free trade, and improvements in transportation. But they realized that more was necessary before substantial changes could be expected in the economic and social structure of the state. People also had to be inculcated with a sensibility that matched the needs and goals of the nascent industrial society, and this meant changes in the kind of education provided to the state's future citizens.[4]

Between 1831 and 1837 the government worked with parliament to reorganize the entire educational system.[5] The first government decree (1834) established a fixed curriculum for the primary schools aimed at improving basic skills in reading, writing, arithmetic, and religion. A few months later two new types of educational establishments were founded: trade schools, intended for the artisan class, and *höhere Bürgerschulen*, or nonclassical secondary schools. The lat-ter offered an alternative to the *Gymnasien* for those who would later be active in the private or commercial sphere of the economy. While not ignoring the importance of a classical education, these schools placed greater emphasis on the *Realwissenschaften*—subjects, such as mathematics, natural science, history, and modern languages, of immediate importance for a life in the world of commerce and trade. As the representative and supreme court judge Josef Merk com-mented during a parliamentary session on education:

> By the future drafting of a school plan, one must especially not forget that the means of communicating between people do not lie in the higher sciences, as they had till now in the Republic of Letters. Rather they are to be found in the general participation of people in a political cosmopolitanism. . . . Therefore knowledge of the modern languages and of that which is of true general welfare will provide the means for young people to take advantage both of this general communication and of the path now being taken by civilization on the whole.[6]

In 1837 parliament also reformed the Gymnasien, establishing natu-ral history, natural philosophy, and mathematics as fixed courses in the curriculum.[7] Moreover, and certainly most impressive, state inter-est in promoting the natural sciences can be seen in the steady in-crease in funds allotted for an education in the *Realwissenschaften*. As table 2.1 demonstrates, through the Vormärz period parliament com-mitted itself more and more to those educational institutions that offered preparation for a nonacademic life, whether it be in trade, commerce, or industry. Furthermore, as columns Va and VIa, and figure 2.1 show, the rate of growth in funds allocated for the *Real-wissenschaften* far surpassed that for the education budget on the whole.[8]

Through these reforms the government hoped, first to create a citizenry capable of understanding and defending modern constitu-tional principles.[9] But this was not the only interest. The reforms were also meant to provide future citizens with those skills neces-sary to modernize a predominantly agricultural economy. The repre-sentatives sought a replacement for what they held to be a degener-ated guild system, and they believed improvements in education provided a possible solution. Ideas, discoveries, inventions, and new methods of production, not rigid government restrictions and high tariffs, were to steer the economy. Carl Nebenius, head of the department of education, argued, for example, that the state's techni-

Table 2.1
State Expenditure for Education in Technology, Trade, Agriculture, and the
Realwissenschaften as Part of the Total Education Budget

YEAR	I	II	III	IV	V	Va	VI	VIA
1831/32	41,240				41,240	1.0	498,438	1.0
1833/34	41,600	12,000			53,600	1.3	536,488	1.1
1835/36	59,727	14,400			74,327	1.8	551,694	1.1
1837/38	58,700	14,000		10,725	83,425	2.0	634,067	1.3
1839/40	51,700	14,221		21,592	87,513	2.1	629,553	1.3
1842/43	60,213	16,087		23,750	100,050	2.4	683,711	1.4
1844/45	66,254	16,784		29,332	112,370	2.7	702,579	1.4
1846/47	67,784	18,709	17,522	34,250	138,365	3.4	880,393	1.8

I = polytechnic school
II = trade schools
III = agricultural education
IV = advanced *Bürgerschulen*

V = Total (Columns I–IV)
Va = Rate of growth (Column V)
VI = Total budget for education
VIa = Rate of growth (Column VI)

Fig. 2.1 Rate of growth in funds allowed for education

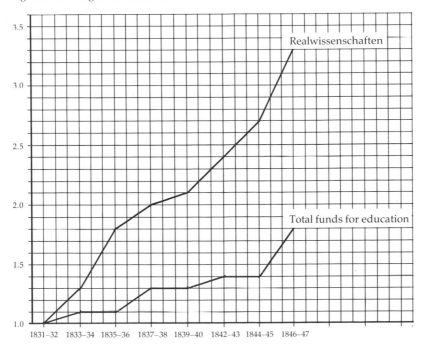

cal school had to train the student to "see with his own eyes, examine, and contemplate." By offering the opportunity for thorough instruction, he added, the government

> finally places [the members of] this class [of producers] in the position to make their own proper observations at the workplace, reflect on what they have observed as well as on phenomena accidentally noticed, and perform well-directed experiments, discovering thereby new truths that can find immediate profitable application in the area of production.[10]

The utilitarian advantage to be gained from this kind of education—that is, the attainment of knowledge that could then be used to stimulate and improve the means of manufacture and production—played an important part in the interest behind these reforms, but the method by which these ideas were to be acquired was anything but the simple transmission of technical information. Rather, these schools were meant as laboratories where students would learn, through active participation, to think for themselves and develop new ideas. The representatives of the Vormärz parliament were intent on creating a new type of citizen, and thereby a new driving force for the economy, and it was within this context that the scientific method and laboratory exercises grew in importance.

Ten to twenty years later laboratories would also become an essential part of university education, but in the early 1830s it was not yet possible to introduce a practical orientation into the higher institutions of learning. This is evidenced by the attempt of a small group within parliament to reform the universities in this very fashion. Led by the factory owner and mayor of Ettlingen, Franz Buhl, and the district councilor, Sander, the members of this group argued that the universities ignored important needs of the state and should therefore receive a smaller dotation. The extra funds could then be used for the establishment of a *bürgerliche* university in which the possible applications of scientific knowledge could be explored, practical exercises could accompany theoretical lectures, and students could have the opportunity to "perform different manipulations, exercises, and handwork themselves."[11] The kind of lesson, Buhl argued, that is ridiculed by Schiller in the parody "He who studies metaphysics / Knows, that he who burns does not freeze" does not suffice for a vocational school. On the contrary, he added,

> We must learn to investigate the richness of the powers contained in the elements, and to apply them to good use. For such a lesson it is

absolutely necessary that practice and theory be combined. The former must demonstrate the correctness of the latter through tests.[12]

A suggestion to move the polytechnical school to Freiburg where a
state university already existed, and to join the two educational establishments together to form a *bürgerliche* university was, however,
rejected by the head of the government ministry. Ludwig Winter,
Minister of State, insisted that universities and technical institutes
had different functions and must therefore be kept geographically
and ideologically distinct from each other. "One," he explained, "has
a scientific goal, and the other a practical one."[13]

Winter's sentiment was shared by Friedrich Tiedemann, professor of anatomy and physiology at the University of Heidelberg,
who expressed his distaste for parliament's "hostile and degrading
attacks."[14] Tiedemann had been one of five professors hired fifteen
years earlier as part of a concerted attempt by the Ministry of Interior to raise the standards of the medical faculty. No doubt inspired
by the founding of the new Prussian university in Berlin (1810), the
university's curator, Sigismund von Reitzenstein, had been looking
for individuals actively involved in research, preferably with European reputations, and in Tiedemann he had found the anatomist
he wanted. The young scholar had not only demonstrated "extraordinary scholarly activity," having published excellent research in
anatomy, comparative anatomy, and zoology, but he had also won
a prize from the famous French Académie des Sciences.[15] These
qualifications suggested that Tiedemann would contribute to the
prestige of the university and thus to the state, and in the years
following his appointment (1815) he more than fulfilled these
wishes. Besides offering courses in anatomy, physiology, comparative anatomy, pathological anatomy, and zoology, he dedicated a
good deal of his time to improving the university's anatomical collection, raising it to "one of the finest in Germany" by 1818.[16]
Furthermore he remained actively involved in research, not only
following his previous interests in anatomical studies but moving
on to physiological chemistry and to the use of chemical, microscopical, and vivisectional techniques. By the early 1830s he had
acquired a reputation as one of the best experimenters in Germany.[17]

Tiedemann did not, however, teach these skills to his students. On
the contrary, his style of teaching, common in the beginning of the

century, kept the process of discovery in the hands of the professors
and a select group of talented students, focusing the educational
process on the transmission of newly acquired information in an or-
derly, packaged system.[18] His students did not learn to look through
microscopes, perform chemical analyses, or do physiological experiments, nor was it expected that they do so: clinical experience and
dissection exercises were neither required courses nor examination
subjects for medical students in Baden. The only requirement for
attaining a license to practice medicine was, in fact, demonstration of
knowledge in the natural sciences and in theoretical medicine. Only
after 1841 were two years of practice required before one could become a state-employed physician, but this did not pertain to private
physicians; nor did it imply that practical experience was to be obtained in the university clinics but, rather, "on the job." Not until 1858
did clinical subjects and laboratory experience become part of the
state medical examination.[19]

Scientific techniques, not only in theoretical subjects but in the
clinical sciences as well, were available by the 1820s, yet the idea that
these skills should be taught to medical students first became popular
a few decades later.[20] The process whereby practical training in the
laboratory and at the bedside became an integral part of medical
education cannot, therefore, be explained by the availability of scientific knowledge alone. Rather, individuals interested in teaching
these techniques, the widespread and inexpensive production of
these instruments, and, as we have already seen, a belief in the value
of practical experience and laboratory training also had to be present.

II

On 21 November 1843 Freiherr von Stengel, a member of Baden's
Ministry of Interior, announced that new talent was urgently
needed if the reputation of the medical faculty at the University of
Heidelberg was to be saved.[21] At that time the faculty consisted of
five full professors, all between the ages of fifty and sixty-five, and,
to make matters worse, Tiedemann had been slowly withdrawing
from university and scientific affairs. In 1835 he had handed over his
courses in physiology and pathological anatomy to the *Privatdozent*
Theodor Bischoff, and in 1837 he had requested a leave of absence
for a year and a half. Personal problems and repeated attacks on the
university by the lower chamber of parliament had been largely

responsible for this withdrawal, but according to Bischoff, "the enormous stimulus that physiology received through the use of the microscope and through the ever-expanding application of physics and chemistry" contributed as well.[22] Tiedemann, already taxed by other problems, did not have the energy to keep abreast of the latest scientific developments.

In his report, sent to the State Ministry, von Stengel showed a particular concern for the decreasing student enrollment brought about by the unpopularity of the medical faculty.

> Privy Councillor Tiedemann is on in years and wishes an easier load. Privy Councillor Puchelt, as much as he distinguishes himself as an honorable scholar and writer, is not very popular as a clinical teacher and many students are leaving the University of Heidelberg because they prefer to attend practical courses in internal medicine at other universities.[23]

Students were indeed choosing other universities. In 1830 Heidelberg had attracted 10 percent (225 students) of all German medical students, but by 1840 this had fallen to 7 percent (140 students) and there was no indication that this decline would cease. The introduction of microscopical and chemical analysis, percussion, and auscultation into the clinic had begun to provide medical education with a practical emphasis, and the new generation of students, not to mention the younger professors skilled in these techniques, were demanding changes in the kind of medical education being provided.[24] By the fall of 1843 attendance at Heidelberg had hit the lowest point in twenty years, with only 32 local and 78 foreign students enrolled, and the university began seriously to reevaluate the situation.[25] The strategy adopted, as a result of negotiations between von Stengel, the medical faculty, and the faculty senate, was to create two new positions—one for anatomy and physiology and the other for the clinical sciences—and to offer them to Jacob Henle and Carl Pfeufer, two men who had already acquired reputations as excellent teachers in modern scientific techniques.

Jacob Henle was born on 19 July 1809 in Fürth, a small city outside Nürnberg.[26] His father, a merchant and a Jew, converted to Protestantism in 1821, and Henle, whose school education focused on classical and modern languages, considered strengthening this conversion by becoming a minister. At an early age, however, he made the acquaintance of Johannes Müller, then professor of anatomy and physiology in Bonn, and decided to pursue a career in medicine. After three years of study in Bonn and one year in Heidelberg, Henle took his doctoral examinations, successfully completing the M.D. in 1832 with a dissertation on the pupil membrane and blood vessels within the eye. A few months later he left for Berlin to take the Prussian state medical examination.

What was meant to be a short stay became, however, a seven-year sojourn, as Müller, having recently been called to Berlin as professor of anatomy and physiology, offered his young protégé the job of prosector in the anatomical institute and the editorship of his *Archiv für Anatomie, Physiologie und wissenschaftliche Medizin*. Henle accepted this immediately, and after completing a habilitation on the epithelium of the intestinal villi in 1837, he began offering courses in general pathology and general anatomy. In the latter course he placed great emphasis on microscopical investigations, but more important, he brought the microscope into the classroom and instructed students in using the instrument. This may have been one of the earliest cases of microscopical technique being taught to students, and the class attained immediate success, attracting sixty students in its first semester.[27]

Henle's decision to make the microscope an essential pedagogical tool had been made possible by recent developments in the construction of the instrument that had improved its quality and reduced its costs. The main problem in early nineteenth-century microscope building—reducing the chromatic aberration caused by the dispersion of light—had been largely solved by the 1830s, and the new microscopes, inexpensive enough to be "paid for out of a student's allowance," permitted observation of clearly definable structures where before only halos and globules had been seen.[28]

As late as 1834 the University of Berlin had, however, only one microscope.[29] As much as Müller may have promoted use of the instrument in scientific research, there is no indication that he, any more than his contemporary Tiedemann, saw its importance for medical education. In 1834, while spending a year in Berlin in order to learn the new research techniques, the Dorpat prosector Bidder expressed his surprise at the teaching style of the great physiologist. "I expected," he wrote in his memoirs,

> that the man who had, in such an outstanding way, attempted to give physiological principles an empirical foundation, would also present

such experience and the method of their [the physiological principles] acquisition in a more concrete way to his students. That was, however, not the case. The students and others in the audience still had to be content with theoretical explanations.[30]

Bidder went on to describe how Müller would be alert for any student who demonstrated talent during the dissection exercises—exercises that went totally unsupervised with ten to twenty students hacking away at a single corpse—whom he would then invite to his private study with the explanation that one "could work better there away from this confusion."[31] Research, though important, remained an activity for the chosen few.

Henle's novelty was in turning the microscope into a significant pedagogical tool. Albert Kölliker, later to become Henle's prosector in Zurich, described his experience in Henle's course in 1839, crediting his teacher with being the first to direct his attention to the microscopical structure of the body.

> I still see the narrow, long hallway in the university building next to the auditorium where Henle, for lack of another room for demonstrations, showed us and explained the simplest things, so awe inspiring in their novelty, with scarcely five or six microscopes: epithelia, skin scales, cilia cells, blood corpuscles, pus cells, semen, then teased-out preparations from muscles, ligaments, nerves, sections from cartilage, cuts of bones, etc.[32]

As mentioned earlier, this would not have been possible without the inexpensive production of good microscopes, but it is obvious from a comparison of Henle's and Müller's teaching styles in Berlin that availability of the instrument and the ability to use it—two conditions that applied equally well to both men—did not suffice to create an appreciation of the pedagogical significance of the microscope. There was needed, in addition, a belief that practical experience was important for all students, not merely for a small elite. They—the average students—were now to be trained in simple microscopical and chemical techniques. Scientific research remained, to be sure, the domain of the professors, assistants, and talented students, but Henle had begun to introduce routine laboratory methods to the students at large.

In a society beginning to develop an interest in modernization, technical culture, and practical experience, Henle's strategy found much acclaim. But the strongly competitive university system in which he wished to establish himself also provided incentive and made it a necessity to develop new strategies. Henle had written home to his parents more than once complaining about the competition among *Privatdozenten*, his frustration with the university's policy of dividing up newly vacated positions among many individuals, and his concern that he be able to dedicate himself fully to academic pursuits without having to supplement his income through private practice. The microscope gave Henle the competitive edge he needed.[33]

In 1839 Henle tried to improve his situation by applying for the chair of pathology in Berlin, made available by Hufeland's death. That a person trained in anatomy and physiology would apply for this position was somewhat unusual, but Henle was anxious to secure a better position, and furthermore, he was convinced that recent developments in these areas were of potential medical significance. In a letter to the State Ministry, Henle argued that his decision to apply was inspired not by the desire to take advantage of an opening in the system but rather by his

> conviction of the intimate connection which anatomy and physiology have to the science of the phenomena of disease. The task of a rational medicine cannot be any other than to comprehend disease symptoms as consequences of the original typical organization of the body and the influences which have an effect upon [the organization]. A combination of both disciplines, however, may be all the more opportune at this moment, because our knowledge of the healthy organism has so increased in the last few years through so many discoveries, particularly microscopical ones, and [our knowledge] is waiting to be applied to pathological processes. In part it has already been applied with some success.[34]

Along with this application Henle submitted a copy of his first major work, *Pathologische Untersuchungen*, which he offered as evidence of his commitment to problems of medical concern.[35] The book contained four separate essays that, taken together, were meant to form "a system of general pathology." In the third essay, "On the Course and Periodicity of Disease," he elaborated upon a central precondition of a scientific or rational medicine—the notion of disease as a physiological process.

In his letter Henle claimed that a rational medicine must view disease as resulting from the interaction of the organized body and the influences acting upon this organization. Implicit in this statement was the rejection of a parasitic theory of disease wherein the disease process was viewed as an entity, and in the third essay

Henle explained why this notion was untenable. From his argument it is evident that he was working completely within what Timothy Lenoir has termed the "teleomechanical tradition" of the Göttingen school, a tradition defined by the inclusion of both teleological and mechanical principles in the study and interpretation of function.[36]

Central to Henle's discussion of the mechanism by which an organism becomes ill was the notion of an organizing principle. The "type," like the *Lebenskraft*, determined the lawful development and, consequently, the particular form of an organism.[37] Subject to the laws of physics and chemistry, the type was nevertheless responsible for the outcome that the semiautonomous structures and organs of the body functioned together to form an integrated whole. Like the teleomechanists, moreover, Henle did not define life merely as the expression of the type but emphasized the role played by the environment in providing the materials, such as nutrients, oxygen, and heat, necessary for the development and maintenance of the organism's activities. It was through the interaction of the type with its environment that life came into being and continued to exist.

Through this interaction the organism could, however, also become ill. In fact it was because of the dependence of the organism on the environment that disease was at all possible. As Henle explained,

> If the organism, the germ, were to carry within itself all the conditions for developing according to its idea [that is, type], then deviations would not be possible. But since these conditions are in part external and independent of it, the possibility exists that it will deviate from the idea, and this is the most general concept of disease.[38]

Given that disease results from the interaction of the type with the environment, there should, logically speaking, be two mechanisms whereby deviations could occur. Either the type could respond abnormally to stimuli or the external stimuli could be directly responsible for the deviations. But Henle denied the first option, arguing that a "Typus irregularis" would be a "contradicto in adjecto."[39] The type, by definition, determined the lawful expression of life's activities. Without this assumption of lawfulness, the entire teleomechanical framework would collapse because if the phenomena of life followed no rules, then a scientific approach to the study of these phenomena would be impossible. Similarly, the science of pathology depended upon the predictability of the disease process, and this was guaranteed by a definition of disease as the response of the "typically organized body" to abnormal conditions, where the lawfulness of the type is given.

> What degree of mechanical or chemical stimulation a being can tolerate without danger, how it is changed through these [stimulations], how long it takes for the normal structure and composition—as far as it is possible—to become healthy again, all this depends upon the original organization of the being and thus, leaving out the breadth of individual fluctuations, upon the type. If, however, the reactions are typical, then so are diseases, because disease is founded . . . in the altered formative activities of the organism in consequence of external influences which the body cannot keep in control.[40]

A parasitic notion of disease, whereby the pathological symptoms would be seen as the expression of a distinct disease entity or, worse yet, as an entity itself, must be denied if one accepts the lawfulness of the type.[41] The idea of a foreign entity carrying out its own life's functions within the affected organism cannot be made consistent with the belief in order and purpose implicit in the notion of the type. This is not to deny that contagions or miasmas could cause disease. The first essay in the *Pathologische Untersuchungen* argued this very point.[42] But they would be only the stimuli for a set of physiological reactions, not the disease itself. The latter is, and can only be, the normal physiological reactions of an organism confronted by abnormal external conditions. As Henle would point out in a later work, "either this principle is correct, or scientific medicine is a chimera."[43]

In his letter to the State Ministry, Henle suggested the advantage of this definition of disease. It permits one to apply the knowledge acquired from anatomy and physiology to the study of the phenomena of disease, thereby helping to bridge the gap between the theoretical and clinical sciences. Furthermore Henle stated explicitly that this should be done through the use of the microscope. Having demonstrated its value in the study of life's normal functions, this instrument would now be used in pathology, allowing one to probe beneath the symptoms to investigate the disturbed organic function.

Henle did not get Hufeland's position, but in 1840 he was offered the chair of anatomy in Zurich.[44] In the four years he spent there Henle continued to develop his ideas for a rational medicine and to promote microscopical research among his students. Furthermore, it was in these years that he met and befriended a young clinician who reinforced his hope that his reform ideas would bring about a change in medical practice. Karl Pfeufer, who had studied under Johannes Schönlein in Würzburg and later worked as his assistant, was highly skilled in the modern clinical techniques of percussion, auscultation, and chemical analysis. Of particular importance for their joint work, moreover, was Pfeufer's fundamental belief in the value of physiology, and especially of pharmacology, for practical medicine. "I found in him," wrote Henle, "a man who is young and energetic enough to throw aside the old beaten track and to accept my views. A man, as I need him to be."[45]

Karl Pfeufer, a physician's son, was born in Bamberg in 1806.[46] When he began his university studies in Erlangen in 1824 he had not yet decided to follow in his father's footsteps but vacillated between a love for literature and a desire to enter the healing profession. It was only after he transferred to Würzburg in 1825 that he decided in favor of the latter. From Pfeufer's letters to his father it is evident that Johannes Schönlein, then professor of special pathology and therapeutics, had inspired him to make this choice. Schönlein, whose name is usually associated with the natural historical school in German medicine, was responsible for introducing the new French diagnostic methods of auscultation, percussion, and pathological anatomy into the German clinics.[47] It was this methodological shift in clinical medicine that would become a central issue in Pfeufer's later lectures and publications.

In 1828 Pfeufer became Schönlein's clinical assistant and began instructing students in the use of the stethoscope.[48] He remained at the clinic until 1831, at which time he received the M.D., passed the state medical examination, and moved to Munich to set up private practice. In the next twelve years Pfeufer tried repeatedly to get a position as *Privatdozent* at the university in Munich, but to no avail. Although both the philosopher Friedrich Wilhelm Schelling and the clinician Philipp von Walther supported these endeavors, Johann Ringseis, then professor in the medical faculty and government advisor, vetoed every application, political and religious differences seeming to have been the determining factor. In 1840, when Zurich offered Pfeufer a professorship in clinical medicine, he asked once more about his chances of getting a position in Munich; obtaining a discouraging reply, he decided to accept the offer.

One month after arriving in Zurich Pfeufer held an inaugural address entitled "Ueber den gegenwärtigen Zustand der Medizin."[49]

In this speech the young professor characterized German, French, and British medicine, discussing the advantages and disadvantages of each. The Germans, he claimed, placed a correct emphasis on careful observations, causal connections, and therapeutics but had too great a tendency to speculate. This trait he attributed to the absence of a clear methodology for investigating the disease process, and advised the Germans to learn from the French, who had already brought a high level of objectivity to diagnosis through the use of the stethoscope, pleximeter, uterine speculum, and vaccination. Pfeufer also credited his neighbors with having integrated pathological anatomy into the clinic, bringing it into closer contact with observations made at the bedside. Nonetheless he had a few words of criticism for the French, arguing that they confused goals and means. Diagnostic techniques and pathological anatomy, he explained, were not ends in themselves but merely methods for uncovering the nature of the disease process—the first step on the way to healing. In short, the Germans had the proper goal but overlooked the way to get there, whereas the French had the means but mistakenly believed it to be the goal.

Like Henle, Pfeufer focused his attention on the need for a method that would permit the scientific investigation of the disease process. To this end he put great emphasis on diagnostic techniques and scientific research, arguing that a solid foundation in medicine would be acquired only when "the anatomical and physiological character of a disease are placed in a true light."[50] It is not difficult to imagine this speech being the event that convinced Henle he had found the man he needed.

Henle—the anatomist qua pathologist—and Pfeufer—the clinician—made a formidable team during the years they were together in Zurich. During this time Henle came to realize that the reform of medicine could be brought about only through the combined efforts of the theoretical and clinical sciences. He gave this conviction clear expression in 1842 when he was offered a teaching position in Tübingen. During the negotiations Henle emphasized that his past success had come about because he had both learned and taught how to apply the methods of physiology to the study of diseased conditions. But in order to remain effective in this area, he added, "I am dependent more than others upon the cooperation and advice of the clinical teacher."

Only with the approval of the latter could I teach with enthusiastic confidence. For my audience to find fruitful the things which I communicate to them . . . depends, because I do not practice, upon the extent to which the head of the clinical institute allows me to participate in his observations.[51]

Henle turned down the position in order to remain in Zurich with Pfeufer.[52] Not long afterward, however, the two friends were given the opportunity to return to the Germanies together. As we have already seen, the University of Heidelberg hired Henle and Pfeufer in 1843 in the hope of breathing new life into the old and unpopular medical faculty. The Baden government had been searching for teachers qualified in the new scientific methods who would be able thereby to draw medical students to Heidelberg, and in these two men the state had found the perfect team. Not only were they skilled in modern techniques, whether in the laboratory working with the microscope or at the bedside doing percussion and auscultation, but they both had outstanding reputations as teachers. Their popularity among students went, moreover, far beyond the articulation of a concrete methodological procedure in which all could take part and by which medical care would presumably be improved. Their wit, youth, liberal views, and the polemical tone of their writings made them immediate favorites among students and younger colleagues involved in the political and social unrest of the forties. "I only wish," wrote Phillip Jolly, assistant professor of physics in Heidelberg and an acquaintance of Henle, "that you and your friend Pfeufer . . . could hear the tone that is dominating among the students since your appointment became known. I have already heard from many who were set on ending their studies at Easter that they want to remain on for at least one semester."[53]

Not only did many students remain, but many more came to Heidelberg specifically to study with Henle and Pfeufer. In the first year after their appointment enrollment increased from 107 to 147. Among the 30 additional students, only 3 were from Baden. The rest came from other German and European lands, and this at a time when every other German university was experiencing declining enrollments in the medical faculty.[54] Heidelberg had made a good choice.

III

Baden's decision to hire Henle and Pfeufer signified more than an attempt to improve the medical faculty; it also reflected a change in the kind of education the state wanted to support. The reforms of the 1830s that had focused on improving practical training in the sciences may originally have been confined to the secondary and technical schools, but in the 1840s the government began to direct its attention to changing the content and structure of university education as well.

Government policy toward the University of Heidelberg in the decade preceding the Revolution of 1848 was liberal and expansionist. Not only were two new positions for full professors created in the medical faculty, but the number of young lecturers was allowed to triple in size (from three to nine) in these years.[55] It was these *Privatdozenten* primarily, along with a couple of younger professors, who introduced the new scientific methods into the curriculum. As early as 1841, for example, two courses were offered at the university that permitted students to learn the new techniques of auscultation and percussion, one in connection with semiotics, taught by the *Privatdozent* Benno Puchelt, and the other in obstetrics, offered by the assistant professor Franz Josef Nägeli. One year later chemical and microscopical investigations were included as an aid in the semiotics course. By 1844 six practically oriented courses were available to the students, five taught by young lecturers and one by Nägeli. The techniques ranged from microscopical exercises to auscultation and percussion as aids in diagnosis. By the late 1840s between five and nine courses were offered every semester emphasizing "practical exercises," "microscopical exercises," "practical use," or simply "*prakticum.*"

In addition to allowing an increase in *Privatdozenten* and to creating positions for Henle and Pfeufer, the government demonstrated its active commitment to practical training in the sciences by increasing its financial support for the university. Between 1840 and 1850 parliament not only raised Heidelberg's yearly dotation from 85,000 to 101,000 gulden but also began investing large sums in the improvement of the institutional facilities.[56]

In the early 1840s discussion began over the inadequacy of the existing laboratory and clinical facilities at the University of Heidelberg. Since 1830 the medical and surgical clinics had been sharing a small building, the former with a total of 50 beds, the latter with 18.[57] In 1842, when the psychiatric asylum moved to the town of Illenau, the government agreed to renovate the vacated building for use as a clinical facility. By 1843 construction was complete, at a total expenditure of 23,160 gulden. The four-story building had space for an auditorium, administrative offices, a surgical assistant, and a dissection room on the first floor; a surgical clinic with 40 beds on the second; and a medical clinic with 170 beds total on the third and fourth floors. When Pfeufer arrived in 1844 the arrangement was modified slightly, and he was given the west wing of the medical clinic with 16 beds and a number of smaller rooms.

The clinical facilities were not the only scientific institutes in need of improvement. Since 1818 chemistry, mineralogy, zoology, anatomy, and botany were all housed in one building, and by the 1840s the situation had become unbearable. In 1845 Leopold Gmelin, professor of chemistry, explained that lectures accompanied by experiments no longer provided an adequate education. "The young chemists, in order to gain a practical education, want to use their own hands everyday."[58] Pfeufer, who began very early to demand more beds for his own section of the medical clinic, also argued along these lines. In a letter to the State Ministry defending the young clinician's demands, the curator of the university, Dahmen, emphasized Pfeufer's claim that the manner in which clinical science was now carried out

> is no longer satisfied with scholarly argumentations of theory but rather applies itself totally to the materials, demonstrations, independent observations and practice. [Consequently], the necessary material is lacking, and with ever increasing enrollment, will be lacking more and more.[59]

The two men, Pfeufer and Dahmen, fought to convince the government that with new institutes, particularly a new hospital, anatomy institute, museum for the natural historical collections, and chemical and physical laboratories, Heidelberg would rank among the best universities in the Germanies, would "soon attract over 1,000 students," and would probably be surpassed in enrollment only by Berlin.[60]

In January 1846 Dahmen met with the medical faculty to discuss plans for a new anatomy institute.[61] Henle's request that a room be added specifically for microscopical investigations met with no objections, and the entire plan was sent to Karlsruhe for approval. At the budget meeting in April the government presented these plans to the lower chamber of parliament, arguing that the old building lacked adequate space, had insufficient equipment, and could not meet the needs of physiology. By the government's estimate a new institute would cost 51,000 gulden, and it requested that these funds be allotted immediately.[62]

A new anatomical institute was not the only item on the list at this meeting. The government also acknowledged the need to provide better facilities for zoology and chemistry, and suggested that the old cloister building be renovated for their use after anatomy moved out. Zoology, in desperate need of more room for its collections, could take over the old anatomy gallery, and chemistry, needing space where "students could perform chemical experiments themselves," would take over the remaining rooms. Expected costs were 16,000 gulden for zoology and 10,000 gulden for chemistry, bringing the total costs for the new scientific institutes to 77,000 gulden.[63]

Parliament responded favorably, praising the government for its interest in improving "those institutes which have a particularly practical value."[64] To the original plans, however, they suggested an alternative: the zoology museum should be included in the new anatomy building. Rather than building only one story, as initially intended, they favored a two-story building with zoology occupying the second floor. This suggestion met with only minimal criticism, and on 3 September parliament approved 65,000 gulden for immediate use in construction.[65]

According to the new plans, anatomy would occupy the first floor with a large lecture hall (1,254 sq. ft.), a room for the anatomical collection, a dissection room (1,280 sq. ft.), a smaller lecture room for physiology and microscopical anatomy (600 sq. ft.), a small kitchen with running water, three rooms for equipment, and workrooms for the directors of anatomy, physiology, and surgery and for the prosector and physiology assistant. On the second floor zoology would have space for the zoological collection (680 sq. ft.), a lecture room (600 sq. ft.), and rooms for the conservator, director, microscopical observations, and materials. The institute, completed in 1849, was, according to Hermann Hoepke, the first in Germany with its own auditorium and with all the necessary equipment for research and instruction.[66]

As a result of these arrangements construction of a chemistry laboratory was made dependent upon completion of the anatomy institute. In the interim, however, the plans broadened from a discussion of chemistry alone to the consideration of a complete natural science institute for chemistry, physics, mineralogy, technology, and archaeology. Improved laboratory space, more room for the presentation of scientific collections, larger auditoriums, and the possibility of live-in quarters for the professors played a central role in the discussions.[67] Furthermore there was interest that this building serve the public good as well as the university. In a letter to the curator, members of the government's building and economics commission spoke out strongly in favor of permitting public use of the scientific collections. It would be desirable, they wrote, "if the building would not be used for the lessons of the individual professors alone, but would be considered as a public institute as well, being open to the public at specified hours."[68]

The new commitment to the construction of scientific institutes at the university was clearly part of the general shift in ideology, begun in the 1830s, which placed greater emphasis upon practical education and scientific knowledge in the education of the state's future citizens. It must, however, be emphasized that this transition occurred before the direct benefits to medicine of laboratory exercises had been demonstrated. Therapeutics cannot be said to have improved until the end of the century, and the few diagnostic gains can hardly explain the enthusiasm that surrounded the calls for a scientific medicine.[69] One must therefore look beyond the medical domain to the broader social context if one is to understand the strength of the conviction that medicine would profit from a greater emphasis on scientific knowledge, laboratory exercises, and bedside experience. It was a faith reinforced by the observable changes in agriculture, manufacture, and transportation—changes that demonstrated the power of such knowledge and led many to believe (or hope) that medicine would soon follow suit. In general, this conviction reflected a belief that the ideological basis of the modern state had to rest in the unification of theory and practice. Neither pure speculation nor raw empiricism alone could promote the intellectual or material interests of the nation. This was a common theme in the 1840s, particularly among the Vormärz liberals, and could be found throughout the many articles published in Brockhaus's *Conversations-Lexikon der Gegenwart* and Rotteck and Welcker's *Staats-Lexikon*, encyclopedias that represented and promoted an ideology of laissez-faire liberalism.[70] The society that found most praise in these texts was one of railroads, electricity, and steamships, and few authors failed to remind their readers that such a society could succeed only through the cooperative efforts of theoreticians and practitioners. "Empiricism and speculation are in like manner necessary," wrote the author of the article "Experience (*Erfahrung*),"

> because both are founded in the nature of the human spirit. The methods related to them, the practical and the theoretical, are therefore worthy of equal respect. Both have the same claim to legitimacy and recognition, and life as well as science can only win when empiricism and speculation stop their hostile confrontations and begin mutually to complement one another.[71]

The desire to strike a balance between speculation and empiricism lay as well at the core of the demands for medical reform that could be heard throughout Germany in the 1840s; it was, in fact, a central issue for Henle and Pfeufer. Shortly after their arrival in Heidelberg they founded the journal *Zeitschrift für rationelle Medizin,* beginning the first volume with an article entitled "Medizinische Wissenschaft und Empirie."[72] It was here that Henle consolidated ideas that he and Pfeufer had been entertaining for years into a polemic for a "rational" medicine. With his criticism directed toward the widespread empiricism flourishing in medicine, Henle campaigned for a balance between fact and theory whereby all hypotheses would be derived from, and tested by, a careful analysis of the natural phenomena. He believed that recent developments in organic chemistry and microscopy would make this possible.

Henle sought a method by which certainty could be brought to medicine, and he believed that this would be possible only by reintroducing theoretical considerations into the study of disease. It was upon these grounds that he criticized the empiricists for consciously abandoning all investigations into the first cause and internal connection of symptoms, and for describing the form of the disease according to external phenomena alone. "The names which the empiric gives to diseases," wrote Henle, "are not definitions but only nomina propria."[73] They say nothing about the disease condition but only represent complexes of material symptoms. In a similar fashion, Henle went on to complain, the empirics care little about the modus operandi of medicaments and thus make use of those remedies that have most frequently had a favorable effect. "Thus the certainty of their different modes of cure," he concluded, "is not determined by internal arguments, but only by a number of medical observations."[74]

Henle believed Louis' numerical method to be the logical consequence of the empirical approach, in fact the only method from which empirical medicine could really benefit, and he praised the Frenchman's caution and distrust of treatments based on a limited number of cases. Nevertheless the numerical method could provide only probable knowledge, and Henle questioned the practical value of such results. Knowing that a certain medicament had a positive effect in the majority of cases could not, for example, tell the physician how to treat the exceptions to the rule. "Shall we adopt it [the treatment] therefore for all cases," questioned Henle, "and therein resign ourselves for the future to sacrifice a certain number of patients? . . . Do we console ourselves, like gamblers, with the prospect that in the end the gain will surmount the loss?"[75] Henle believed the only possibility for achieving the certainty he wanted was through analysis of the internal connections of the symptoms, and this demanded going beyond the mere collection of data to the construction of theories.

The use of theory had, of course, been carried to an extreme by nature philosophers at the beginning of the century, and Henle realized that empiricists were reacting against this excess. He nevertheless defended the former's conception of organic nature, their recognition that matter and force are not separable, and their emphasis on the development of organic beings, and thus on comparative anatomy and embryology. He praised highly the search for relations between phenomena and causal explanations, but he did not hesitate to point out that however fruitful nature philosophy may have been for embryology and comparative anatomy, its influence on pathology and practical medicine had been a disaster, in part because of the false application of theories to the explanation of empirical data, and in part because of the a priori construction of empirical knowledge.[76] His alternative approach, which "stood to a certain extent in the middle of these two [the empirical and philosophical systems]," sought on the one hand to retain the philosophical interest in causal connections while, on the other hand, abandoning the use of a priori theories and making use of the empirical methods of the natural sciences. "I want to name this method rational," he wrote, because it aims to give an account of the causes of phenomena as well as of the manner of operation of remedies. It strives to understand the symptoms in their dependence upon one another and in their connection to internal organic changes, and it considers these changes as the result of the interaction of abnormal external influences on organic matter endowed with specific forces.[77]

The means for acquiring this information would be pathological anatomy, microscopy, chemistry, clinical observation, and experiment. Theories would not be constructed a priori; rather, hypotheses would be derived from analysis of the data and then tested.

In his own research Henle did not always live up to his prescriptions. Many of his studies offered little more than pure descriptions of anatomical structures where others, particularly his textbooks, often retained a strong speculative flair. But even those contemporaries who criticized Henle's philosophical tendencies did not hestitate to praise his microscopical skills and, of equal importance, his methodological intentions. The young experimental physiologist Carl Ludwig even went so far as to speak of Henle's "microscopical school"; and Rudolf Virchow, in an attempt to convince the Prussian ministry to build an institute for pathological anatomy, described his own work as being in "Henle's spirit."[78] By this he was referring to a methodological approach to the study of disease which used microscopy, chemistry, and experiment to investigate the conditions under which disease occurred and the laws governing this process.

Henle actively sought to promote his reputation as a reformer. In 1845, just before completing his *Handbuch der rationellen Pathologie*—a text that represented the fulfillment of the program he had laid out in the introductory article of his journal—Henle wrote to his publisher that he "wanted to pave the way for a new direction" in medicine; and on the day he finished the book, he predicted that it would "cause a revolution in medicine, making me an enemy of the old, and binding me to the young."[79] As the statistics in table 2.2 show, the "young" certainly were attracted to the two new professors. Enrollment, falling in all other German medical departments, did not cease to increase at the University of Heidelberg until the troublesome times just before the Revolution of 1848.

"Rational" medicine was a reform program for the younger generation, and those students coming to Heidelberg could expect to be indoctrinated in its principles and methods. In the eight years Henle and Pfeufer spent at the university (1844–1852) they offered courses

Table 2.2
Enrollment at the University of Heidelberg, 1842–1848*

Year	Baden Students	Foreign Students
1842–1843	29	84
1843–1844	30	87
1844–1845	33	114
1845–1846	31	124
1846–1847	36	129
1847–1848	30	89

*Statistics are compiled from enrollment reports printed in *Regierungs-Blatt*, 1842–1848.

in, among others, general and special pathology, general and special therapeutics, general anatomy, physiology, and rational pathology. Henle was, in fact, the last professor at Heidelberg to teach both physiological and pathological subjects. (Upon his departure in 1852 general pathology and pathological anatomy became the responsibility of the clinical professor.[80]) His lectures, drawn primarily from his textbooks on general anatomy and rational pathology, provided students with the theoretical principles of a scientific medicine, and in the clinic and laboratory these same students began to work with the tools of the trade.

Beginning in 1846 every semester Henle and his assistant Bruch offered a course entitled "Exercises in the Use of the Microscope."[81] Of most importance to Henle was that each student have his own instrument with which to work. With only three microscopes initially at their disposal, Henle and Bruch contributed their private instruments to the collection, raising the total to five. In the first semester, however, over twenty students signed up for the course, and the two instructors had to divide the class into three groups to ensure that each student had a microscope available. Surprised at the large turnout, Henle wrote immediately to the curator requesting money for more instruments. At first he received only 175 gulden—probably just enough for one microscope—but repeated requests throughout the years permitted him to acquire eleven microscopes by the time of his departure in 1852.[82]

In 1850 Henle and Bruch expanded their course to include "physiological experiments." Unfortunately, little is known about the nature of these experiments, but it can be surmised from the list of instruments in the institute's collection that nothing more than the simplest vivisectional experiments could have been carried out. Other than the eleven microscopes mentioned earlier, by 1852 the institute possessed one galvanometer, one balance, two thermometers, and a series of knives and instruments for cutting nerves and bones.[83]

Nevertheless it seems likely that more than mere demonstration was occurring, at least during the microscopical exercises. Given that each student had his own instrument, it may be assumed that he was being taught to work with the microscope, learning to see and identify the objects at the other end of the ocular. Moreover these students did not comprise an elite group, selected by the professor because of demonstrated talent. They were self-selected: any interested person could sign up for the course.

One of the consequences of this shift in the nature of medical education had been addressed by Pfeufer in his Zurich speech of 1840: the use of scientific methods altered the practice of medicine by introducing standardization and routine into the complicated domain of diagnosis. As Pfeufer explained to his audience:

> Since the first appearance of the *Traité de l'auscultation,* in which Laennec—this Herschel of the human thorax—published his discovery, the doctrine of the diseases of the organs of respiration has made greater progress than in the previous thousand years. With this a new era in objective diagnostics begins, in which the less gifted can also diagnose such diseases whose diagnosis previously was a sort of private possession (although still very unsure) of a few exceptional men.[84]

Pfeufer's comment must be viewed within the broader social and political context of the 1840s. In many ways it could not have been more typical of that decade. The enemy was the elite, but the intent was not merely to substitute one privileged group for another. Rather the goal was to broaden access to this select community, and the way to accomplish this was to standardize the requirements for entry. The "objectification" of medicine, Pfeufer believed, permitted one to replace talent and intuition by routine methods. In the future young medical students had merely to learn the techniques of auscultation, percussion, microscopy, and chemical analysis to become successful physicians. To accomplish this no particular aptitude or insight was necessary: scientific methods were something that could be taught even to the "less gifted."

Extending education to the "less gifted"—that is, to a broader spectrum of the population—had been one of the central goals of the educational reforms of the 1830s. As we have seen, parliament appreciated the power of education as a tool for replacing old traditions with those skills and perspectives necessary for changing the economic and political structure of the state. The reforms thus embodied an essential tension promoting, on the one hand, a certain democratization of society (by providing education for all social classes) but on the other hand permitting increased state encroachment in, and control of, the lives of its citizens.

Standardization and control—these two components were present as well in the changes in medical education in Baden in the 1830s and 1840s. The shift from the lecture hall to the laboratory and clinic—and I wish to emphasize once again that this occurred before the practical benefits of such a pedagogical shift had been demonstrated—gave the run-of-the-mill student access to an activity that had previously been restricted to an elite. The medical student's academic training was thereby becoming more routine and technical, but it was also coming under greater control. In 1841 the Baden government passed legislation requiring two years of practical experience for all physicians interested in state-employed positions, and a few years later parliament began debating whether to add a "practical clinical examination" to the state licensing examination. This trend would culminate in 1858 in a total revamping of the state medical examination. Thereafter anyone wishing to practice medicine would have to demonstrate skills not only at the bedside but in the laboratory as well.[85]

Henle and Pfeufer had argued as early as 1840 that a connection between anatomy and physiology on the one hand and pathology on the other had been made all the more possible by microscopical discoveries and new diagnostic techniques. By 1850 this conviction had received wide institutional support: thirteen of the nineteen German universities were providing practical instruction in the use of the microscope, and almost every medical department offered courses in auscultation and percussion.[86] The use of new instruments, not only for diagnosis but for increasing understanding of the disease process as well, had begun to find a place in the medical curriculum. The process by which this had come about was, however, complex. Direct medical benefits aside (and certainly in the 1840s they were still few), the institutionalization of scientific medicine depended upon a constellation of factors: the presence of a younger generation anxious both to teach and to learn the new techniques; broader social and economic changes, characterized by the beginning of modernization, that had begun to evaluate more highly the acquisition of scientific knowledge and practical experience; and, last, the success of the natural sciences in other branches of the economy, which had generated faith that medicine would soon benefit. In the mid-1850s many universities would begin constructing new research institutes equipped with laboratories intended specifically for student instruction. This would not, however, be a consequence merely of the internal dynamics of the German academic system. Rather, it would also reflect the changing function of the university in a society that was beginning to demand new forms of knowledge and expertise from its academic elite.

NOTES

This essay is part of a dissertation entitled *Science, Medicine and the State: The Institutionalization of Scientific Medicine at the University of Heidelberg* (Ph.D. diss., University of Wisconsin-Madison, 1985). I wish to thank the Fulbright Foundation for its generous support of my doctoral research.

I am grateful to a number of individuals for their critical comments on earlier drafts of this paper. William Coleman, Gerald Geison, Frederic L. Holmes, Russell Maulitz, and David Vampola asked many difficult questions, and I only hope that I have answered them to their satisfaction. I am, moreover, especially indebted to Timothy Lenoir for helping me to understand better the broader social context in which the experimental sciences flourished during the nineteenth century. Our ongoing conversations during the year we both spent in Berlin proved invaluable for my understanding of the interplay between cognitive and institutional factors in the development of scientific concepts.

1. Helmut Schelsky, *Einsamkeit und Freiheit. Idee und Gestalt der deutschen Universität und ihrer Reformen*, 2d ed. (Düsseldorf: Bertelsmann Universitätsverlag, 1971); R. Steven Turner, "University Reformers and Professorial Scholarship in Germany, 1760–1806," in *The University in Society*, ed. Lawrence Stone, 2 vols. (Princeton: Princeton University Press, 1974), 2: 495–531.

2. Joseph Ben-David, "Scientific Productivity and Academic Organization in Nineteenth-Century Medicine," *American Sociological Review*, 25, no. 2 (1960): 828–843; Awraham Zloczower, *Career Opportunities and the Growth of Scientific Discovery in Nineteenth-Century Germany, with Special Reference to Physiology* (Ph.D. diss., Hebrew University, 1960); Joseph Ben-David, "Scientific Growth: A Sociological View," *Minerva* 2, no. 4 (1964): 455–476.

3. Thomas Nipperdey, *Deutsche Geschichte, 1800–1866. Bürgerwelt und starker Staat* (Munich: C. H. Beck, 1984), pp. 185–191. Also see F.-W. Hen-

ning, *Die Industrialisierung in Deutschland, 1800–1914* (Paderborn: Ferdinand Schöningh, 1973).

4. Loyd E. Lee, *The Politics of Harmony. Civil Service, Liberalism, and Social Reform in Baden, 1800–1850* (Newark: University of Delaware Press, 1980), chap. 5.

5. Parliamentary discussions concerning these reforms were published in the proceedings of the lower chamber of the Baden parliament: Baden, Ständeversammlung, 2. Kammer, *Verhandlungen der Stände-Versammlung des Großherzogthums Baden. Protokollhefte und Beilagenhefte der 2. Kammer für die Jahre 1831 bis 1837*. (Hereafter cited as *Verhandlungen*.) The government's decision to establish trade schools and burger schools was published in the *Großherzoglich Badisches Staats- und Regierungs-Blatt* 26 (1834): 201–226. (Hereafter cited as *Regierungs-Blatt*.).

6. Josef Merk, *Verhandlungen*, 87 sess., 2 September 1831, Protokollheft 21, p. 91.

7. *Regierungs-Blatt* 8 (1837): 53–64.

8. Financial statistics are from the "Vergleichung der Budgets-Sätze mit den Rechnungs-Resultäten für die Etats-Jahre 1831 bis 1847," *Verhandlungen* (usually, but not always, in Beilagenheft 2). Rate of growth was calculated by setting the value for the first year at one and dividing each successive year by the first year's value.

9. See, for example, a report by the finance committee in *Verhandlungen*, 1831, Beilagenheft 10, p. 219. The Grand Duke of Baden had granted his citizens a constitution in 1819, being one of the first German rulers to do so. See Wolfram Fischer, "Staat und Gesellschaft Badens im Vormärz," in *Staat und Gesellschaft im deutschen Vormärz, 1818–1848*, ed. Werner Conze (Stuttgart: Ernst Kett, 1962), pp. 143–172.

10. C. F. Nebenius, *Ueber technische Lehranstalten in ihrem Zusammenhange mit dem gesammten Unterrichtswesen und mit besonderer Rücksicht auf die polytechnische Schule zu Karlsruhe* (Karlsruhe, 1833), p. 52. This passage was also cited during the parliamentary meetings. See the report from the parliamentary representative Kröll: "Commissionsbericht über die Errichtung von höhern Bürger- und Gewerbschulen," *Verhandlungen*, 66 sess., 24 September 1833, Beilagenheft 5, pp. 252–254.

11. The quotation is from Friedrich Walchner, head of the chemistry-technology branch of the polytechnical school in Karlsruhe, in *Verhandlungen*, 85 sess., 18 October 1833, Protokollheft 18, p. 16.

12. Franz Buhl, *Verhandlungen*, 137 sess., 17 November 1831, Protokollheft 30, pp. 246–247.

13. Ludwig Winter, *Verhandlungen*, 137 sess., 17 November 1831, Protokollheft 30, p. 253.

14. Tiedemann's comment is in a letter from him to the State Ministry in File 205/524, Badisches Generallandesarchiv Karlsruhe [Baden State Archives], Karlsruhe, Federal Republic of Germany (hereafter Badisches Archiv), 18 November 1832.

15. "Die Wiederbesetzung der Lehrstelle der Anatomie und Physiologie zu Heidelberg betrf.," in File 235/3133: Die Lehrstellen bei der medizini-

schen Fakultät und deren Besetzung, Badisches Archiv, 6 December 1815. The reform of the medical faculty in general is discussed in Eberhard Stübler, *Geschichte der medizinischen Fakultät der Universität Heidelberg, 1326– 1925* (Heidelberg: Winter, 1926), pp. 239–266. Reitzenstein's specific interest in Tiedemann's appointment is mentioned in Theodor Bischoff, *Gedächtnißrede auf Friedrich Tiedemann.* Read at the public meeting of the Königliche Akademie der Wissenschaften on 28 November 1861 (Munich, 1861), p. 11.

16. Tiedemann's courses are listed in the *Anzeige der Vorlesungen auf der Großherzoglich Badischen Ruprechts Karolinischen Universität zu Heidelberg, 1822– 1849.* (Hereafter cited as *Vorlesungen.*) (Unfortunately, printed accounts of courses being offered did not begin until 1822.) The quotation is from a ministerial report in File 205/524, Badisches Archiv, 30 October 1818.

17. See, for example, Friedrich Tiedemann and Leopold Gmelin, *Versuche über die Wege, auf welchen Substanzen aus dem Magen und Darmkanal in's Blut gelangen, über die Verrichtung der Milz und die geheimen Harnwege* (Heidelberg, 1820); idem, *Die Verdauung nach Versuchen* (Heidelberg, Leipzig, 1826).

It was because of Tiedemann's reputation as an experimenter that Prussia offered him the chair of anatomy and physiology in Berlin in 1833. See Manfred Stürzbecher, "Zur Berufung Johannes Müllers an die Berliner Universität," *Jahrbuch für die Geschichte Mittel- und Ostdeutschlands* 21 (1972): 184–226, here p. 193.

18. Tiedemann's teaching style is discussed in Adolf Kussmaul, *Jugenderinnerungen eines alten Arztes* (Stuttgart, 1899), pp. 193–199. For a general discussion of teaching styles in nineteenth-century Germany, see Hans H. Simmer, "Principles and Problems of Medical Undergraduate Education in Germany during the Nineteenth and Early Twentieth Centuries," in *The History of Medical Education,* ed. C. D. O'Malley (Berkeley and Los Angeles: University of California Press, 1970), pp. 173–200, esp. p. 187.

19. *Regierungs-Blatt,* 5 August 1828, 5 July 1841. Also "Prüfungsordnung für die Kandidaten der Heilkunde," *Aerztliche Mittheilungen aus Baden* 12 (1858): 17–20. (Hereafter cited as *Mittheilungen.*)

20. Leopold Auenbrugger had, for example, published his treatise on percussion in 1761; René Laënnec had published his book on auscultation in 1819 in which he discussed his invention of the stethoscope; and relatively inexpensive microscopes were available by the late 1820s. See Stanley Joel Reiser, *Medicine and the Reign of Technology* (Cambridge: Cambridge University Press, 1978).

21. Report from the Ministry of Interior to the State Ministry in File 235/ 3133, Badisches Archiv, 21 November 1832.

22. Bischoff, *Gedächtnißrede auf Friedrich Tiedemann,* p. 17. See also the letter from Tiedemann to the State Ministry, in File 205/524, Badisches Archiv, 23 December 1837.

23. Report from the Ministry of Interior to the State Ministry in File 235/ 3133, Badisches Archiv, 21 November 1832.

24. Statistics have been compiled from enrollment reports printed every year in *Regierungs-Blatt,* 1830–1840. For the introduction of the new tech-

niques into the clinics, see Konrad Kläß, *Die Einführung besonderer Kurse für Mikroskopie und physikalische Diagnostik (Perkussion und Auskultation) in den medizinischen Unterricht an deutschen Universitäten im 19. Jahrhundert* (Ph.D. diss., Göttingen, 1971).

25. *Regierungs-Blatt* for the year 1843. "Foreign" students are those who were not from the state of Baden.

Although falling enrollments in the early 1840s reflected a general trend in the medical faculties throughout Germany, enrollments at Heidelberg fell more sharply than at other universities. See Franz Eulenberg, *Die Frequenz der deutschen Universitäten von ihrer Gründung bis zur Gegenwart* (Leipzig: B. G. Teubner, 1904), p. 255. Thus for Heidelberg the loss was not only in absolute numbers but relative to other schools as well.

26. Biographical information is from Fr. Merkel, *Jacob Henle. Ein deutsches Gelehrtenleben* (Braunschweig, 1891); W. Waldeyer, "J. Henle. Nachruf," *Archiv für mikroscopische Anatomie* 26 (1886): I–XXXII.

27. Merkel, *Jacob Henle*, pp. 154–155; Waldeyer, "J. Henle," p. III. Henle claimed he was the first to bring a microscope into the classroom. Cited in Hermann Hoepke, "Jakob Henles Gutachten zur Besetzung des Lehrstuhls für Anatomie an der Universität Berlin 1883," *Anatomischer Anzeiger* 120, no. 8 (1967): 221–232. It seems probable, however, that Henle was not alone in turning the microscope into a pedagogical tool at this time. Unfortunately, little is known about the exact nature of scientific instruction in the early nineteenth century. When the university course listings advertised an anatomy or physiology lecture accompanied by "microscopical demonstrations" or "microscopical investigations"—and these were very common by the late 1830s—it is not clear to what extent students were involved actively in using the instrument. By 1839, however, at least two other individuals (August Meyer in Bonn and Wilhelm Grube in Tübingen) were providing "instruction in the use of the microscope" (Uebung im Gebrauch des Mikroskopes), and this is probably a low estimate. See Kläß, *Die Einführung besonderer Kurse für Mikroskopie*, pp. 53, 245. Henle, for example, did not state explicitly in his course description that he would be showing students how to work with the microscope. There is therefore every reason to believe that at other universities as well some individuals were beginning to introduce students to microscopical techniques.

28. For information on early microscopes, see E. Hintzsche, "Das Mikroskop," *Ciba Zeitschrift* 115 (1949): 4238–4268; K. Fischer, "Die utrechter Mikroskope," *Zeitschrift für Instrumentenkunde* 55 (1935): 239–300; Viktor Patzelt, "Die Bedeutung des Wiener Optikers Simon Plössl für die Mikroskope," *Mikroskopie* 2 (1947): 1–64; Josef Holzl et al., "Simon Plössl—Optiker und Mechaniker in Wien," *Blätter für Technikgeschichte (Wien)* 31 (1969): 82; S. Bradbury, *The Evolution of the Microscope* (Oxford and New York: Pergamon Press, 1967), pp. 174, 200.

The quotation is from J. Henle, "Theodor Schwann. Nachruf," *Archiv für mikroscopische Anatomie* 21 (1882): I–XLIX, here p. II.

29. From a report by the Dorpat prosector Friedrich Bidder, written after

his visit to Berlin in 1834. Reprinted in the following article: P. Morawitz, "Vor hundert Jahren im Laboratorium Johannes Müllers," *Münchener Medizinische Wochenschrift* 82 (1934): 60–64.

30. Ibid., p. 63.

31. Ibid., p. 62.

32. Albert von Kölliker, *Erinnerungen aus meinem Leben* (Leipzig, 1899), p. 8.

33. Herman Hoepke, "Jakob Henles Briefe aus Berlin 1834–1840," *Heidelberger Jahrbücher* 8 (1964): 57–86, here p. 60; Merkel, *Jacob Henle*, p. 156; Max Lenz, *Geschichte der königlichen Friedrich Wilhelms-Universität zu Berlin*, 4 vols. in 5 (Halle: Buchhandlung des Waisenhauses, 1910–1918), vol. 2, pt. 1, pp. 452–453.

34. Letter from Henle to the State Ministry on 31 August 1839. In the Darmstaedter collection, File 3c1844(4). This collection is in the possession of the Staatsbibliothek Preußischer Kulturbesitz zu Berlin, Federal Republic of Germany.

35. Jacob Henle, *Pathologische Untersuchungen* (Berlin, 1840).

36. Timothy Lenoir, *The Strategy of Life. Teleology and Mechanics in Nineteenth Century German Biology* (Dordrecht: D. Reidel, 1982).

37. Jacob Henle, "Ueber Verlauf und Periodicität der Krankheit," in *Pathologische Untersuchungen*, pp. 166–205. Henle's discussion of the "type" is found on pp. 170–182.

38. Ibid., p. 182.

39. Ibid., p. 179.

40. Ibid., pp. 170–171.

41. Ibid., pp. 166, 184.

42. Jacob Henle, "Von den Miasmen und Contagien," in *Pathologische Untersuchungen*, pp. 1–82. Because of this article Henle is often seen as one of the earliest proponents of a germ theory of disease. It must be pointed out, however, that although Henle believed that living organisms could stimulate the disease process, he never accepted an ontological definition of disease. In this regard his views differed radically from those of Koch and others who argued for discrete disease entities.

43. Jacob Henle, *Handbuch der rationellen Pathologie*, 2 vols. (Braunschweig: F. Vieweg, 1846–1853), 1: 93.

44. Guido Gozzi, *Jakob Henles Zürcher Jahre, 1840–1844* (Zürcher Medizingeschichtliche Abhandlungen, Neue Reihe Nr. 103, 1974).

45. Cited in Merkel, *Jakob Henle*, p. 167.

46. Biographical information is from Josef Kerschensteiner, *Das Leben und Wirken des Dr. Carl von Pfeufer* (Augsburg, 1871).

47. Johanna Bleker, *Die Naturhistorische Schule, 1825–1845. Ein Beitrag zur Geschichte der klinischen Medizin in Deutschland* (Stuttgart: G. Fischer, 1981).

48. Kerschensteiner, *Das Leben und Wirken des Dr. Carl von Pfeufer*, pp. 9–15.

49. Carl Pfeufer, "Ueber den gegenwärtigen Zustand der Medizin. Rede gehalten bei dem Antritt des klinischen Lehramts in Zürich den 7. November 1840." Reprinted in the *Annalen der städtischen allgemeinen Kran-

kenhäuser in München (ed. H.v. Ziemssen) 1 (1878): 395–406, here pp. 398–403.

50. Ibid., p. 400.

51. Cited in Gozzi, *Jakob Henles Zürcher Jahre*, p. 55.

52. Merkel, *Jacob Henle*, p. 186.

53. Cited in Werner Goth, *Zur Geschichte der Klinik in Heidelberg im 19. Jahrhundert* (Ph.D. diss., University of Heidelberg, 1982), p. 128.

54. Richard Riese, *Die Hochschule auf dem Wege zum wissenschaftlichen Großbetrieb* (Stuttgart: Ernst Kett Verlag, 1977), pp. 23–24; Eulenberg, *Die Frequenz der deutschen Universitäten*, p. 255.

55. Compiled from the lists of courses and teachers in *Vorlesungen*. The following information is taken from this source.

56. From the "Vergleichung der Budgets-Sätze mit den Rechnungs-Resultaten für die Etats-Jahre 1840 bis 1850," in *Verhandlungen*. Until 1858, 1 gulden equaled 0.67 taler, or 2.01 marks. After 1859, 1 gulden equaled 0.56 taler, or 1.68 marks. See Frank R. Pfetsch, *Zur Entwicklung der Wissenschaftspolitik in Deutschland 1750–1914* (Berlin: Duncker und Humblot, 1974), p. 45.

57. The following information is from Stübler, *Geschichte der medizinischen Fakultät*, pp. 289–294.

58. Letter from Gmelin to the curator in File 235/571: Betr. den Neubau des Anatomie- und Zoologiegebäudes, 1847, Badisches Archiv, 25 March 1845. The generally poor state of the clinical faculties is discussed in Stübler, *Geschichte der medizinischen Fakultät*, pp. 225–227. In a report from the medical faculty in 1846 it is mentioned that discussion of improving the natural science institutes had begun in 1844. See File 235/571, Badisches Archiv, 14 November 1846.

59. Letter from Dahmen to the State Ministry on 14 March 1845, in Goth, *Zur Geschichte der Klinik*, pp. 171–174. For Pfeufer's complaints about inadequate clinical space, see p. 160.

60. Letter from Dahmen to the State Ministry on 15 March 1845, in ibid., pp. 171–174; letter from Pfeufer to the State Ministry on 19 March 1845, in ibid., pp. 165–166.

61. Minutes of the medical faculty meetings from 8 January 1846, in Ano. 1846, III,4a,89. These minutes are in the possession of the University of Heidelberg, Federal Republic of Germany.

62. *Verhandlungen*, 1846, Beilagenheft 4, pp. 292–294.

63. Ibid. The history of Baden's interest in promoting chemical research is dealt with in great detail in Peter Borscheid, *Naturwissenschaft, Staat und Industrie in Baden, 1848–1914* (Stuttgart: Ernst Kett Verlag, 1976). Borscheid argues that state support for the experimental sciences, and especially for chemistry, increased in the 1850s because the government, convinced that a major cause of the revolution of 1848 had been the poverty and destitution resulting from numerous crop failures, decided to invest money and energy in improving the quality of the land.

64. Representative Bissing in *Verhandlungen*, 33 sess., 13 July 1846, Protokollheft 5, p. 227.

65. *Verhandlungen,* 1846, Beilagenheft 8, pp. xxxiv–xxxvii. See also Dahmen to the Ministry of Interior in File 235/571, Badisches Archiv, 4 September 1846.

66. Hermann Hoepke, "Zur Geschichte der Anatomie in Heidelberg," *Sonderdruck aus Ruperto Carola,* vols. 67–68, pp. 115–120. The architectural plans are included in a report from the medical faculty in File 235/571, Badisches Archiv, 14 November 1846.

67. In a letter from Dahmen to the Ministry of Interior in File 235/352: Der Neubau für die naturwissenschaftlichen Institute der Universität Heidelberg—"Friedrichsbau," Badisches Archiv, 15 February 1847.

68. In a letter from the Bau und Oekonomie Commission to Dahmen in ibid., 4 August 1847. The grandiose plans for a natural science institute did not come to fruition until 1863. A number of factors contributed to this delay, foremost being the social and political unrest of the late 1840s. This directed the government's attention and funds to measures of a more immediate and pragmatic nature—the construction of a chemistry laboratory to help alleviate the state's serious agricultural crisis. See Borscheid, *Naturwissenschaft, Staat und Industrie.*

69. See Erwin H. Ackerknecht, *Therapeutics. From the Primitives to the Twentieth Century* (New York: Hafner Press, 1973), chaps. 10, 11; Paul Diepgen, *Geschichte der Medizin,* 2 vols. in 3 (Berlin: Verlag de Gruyter, 1951), 2(1): 163–166.

70. See the articles "Materielle Interessen (1840)" and "Baden (1838)," in F. A. Brockhaus, *Conversations-Lexikon der Gegenwart* (Leipzig, 1838–1841). Also see the articles "Erfahrung (1837)," "Ideen, politische und Ideologie; ideelle und materielle Interessen (1839)," and "Praxis und Theorie (1841)" in Karl von Rotteck and Karl Welcker, eds., *Staats-Lexikon oder Encyclopädie der Staatswissenschaften* (Heidelberg). (Hereafter cited as *Staats-Lexikon.*).

71. "Erfahrung," *Staats-Lexikon* 5 (1837): 253.

72. Jacob Henle, "Medizinische Wissenschaft und Empirie," *Zeitschrift für rationelle Medizin* 1 (1844): 1–35.

73. Ibid., pp. 15, 18.

74. Ibid., pp. 18–19.

75. Ibid., pp. 18, 34.

76. Ibid., p. 4.

77. Ibid., p. 23.

78. Carl Ludwig to Jacob Henle on 22 November 1848, in Astrid Dreher, *Briefe von Carl Ludwig an Jacob Henle aus den Jahren 1846–1872* (Ph.D. diss., University of Heidelberg, 1980), p. 57. Rudolf Virchow, "Ein alter Bericht über die Gestaltung der pathologischen Anatomie in Deutschland, wie sie ist und wie sie werden muss," *Archiv für pathologische Anatomie und Physiologie und für klinische Medizin* 159 (1900): 31.

79. Cited in Walter Artelt, "Jacob Henle," in *Geschichte der Mikroskope, Lehren und Werk großer Forscher,* ed. Hugo Freund and Alexander Berg, 3 vols. (Frankfurt-am-Main: Umschau Verlag, 1964), vol. 2: *Medizin,* pp. 147–159. Here p. 155.

Henle's interest in uniting with the younger generation against his older colleagues is particularly evident in the following letter, written shortly after his arrival in Heidelberg: "Nothing is left here but to let that which is old wither and to ground a new colony. The government and students seem to want to help that come to power. The government, whose eyes are now opened, is astonished at how the faculty has used Heidelberg's reputation and beautiful setting in order to grow fat in luxurious tranquility and to seclude itself from intruders. . . . The students already notice quite well, however, that something new and capable of developing is being offered them now. They are full of enthusiasm for our rational medicine and subsequently furious at the boredom in which they have been educated." Cited in Merkel, *Jacob Henle,* p. 214.

80. *Vorlesungen,* 1853. Henle's and Pfeufer's courses are listed in the *Vorlesungen,* 1844–1852. I am also grateful to Professor Johanna Bleker for allowing me to use the unpublished lectures of Henle and Pfeufer, which are in her private possession: Jacob Henle, *Physiologie der Menschen,* SS/1846, Heidelberg. Carl Pfeufer, *Vorlesungen über specielle Pathologie und Therapie,* SS/1847, Heidelberg. Both notebooks are from the student C. Rauschenbusch.

81. *Vorlesungen,* 1846–1852.

82. Henle to "Geheimen Rath" (this was either the curator or the minister of interior) in File 235/604: Das physiologische Institut, Badisches Archiv, 11 April 1847. Henle's repeated requests for more microscopes can be found both in this file and in File 235/559: Das anatomische und physiologische Institut respective Sammlung, 1807–1865, Badisches Archiv.

83. A description of the instruments found in Henle's institute in 1852 is offered in Friedrich Arnold, *Die physiologische Anstalt der Universität Heidelberg von 1853 bis 1858* (Heidelberg, 1858).

84. Carl Pfeufer, "Ueber den gegenwärtigen Zustand der Medizin," p. 402.

85. The 1841 ruling was published in *Regierungs-Blatt,* 5 July 1844. The 1844 debate can be found in *Verhandlungen,* 67 sess., 13 May 1844, Protokollheft 5 (1843–1844), pp. 182–183.

After 1858 the following courses were required of students wishing to take the state medical examination: two courses in anatomical dissection, a half year in the chemistry laboratory, a half year in the physiology laboratory, and one year in the medical, surgical, and obstetrical clinics. See "Prüfungsordnung für die Kandidaten der Heilkunde."

86. See Kläß, *Die Einführung besonderer Kurse für Mikroskope.*

CHAPTER THREE

The Paris Academy of Medicine and Experimental Science, 1820–1848

John E. Lesch

Among the institutional connections of science, few have as long or as variegated a history as those with medicine. At least since the Hippocratic school, a vocal minority of physicians in successive periods of Western history have become engaged with prevailing modes of scientific or philosophical thought, to the benefit of physiology and anatomy as well as more specifically medical fields such as pathology. The maintenance of an esoteric body of knowledge has usually served not only to inform or rationalize practice but also to legitimize the physician's authority and social position. Especially since the rise of the profession in association with the universities in the thirteenth century, special knowledge has gone far to define the doctor and his role. Since the Renaissance medically trained individuals have taken a prominent part in the construction of modern science.

Yet the association of medicine and theoretical knowledge has often been subject to tensions and contradictions. The central aims of medicine—the cure, palliation, or prevention of disease—are practical. The practicing physician typically deals with individuals in specific circumstances, not with the general laws and idealized cases of science. The majority of practitioners at any given time have only limited and routinized contact with theoretical medicine and may tend to view it with indifference, suspicion, uneasiness, or hostility, or to regard it as merely irrelevant. To a remarkable degree the problematic aspects of the relationship between medical theory and practice display a resemblance over widely separated historical periods. In the ancient world empirics were already challenging the claims of abstract theory in medical practice, a challenge that has recurred in later times.[1] William Harvey's scientific achievements were used by members of London's College of Physicians to shore up the college's position vis-à-vis empirics and apothecaries but were also attacked—along with the ideal of the "anatomical physician" Harvey represented—as irrelevant to practice.[2] The emergence of the preclinical fields as specialized sciences and as components of medical education has raised the issues anew in the nineteenth and twentieth centuries.[3]

The Paris clinical school of the first half of the nineteenth century offers an especially noteworthy case of the interaction of medicine and science in both its synergism and its tensions. Parisian physicians have rightly been credited with innovations that were constitutive of modern medicine, including the reunion of medicine and surgery, the consolidation of hospital-based training and practice, and the development of methods of physical diagnosis and pathological anatomy. Yet the very clinical preoccupations of the school have also been seen as inimical to the laboratory sciences, which are more readily associated with the German universities of the second half of the century.[4]

I have argued elsewhere that the Paris clinical school, in association with the Paris Academy of Science, provided an environment favorable to the development of the laboratory sciences, in particular experimental physiology, organic analysis, and pharmaceutical chemistry.[5] Here I would like to extend that argument by examining the place of experimental science in the life of what for a time was the foremost medical assembly not only in France but the world: the Paris Academy of Medicine.

From the 1820s to the founding of the Société de Biologie in 1848, experimental science found a growing constituency among the leadership of the Parisian medical community, gathered in the Academy of Medicine. In spite of shortages of funds and facilities and occasional reservations, resistance, or indifference on the part of some members, the academy was receptive to and encouraged the cultivation of the sciences, including experimental physiology and pharmacology, in their bearing on clinical practice. This positive relationship to science is reflected in the stated goals and formal organization of the academy, in the overlap of its membership with those of the Academy of Science and Société de Biologie, in the experimental investigations conducted by its members, in the role accorded experimental findings in its debates on medical issues, and in the extent to which the values of experimental medicine, as later defined by Claude Bernard, were explicitly formulated and acted upon by its members.

The academy's embrace of experimental science had its critics and its limitations, foremost among the latter a tendency to turn investigation into channels that promised quick returns to practice. It was against this impatient utilitarianism that the founders of the Société de Biologie defined their program for a science of life freed from immediate practical demands. Even as they did so, however, they drew upon a well-established tradition of openness and engagement in the academy's relationship with experimental science.

I

The Academy of Medicine was brought into existence by a royal ordinance of 20 December 1820. Louis XVIII had been persuaded of the need for this move by the redoubtable Antoine Portal, who had become the king's friend and confidant after his appointment as first physician in 1818. Professor at the Collège de France and member of the Academy of Science, Portal had been involved for many years in efforts to create an organization that would offer technical counsel to the government and act as supreme arbiter of medicine in France. His models, the Royal Academy of Surgery and the Royal Society of Medicine, had suffered the fate of the Old Regime of which they were a part. Portal, whose own Old Regime provenance was evident in his anachronistic dress, judged correctly that the Restoration government might be receptive to their revival in a form more appropriate to the times. Portal's hand is visible not only in the academy's instigation but also in the selection of its first members, the framing of its regulations, and the design of its administration.[6]

The founding statutes of the Academy of Medicine and its goals as stated in Etienne Pariset's inaugural address of 6 May 1824 refer directly to the two Old Regime models, and the parallels are borne out by the structure and duties assigned to the academy. Besides promoting the advancement of the medical sciences, the academy was to respond to the demands of the government in all that concerns the public health, and primarily epidemics, the diseases peculiar to certain countries, the epizootics, different cases of legal medicine, the propagation of the vaccine, the examination of new and secret remedies whether internal or external, natural or active mineral waters.

The archives of both the Royal Academy of Surgery and the Royal Society of Medicine were turned over to the Academy of Medicine, which also absorbed the records and functions of government units responsible for the oversight of medicinal baths and vaccination.[7]

Deference to political sensitivities helps to explain Portal's and Pariset's emphasis on Old Regime models, and also their failure to credit postrevolutionary organizations on whose experience and resources the academy drew. Of these the most important was the Société de l'Ecole de Médecine. Founded on 12 fructidor an VIII—30 August 1800—by ministerial order, the Société's membership included the professors of the medical school, and the *procès-verbaux* of the Société's regular meetings were published in the medical school's *Bulletins*. Most members of the Société were named members of the academy in 1820, and the Société was then dissolved.[8]

The major point of difference between the academy and its Old Regime models was its union of medical, surgical, pharmaceutical, and veterinary professionals in a single corporate body. This was not accomplished without resistance from a minority of physicians and surgeons who wished to restore the old separation, and concessions to those views are visible in the internal division of the academy into three classes—medicine, surgery, and pharmacy—each with its own officers and meetings. Each section met twice a month. The academy held a general meeting every three months, and each section held an annual public meeting. Even this degree of separation proved impractical, however, and a new royal ordinance of 1829 prepared by Pariset abolished the three classes. They were replaced by eleven sections the definitions of which either corresponded to scientific specialties or otherwise cut across the traditional professional divisions. At the same time the statutory number of members was sharply reduced, and a subsequent ordinance of 1835 abolished distinctions of title among members. Portal served as permanent honorary president until his death in 1832; he was not replaced. The academy's administrative council at first consisted of a president and vice-president, a permanent and an annual secretary, a treasurer, the dean of the Faculty of Medicine ex officio, and the presidents and secretaries of the three classes. When the classes were abolished their officers were replaced by three annual members elected by the academy at large. Representatives of the state took the occasion of the 1829 ordinance to affirm the unity of medical science and the privileged status of the academy as its sole official representative.[9]

From the beginning science had an important place in the academy's activities. Portal himself had been scientifically active and was a long-standing member of the Academy of Science. The founding statutes that he helped to frame give as one of the academy's principal goals "the perfecting of medical science," and the same ordinance directs that the academy is to "occupy itself with all the objects of study and research which may contribute to the progress of the different branches of the art of healing." Among the criteria to be used in the selection of members and *associés libres* was their successful cultivation of the "sciences accessory to medicine." To be included among the academy's archives with the printed or manuscript works and their illustrations were instruments and machines, anatomical pieces, objects of natural history, and chemical products. The ordinance of 1829 states the academy's intention to maintain a *chef des travaux chimiques* and a chemical laboratory. Both the original and the 1829 ordinances call for the academy to propose "every year, as prize subjects, questions on matters that, as much as possible, may be investigated by experiments (*expériences*), observations, and positive research."[10]

In October 1829 Minister of the Interior La Bourdonnaye wrote to the king, in reference to the academy's impending reorganization, that

> the most enlightened minds recognize that the division of the Academy into sections of medicine, surgery, and pharmacy can only be considered as the outline of a more complete division. They think that if it were, like the Academy of Science, divided into classes or sections corresponding to the essential specialties of the medical sciences, this mode of organization would offer . . . the guarantee of a better elaboration and a more enlightened judgment.

Pariset's most enlightened mind did look to the Academy of Science as a model, and the sections established—anatomy and physiology, medical pathology, surgical pathology, therapeutics and medical natural history, operatory medicine, public hygiene, legal medicine and medical police, veterinary medicine, medical physics and chemistry, and pharmacy—incorporated scientific as well as peculiarly medical specialties.[11]

The academy's *Mémoires*, which appeared from 1828, published substantial pieces of research in medicine and related sciences along with *éloges*, programs of prizes, texts of speeches at annual meetings, and other matters bearing on the history of the academy. *Procès-verbaux* of meetings, including frequent reports and debates on medical-scientific research, were printed in the *Bulletin*, which was published from 1836. Both publications give ample evidence of the scientific interests of the academy as a body and of its members as individuals.[12]

The late start of the *Mémoires* and the *Bulletin*—eight and sixteen years, respectively, after the academy's founding—is one indication that the academy's reach often exceeded its grasp. The original legislation had not provided for suitable physical accommodations, and at first closed meetings were held in the amphitheater of the Faculty of Medicine and public meetings in the Palais du Louvre. After considering and rejecting several alternatives, the academy finally settled for a building at 8 rue de Poitiers, which had previously housed the Comité de Vaccine.

The new quarters were formally inaugurated on 6 May 1824. The building was not ideal, and budgetary constraints soon forced the academy to confine itself to the ground floor. In this restricted space there was no room for the anatomical collections or the physical and chemical laboratories with experimental apparatus that the academy had hoped to install. The meeting room was so small that visitors and journalists had to be excluded. Though thought to be provisional, this arrangement persisted for a quarter of a century, until termination of the academy's lease in 1850 forced it to move to a new set of inadequate quarters in the former chapel of the Charité hospital.[13]

Constraints of lodging and finance could limit but not prevent the effort for the advancement of medical science that was affirmed to be the academy's major goal by its permanent secretary, Etienne Pariset. Known for work in epidemiology and for his eloquence as a speaker and writer, Pariset collaborated closely with Portal in shaping and running the academy in its early years, and until 1847 served as permanent secretary. He gave voice to the academy's aspirations and self-image through his many *éloges*, and especially in the address he gave to assembled members and dignitaries at the inauguration of the academy's new quarters in May 1824.[14]

The most striking quality of Pariset's speech was its insistence on the privileged place of science in the life of the academy. Reminding his colleagues that the government looked to them above all for "the perfecting of the medical sciences," Pariset grounded the legitimacy of the enterprise in the proven success of earlier academies. Although he included in this exemplary past the Academy of Surgery and the Royal Society of Medicine, it is clear that the scientific academies were uppermost in his mind. Academies, he said, had stimulated love of learning and had taught by example to bring precision and rigor to the investigation of natural facts. Because knowledge is "constantly in flux and progress," it was important, in Pariset's view, to keep its oscillation within narrow limits so that it moved, if not toward the truth, at least toward the strongest probabilities. Such, he said, was the great achievement of the modern European academies, which, in contrast to the "endless contention" of the Greek schools, brought about scientific consensus.[15]

Just as medicine stood to be enriched by the model of academic science, so too would it be impoverished if it failed to call upon the help of physiology, natural history, botany, physics, and chemistry, "sciences which almost all are born from medicine, which draw their principal importance only from their relation with the conservation of man, that is to say, with medicine itself; which, consequently, cannot be separated from it, and must always identify themselves with it." Pariset here defines what may be termed an incorporative view of the relations of science and medicine. According to this view not only do the sciences have their origins in medicine and derive from it their highest goal, but the broad cultivation of scientific knowledge, not just a narrow utility, is part and parcel of the medical enterprise. The implications of such a view are double-edged. For if, on the one hand, medicine embraces the sciences, seeks to support and advance them, and makes use of their results, it seeks, on the other hand, to subordinate them by defining their "highest" goals and—at least implicitly—laying claim to a kind of proprietary right and authority.[16]

For Pariset the incorporation of the sciences into medicine was paralleled by—in fact, demanded—the closest alliance among the healing arts. The class of pharmacy, for example, was joined to those of medicine and surgery not merely because the academy had been charged with the inspection of mineral waters and the judgment of new remedies, or because it wished to advance the gathering and preparation of medicines, but because through pharmacy the academy gained access to the new chemistry. Pharmacy, Pariset noted, "assembles around it all the productions of the three kingdoms; and thanks to analysis, it enters as if by enchantment into the interior of bodies." Separating their principles, molecules, and elements, "it gives them a new order, new connections, new appearances, new properties; and from these happy metamorphoses it finally causes to emerge beings more appropriate to our needs."[17] Pariset took to task those who would resist innovation in pharmaceutical chemistry on the grounds that therapeutics was already overburdened by "a horde of superfluous medicines," and that a few remedies, already known, sufficed in many cases. To these voices of therapeutic skepticism Pariset responded with a version of the moderate program for reform of the *materia medica* and drug therapy already formulated by François Magendie and the Paris pharmacists. Because we cannot admit everything, he pointed out, does not mean that we must reject everything; and if we are ever to know the subtle changes in the body that determine health and disease, it will be through chemistry.[18]

Pariset's remarks reflect a clear sense of the importance and promise of experimental physiology as it was practiced by Magendie, Pierre Flourens, and others in the 1820s. He rightly identified the nervous system, in particular nervous control of sensation and movement, as the center of then current interest. On the whole, his notion of research methodologies—animal experiment, pathological observation, comparative anatomy—and their relative importance might have been lifted from the pages of Magendie's contemporary *Journal de physiologie expérimentale et pathologique*. Without using the phrase, he captured the essence of Magendie's idea of pathological physiology in viewing diseases as "so many physiological experiments made by nature." To realize its brilliant future, Pariset told his colleagues, physiology needed only to put into its experiments "more order, connection, and coordination." The natural locale for this project, he added, was the Academy of Medicine.[19]

Just as medicine's conceptual and methodological need for chemistry impelled a professional and institutional alliance with pharmacy, so too, in Pariset's view, did its reliance on physiology require a league with veterinary medicine. For if the primary methodological base of physiology was animal experiment, it was in the "justly celebrated" veterinary school of Alfort that the academy would find the necessary facilities for those experiments and among the "most able professors" of that school that the experimenters of the academy would find their natural colleagues. Physiology, "the most attractive and most delicate of the medical sciences," was the proper domain of the Academy of Medicine, but only of an academy in which human and animal medicine were treated as a unity."[20]

Beside his enthusiasm for chemistry and physiology Pariset's remarks on normal and pathological anatomy, though positive, seem scant and bland. In his view the normal anatomy of the adult had reached a state of near perfection to which little beyond information on variations related to such factors as country, region, occupation, or age need be added. The anatomy of development left more room for improvement, and chemical analysis, Pariset pointed out, even provided anatomists with a chance to understand the composition of the body's fluids. It is clear, however, that for Pariset scientific glory did not lie in these directions. His case for pathological anatomy was somewhat better in that he acknowledged that its recent flourishing had thrown much light on diagnosis and on surgical—and some medical—treatments. Yet he stressed pathological anatomy's limits—the easy confusion of cause and effect, the difficulties in interpreting observations—as much as its success. Pathological anatomy might be—indeed, was—on its way to a preeminent place in the Paris clinical school. For the first permanent secretary of the Academy of Medicine, however, it was the experimental sciences of physiology and chemistry that held the keys to medicine's future.[21]

II

Pariset's plea for science must have found a receptive audience among the members and dignitaries assembled for the inauguration of the academy's new quarters. For if membership in the Paris Academy of Science at some time in a career is taken as an indicator of serious scientific interest and activity, a significant fraction—14 percent of the broad membership, 24 percent of the titular members—of the original Academy of Medicine was scientifically active and recognized as such by the elite of the scientific community. Original titular members of the Academy of Medicine who also belonged to the Academy of Science included Portal and Pariset (the latter a *membre libre* of the Academy of Science), the physician and physiologist François Magendie, the physician and comparative anatomist André Dumeril, the surgeon and pathologist Guillaume Dupuytren, and the pharmacist and chemist Pierre-Joseph Pelletier. The pattern was to continue through the first half of the century. Twenty percent of those promoted to full membership or elected as new members between 1820 and 1848 were at some time members of the Academy of Science. Sixteen percent of all members in 1849 had the same distinction at some time in their careers.[22]

In the period covered by this study, distinction in the Paris medical community was correlated with a still higher degree of scientific activity. Of the sixty individuals who served between 1820 and 1848 as members of the Paris Faculty of Medicine, an overwhelming majority—fifty-five, or 92 percent—were at some time in their careers members of the Academy of Medicine. Yet at any given time they constituted only a minority of the academy's membership. In 1849 they made up 26 percent of the members. The Faculty of Medicine was therefore an elite within an elite and may be taken as the heart of the Paris clinical school and medical establishment. Of the sixty holding Faculty of Medicine positions at some time between 1820 and 1848, a very substantial minority—twenty-two or 37 percent—were at some time in their careers members or correspondents of the Academy of Science. Among those so honored were Gilbert Breschet, who held the Faculty's chair of anatomy from 1836 to 1845; Jean-Baptiste Dumas, who held the chair of organic chemistry from 1838 to 1852; and Jean Bouillaud, who served as dean of the Faculty in 1848. Of the thirty-one individuals who were members of the Academy of Medicine in 1849 and also at some time in their careers members of the Faculty of Medicine, a comparable fraction—thirteen, or 42 percent—were also at some time members of the Academy of Science.[23]

Although the academy held a preeminent place in the professional organization of French medicine, it began to be joined in the 1830s by new societies responding to more specialized interests. These included the Société Médicale d'Observation (1837), the Société de Chirurgie (1843), the Société de Biologie (1848), and the Société Médicale des Hôpitaux (1849). As its name indicates, it was the Société de Biologie that went furthest in formulating a program for a scientific medicine. Eleven individuals, or 9 percent of the Academy of Medicine in 1849, were among the founding members of the Société de Biologie. All eleven were also at some time members of the Academy of Science. A minority of members of the Academy of Medicine, therefore, were founders of the Société de Biologie. This is to be expected in a more specialized society. If we look at the Société de Biologie, however, it is clear that a substantial majority of its original members were at some time members of the Academy of Medicine (thirty-four of fifty-five, or 62 percent of the broad membership; seven of eight, or 88 percent of the officers; thirteen of fifteen, or 87 percent of the honorary members; fourteen of thirty-two, or 44 percent of the titular members). The Société's first president, Pierre Rayer, would later (1862–1864) be dean of the Faculty of Medicine. The Société de Biologie may be regarded as initially dominated by those who were or would become part of the elite of the Parisian medical community.[24]

These figures have their limitations, and conclusions based on them must be qualified. Membership in the Academy of Science does not tell us the nature of the science involved, which could and did range from normal and pathological anatomy through chemistry, comparative anatomy, and experimental physiology to microscopy and other fields. It does not tell us anything directly about attitudes toward any specific field of science or its relevance for medicine. An individual might be active in research in anatomy, for example, and yet be skeptical about the reliability of experimental physiology or its bearing on diagnosis, etiology, or therapeutics. Figures given here do not indicate when, and for how long, individuals who became members of the Academy of Science were scientifically active. The date of election alone can be misleading. Dupuytren, for example, had given up experimental physiology—though not pathological anatomy—for surgery by the time he was elected in 1825. Finally, these figures do not account for those members of the Academy of Medicine who, because their level of scientific activity never reached the necessary threshold or for some other reason, were never elected to membership in the Academy of Science. Many may nevertheless have engaged in scientific research and recognized the utility of science in medicine in some form. Those so neglected in the 1849 membership include such scientifically significant names as Joseph Caventou and Jean-Louis Poiseuille, and such vocal and prominent members as Jean Amussat, Jean Cruveilhier, Pierre Nicolas Gerdy, Pierre Louis, and Pierre Piorry.

What cannot be doubted is that the membership figures indicate a substantial involvement in science among the elite of the Parisian medical community from the 1820s through the 1840s. They strongly suggest at least a receptive attitude toward the experimental sciences and their bearing on medicine. For membership in the Academy of

Science meant participation in a body in which experimental physiology and pharmaceutical chemistry were held in high regard, a body that indeed had been partly responsible for the development of those fields. It would be difficult for a member to escape those attitudes.

III

In the academy's activities experimental investigation held a limited but significant place. One indication of this role may be found in the academy's definition of prize subjects. Title 6 of the original regulations specified that "prize subjects should, so far as possible, be susceptible to investigation by experiments (*expériences*), observations, and positive research." There were to be four prizes per year: one each for medicine, surgery, and pharmacy, and a fourth for subjects of interest to several classes.[25] These numbers and the distribution by classes were not adhered to—the classes themselves were abolished in the reorganization of 1829—but the stricture on content was evidently taken seriously. By 1843 the academy's practice and separate endowments by individuals had brought the list of prizes to five. In that year Frédéric Dubois d'Amiens described these as one supported by the academy and subject only to the restriction noted earlier; one set up by Antoine Portal, to be concerned with organic diseases; one endowed by Madame Bernard de Civrieux having to do with "nervous overexcitation"; a fourth owing to the Marquis d'Argenteuil, devoted to diseases of the ureter or urinary tract; and a fifth set up by Jean Itard, to be awarded every three years for the best work in applied medicine or practical therapeutics.[26]

A few examples of subjects proposed by the academy for its own prize suffice to indicate the center of its interests. "What is to be understood by laryngeal phthisis? What are its organic alterations, its causes, its terminations, and what is its treatment?" was the question posed for 1834.[27] For 1838 contestants were to "do the physiological history of menstruation; make known the influence that this function exerts on diseases, and that which diseases exert on it."[28] For 1848 authors were to "make known the composition of the bile in the physiological state; describe the principal alterations to which this liquid is susceptible and the chemical methods by which to ascertain them; indicate the causes of these alterations and the morbid modifications they can exercise on the body's economy, the semiological means of assessing them, and their appropriate treatment."[29] Scope was offered for normal anatomy and physiology, but only in conjunction with a predominant interest in problems of the origin and course of disease, its diagnosis and treatment,

The same distribution of emphasis may be observed in the academy's *Mémoires*. From volume one (1828) through volume fourteen (1849) the academy published 177 of these formal papers, not all authored by its own members. These may be grouped under twelve categories (in descending order of frequency): pathology, surgery, psychiatry, public health, therapeutics, pharmacy, anatomy, physiology, veterinary medicine, chemistry, history of medicine, and nutrition.[30] Two of these, pathology and surgery, dominate, together accounting for 48 percent of the total. Characteristic of this group are memoirs by René Prus, physician at the Salpêtrière, "On Two Diseases Known by the Name of Meningeal Apoplexy," and by Hippolyte Larrey, professor of surgical pathology at the Val-de-Grace, "On Penetrating Wounds of the Abdomen, Complicated by Protrusion of the Omentum," both published in 1845. Each involves the description and analysis of clinical cases, with an attempt to understand the underlying pathology and to specify implications for therapy.[31] A middle group, consisting of psychiatry, public health, therapeutics, and pharmacy, contribute another 37 percent. The remaining 15 percent comprises small numbers from anatomy, physiology, veterinary medicine, chemistry, history of medicine, and nutrition.

A cursory survey of memoirs from all categories reveals that twenty-six, or 15 percent of the total, contain reports of chemical analysis or animal experiments, or are based on experimental investigation in some significant way.[32] In many cases these memoirs brought the techniques of experiment to bear on problems of therapeutics or pathology. In 1845, for example, Henri Onésime Delafond, a professor of pathology and legal medicine at Alfort, published a systematic and detailed account of experiments he had made to determine whether urinary secretion was suppressed in arsenic acid poisoning.[33] The following year, to give one more instance, physicians H. de Castelnau and F. M. Ducrest published reports of experiments in which pus and other substances were injected into dogs and the sequence of events carefully followed to study the formation of multiple abcesses. Consideration of both memoirs and prizes indicates that although the academy's interests inclined sharply toward pathology and therapeutics, including surgery, normal anatomy and physiology were never lost from sight, and experimental methods of investigation were not only honored but also used in a significant fraction of published studies.[34]

Different access to the status of experimentalism within the Academy of Medicine is provided by the academy's *procès-verbaux*, which record debates on medical issues in which experimental science served as a prominent and respected, though by no means exclusive, source of evidence. Typically experimental research entered into discussion in the company of other information drawn from medical and surgical practice, pathology, veterinary medicine, and statistics. Examples of such debates pursued to some length—though not necessarily to a final resolution—are those on the introduction of air into the lungs in the operation of empyema and on the introduction of air into the vascular system. These debates are worth considering in some detail, for they display in clear relief the strengths, tensions, and limitations of experimentalism in the thought and action of the leaders of the Paris medical community.

In October 1836 the Academy of Medicine began discussion of the surgical operation performed in cases of empyema, a condition in which pus collects in the pleural cavity as a result of pleurisy, or inflammation of the pleural membrane. One question was of special interest: was the introduction of air into the pleural cavity which could occur in this operation always fatal? The talk was lively and drew in a variety of speakers, including the physicians Jacques Rochoux, Alfred Velpeau, and Louis, the surgeons Dominique Jean Larrey and Amussat, and the veterinarians Eloi Barthélemy and Jean Dupuy. Louis provided statistics in the form of summary remarks on approximately five hundred cases. Larrey described his surgical procedures in detail, and Dupuy and Barthélemy reported observations from veterinary practice and from experiments on horses.[35]

As the debate proceeded, however, it came to center on animal experiments performed by Amussat and by the physicians Cruveilhier and Piorry. Cruveilhier had made openings in both lungs of a dog and had maintained these openings for eight minutes. He reported that although the animal's respiration was extremely laborious during the operation, breathing returned to normal as soon as the animal was left to itself. Repeating the experiment several times, he concluded that the introduction of air into the pleural cavity was not invariably fatal. Amussat and Piorry replied that their own experiments had yielded contrary results, and that they even used the large opening of both pleural cavities as the quickest and most humane way of shortening the sufferings of experimental animals. "Wishing to escape this uncertainty," Piorry said, "I began my experiments again." Since his results were still different, Piorry thought that "there must be some cause of this difference that escaped us." He tried opening the chest of a rabbit further down than in the earlier trials, at a point just above the diaphragm. In this case the diaphragm, in raising itself, closed the wound and saved the animal. Piorry concluded that when the chest is opened high up the operation is "essentially mortal." When it is lower "life is not necessarily compromised."[36]

To Cruveilhier's suggestion that the disparate results were attributable to differences in operative procedure, Amussat replied that he did not think that Cruveilhier had operated differently, but he did think that "it is probable that he did not do completely the experiment in question, and that above all he did not repeat it, as I indicate, in agreement on this point with M. Magendie and all experimenters." From his own experiments Amussat concluded "that the introduction of air by a wound in the lung causes the lung to collapse; that this collapse is troublesome and painful; that the air contained in the lung prevents it from dilating; and that to assist nature the best means is to occlude the opening, after a strong expiration, and to compress the thoracic walls." Cruveilhier promptly complained that "it is supposed that I do not take enough care with my experiments, and it is because of the weakness of the experimenter that the difference of results is rejected." Describing his experiment again, Cruveilhier continued, "I for my part suspect that the experimenters who are not in accord with me have operated on dogs already exhausted by illnesses or by other experiments. If these suspicions have some foundation, we should not be surprised that these animals succumbed so promptly."[37]

Finally the disputants resorted to direct confrontation in the laboratory. "Well persuaded that facts are contradictory only when they comprise different elements not yet perceived, and in order to escape from this state of perplexity always created by an unresolved question of fact," Cruveilhier reported, "I invited M. Amussat to come to my laboratory, where we should repeat the experiment, each in his own way." In so doing Cruveilhier had to admit his error. He had been misled because in struggling his experimental animal had succeeded in intermittently closing the openings in its pleural cavities. When these were kept constantly open, the animal died. The pertinence of these results to the surgical operation in question could not be doubted. "Whatever reservations must be made in the use of the facts of comparative physiology," Cruveilhier noted, "nevertheless no one can contest the legitimacy of the application of the results of these experiments to man." In support of this contention Cruveilhier cited a case from Larrey's military surgery, and, in a subsequent meeting, described in detail another clinical case. Both of these he held to be consistent with the experimental findings that had issued from the debate in the academy.[38]

Even before he debated Cruveilhier on the matter of air in the pleural cavity, Amussat was pursuing experiments prompted by another hazard of surgical practice. In a memoir on traumatic hemorrhage read at the academy's annual meeting in July 1835, he called his colleagues' attention to an accident still more formidable than bleeding: the spontaneous introduction of air into wounded veins neighboring the heart. Whenever this had happened in man, he noted, it had always been quickly fatal. Many experiments on animals had shown, he said, that the opening in the vein need not be wide, and that when air penetrates, it does so with a "quite peculiar" sound. The same experiments had shown that the best means of assistance in such cases consisted of first closing the vein, then rapidly and in succession compressing the chest and abdomen, while placing a finger on the opening of the vein in each interval between compressions. By this means Amussat claimed to have recalled to life a great number of animals, while those not so treated in similar circumstances had died. For this technique might be substituted aspiration of air by mouth through a tube inserted in the vein, or, "as M. Magendie proposes," with a syringe and a flexible sound. If these methods are used, Amussat noted, the operator must immediately afterward apply ligature or torsion to the wounded vein.[39]

Taking courage from his experiments, Amussat ventured to apply his countermeasures when the accident befell one of his own patients. In the academy's meeting of 4 July 1837, he described an operation in which he removed the cancerous right breast of a forty-seven-year-old woman. At the moment he cut a group of suspicious granulations below the clavicle, he heard a "broken" and "zigzag-like" sound, which he took to be that of air that had penetrated a vessel. Mastering his own anxiety, he compressed the chest several times while leaving the vessel open, then directed an aide to press the point from which the sound came with his hand. He finished the operation, twisted several arteries, and ligatured the vein at the point from which the sound had issued. He dressed the wound and returned the patient to her bed. Amussat remarked that although this was not the first such case that had been observed, it was, perhaps, the only one that had not been fatal.[40]

Unlike many clinical observations that made a momentary appearance before the academy and then vanished into obscurity, this one provoked a discussion that lasted seven months, involved several of the academy's leading members in heated debate, and led to the formation of a commission that carried out its own experimental studies of the problem. Like the debate previously described, this one was revealing of the academy's receptivity to experimentalism.

Velpeau set the tone of the debate by quickly recognizing the importance of the issues raised by Amussat while questioning Amussat's interpretation of his observations. Although a score of accidents in surgical operations had been attributed to the introduction of air into the veins, Velpeau noted, several of these attributions were inconclusive in light of current physiological knowledge. Xavier Bichat, he pointed out, had thought that it was sufficient to let a few bubbles of air into the veins of an animal to kill it and that death occurred first in the brain. Pierre Nysten had shown, on the contrary, that to kill an animal enough air must be introduced to fill the right cavities of the heart, and that the animal died by arrest of the circulation. Nysten's experiments, Velpeau continued, had been repeated by many, including Magendie, always with the same result. Pierre Bérard had shown that at the root of the neck the great veins are stretched and that air can penetrate them as soon as they are opened. Poiseuille, however, had shown that this was possible only over the distance of a few centimeters. Now, Velpeau pointed out, in most known clinical cases several of these conditions were lacking. In a fatal case reported by Dupuytren, for example, only a few bubbles of air were found in the heart at autopsy. In other cases it appeared that either so little air got in, or the operation was far enough from the danger area, that "physiological experiments do not permit admitting death by the introduction of air." Amussat was also mistaken, Velpeau noted, in thinking that his patient was the first such case to be saved. Four or five other instances were known, including one of Velpeau's own in which air may have entered the veins, yet the patient survived without compression of the chest.

Velpeau concluded that the question was an open one that required more investigation.[41]

Velpeau's remarks prompted other comments in the meeting of 4 July. Attempting to clarify the confusing clinical picture, Pierre Ségalas suggested that if a large quantity of air is introduced, but slowly, the animal—or, by implication, the patient—may live; if the introduction is abrupt, it will die. The veterinarian Dupuy was inclined to support Amussat. He noted that if veins near the heart are opened in a horse and the hand is brought to the opening, it is strongly pulled. Dupuy reported that when Magendie—who often experimented at the veterinary school of Alfort—made injections in the veins of horses, the right heart was always filled with a frothy liquid, which stopped its movements. From these experiments Dupuy thought that he could draw rules of treatment in certain diseases, such as typhoid fever in cattle.[42]

When the discussion reopened a week later, Amussat reaffirmed his position, stating that "the experiments I have made on this subject are decisive and do not admit the least doubt." Velpeau's uncertainties had led him, if anything, to sharpen his thesis. "Every time," he continued, "on an animal placed in the same conditions as a man on whom one operates, one opens a vein next to the heart, the jugular, for example, at a point in its extent where the flux and reflux of the blood takes place, one hears immediately afterward a distinct sound." This sound, "which announces the introduction of the air, is consistently followed by death, generally after one minute or less." Opening the cadaver, Amussat noted, one always finds the right heart to be distended by a great quantity of air mixed with blood which is lighter than usual. The left cavities, in contrast, are collapsed and empty, as in cases of death by hemorrhage.

"But the important part of my experiments," Amussat continued, "was to see whether there was not a remedy against an accident that is almost always fatal." To this end he had compressed the chests of several animals immediately on hearing the sound indicating entry of air into the veins. Made "by fits and starts" this compression expelled the introduced air and recalled the animals to life. This technique could be easily and practically applied under any circumstances. This was important in "rapidly dangerous cases, because rarely has one sufficient foresight to have at one's disposition Magendie's instruments, which are moreover difficult to use." Amussat acknowledged that other members of the academy did not share his convictions on these points. He suggested that because the question of the introduction of air into the chest cavity had recently been resolved in a definitive manner, that of the introduction of air into the veins should be handled in the same way—that is, by repeating several experiments on animals in the presence of members of the academy.[43]

The commission was appointed by the academy in response to Amussat's appeal and consisted of Bouillaud, Velpeau, Gerdy, Philippe Blandin, Barthélemy, Nicolas Adelon, and François Moreau. It took four months to do its work. During this time open debate was largely silenced, but some indication of what the issues would be can be seen in the comments that followed Amussat's at the 11 July meeting. Blandin, Rochoux, and the surgeon Philibert Roux all doubted whether the introduction of air was invariably fatal. Velpeau, who congratulated himself for provoking the discussion, nevertheless was unconvinced that air was lethal in the clinical cases so far described, citing hemorrhage, pain, and exhaustion as other factors to be considered. The veterinarian Barthélemy pointed out that horses with glanders used to be killed by opening the jugular and injecting air, in the hope of preventing the contagion risked by bleeding. He therefore thought that a certain quantity of air, as yet undetermined, could cause death when introduced into the veins. Blandin, Roux, and Gerdy were not convinced of the usefulness of compressing the chest after the accident, and Gerdy added that he also placed little confidence in the insertion of sounds into the heart. Better, Gerdy said, to prevent the accident, perhaps by restricting the patient's breathing by a large chest bandage at the most dangerous point of the operation. Gerdy urged his colleagues to resist the temptation to rush to the first plausible explanation out of horror of sudden, unexplained death, and instead to subject its possible causes, including the introduction of air into the veins, to rigorous scrutiny.[44]

The commission reported through its spokesman Bouillaud on 21 November. The pains taken over the report were reflected in its formal, methodical structure. Following introductory remarks a first part summarized research and opinions prior to Amussat and restated his assertions; a second part described the commission's research and conclusions. The second part was itself divided into introductory remarks, a first section describing the commission's experiments in a consistent format, and a second section explaining the commission's conclusions. The first and second sections of the second part were themselves carefully subdivided.[45]

Bouillaud introduced the problem with appropriate gravity. The question posed by Amussat is a complex one, he said, in part because "it is at the same time a question of experimental physiology properly speaking and a question of practice, I almost said of surgical physiology." Its investigation must include rigorous study of the principal means by which air may enter the veins and the effects of the air once in the body. Variations in conditions or circumstances, such as the species and strength of the animal, the quantity of air introduced, and the speed of introduction of air, must all be carefully considered. Finally, Bouillaud continued, since Amussat had claimed novelty for his views, the commission had surveyed the past state of knowledge on the introduction of air into the veins.[46]

Bouillaud reported that several physiologists, and especially Barry and Poiseuille, had shown that air could spontaneously—that is, without injections or tubes—enter an open vein. Poiseuille had found that inspiration tends to push venous blood away from the chest cavity, while expiration has the reverse effect. Both effects, Poiseuille argued, diminish to zero at a determinable distance from the heart. Given, in Poiseuille's view, that the tugging effect isochronous with expiration was what drew air into the veins, the latter effect was to be feared only within a restricted radius around the heart. Nysten's experiments had shown that, contrary to Bichat's opinion, the introduction of small quantities of air into the veins is not necessarily fatal. As the quantity of air introduced is increased, Nysten found, death does occur, but it is not always rapid. Whereas Bichat had located the air's fatal action in the brain, Nysten placed it in the lungs. Magendie's experiments confirmed Nysten's in finding that air in the veins is not necessarily fatal, but ascribed its killing action when it was fatal to distension of the right heart by gas or foamy blood. Concluding the commission's survey of earlier work, Bouillaud described six clinical cases taken from the roughly thirty then in the literature in which autopsy revealed the presence of air in the veins or heart following death during or after a surgical operation.[47]

Reminding his colleagues of Amussat's initial claims of July 1837 and the partially skeptical response of some members, Bouillaud recalled that "since the truth did not burst forth clearly enough from the clash of these opinions to carry the conviction of the Academy, a member proposed to send the question back to its natural judge, that is experimentation, and to name a commission to witness the new experiments made by M. Amussat." The question at hand was very serious in itself, he said, but "after having been agitated in the heart of the Academy, it presents a still more imposing character, and has, if I dare say so, acquired more grandeur and dignity."[48]

Having disposed of preliminaries, Bouillaud turned to the second part of his report. The commission had carried out forty experiments, twenty-nine of these on dogs, the rest on horses and a mule. In doing so it had attempted to adhere to rules that it took to govern physiological experimentation. Quoting Albrecht Haller, Bouillaud stressed the experimenter's need to set aside preconceptions, to draw conclusions only on the basis of experiments repeated many times with constant result, and to vary experimental conditions. Variations were of several kinds. The commissioners opened different veins in the upper chest. Sometimes they maintained the surrounding parts in their normal state; sometimes they arranged them such that the walls of the opened vessels were more favorably disposed for the introduction of air. They followed experiments on the spontaneous introduction of air with those in which air was introduced by injection with a syringe or insufflation. Some experimental animals were weakened by preliminary bleeding or previous experiments in order to approximate the conditions of a surgical operation, whereas others were not. Some were operated upon while in a horizontal position, others while vertical, again better to approximate the conditions of the parallel surgical procedures in humans.[49]

The commission gave a separate numbered description of each experiment and arranged these analytically so as to display the major subdivisions of the problem and the systematic variation of experimental conditions. It subdivided the first series, on dogs, into four categories, the first on the spontaneous introduction of air, the second on introduction by sounds or artificial injection, a third on introduction by insufflation, and a fourth on attempts to remedy the effects of these measures. The second series on horses and a mule they similarly subdivided into experiments on the spontaneous introduction of air and those on insufflation. The commission fitted its descriptions to a consistent format: number, date (sometimes missing), kind and approximate size of animal, time of start of experiment, and description of observations and procedures including times of the most important ones, autopsy.[50]

Finally Bouillaud turned to the commission's conclusions, which he called "a reasoned exposition of the principal results furnished by the preceding experiments," and which he presented in five articles. The first article treated the mechanism of the so-called spontaneous introduction of air into the veins and its signs. The commission had found that whenever a jugular vein is opened to a sufficient extent in its inferior portion where, when the veins are laid bare, a phenomenon of flux and reflux isochronous with respiration is observed, atmospheric air is soon introduced through this opening and penetrates the right cavities of the heart. The sign of this, Bouillaud continued, is a particular sound which in dogs exactly resembles the sound of lapping, and in horses the sound of gargling or gurgling. The principal cause of the introduction of air is evidently inspiration [sic] which is isochronous with the sound.[51] A contributing cause is the systole and diastole of the right cavities of the heart. Another sign of the introduction of air is the sound of bellows (or breath: both *soufflet* and *souffle* are used here) with or without gargling which occurs in the right heart. This sound persists long after the introduction of air has ceased and is isochronous with movements of the heart and with inspiration and expiration. Bouillaud remarked that although other physiologists, including Poiseuille, had studied these phenomena, "Amussat was the first to show in the most precise, and in a sense the most mathematical way this fact, namely, *that in the cases in which one makes a sufficiently large opening in the jugular veins where the movement of flux and reflux is visible, air is always introduced into the vascular system.*" Moreover, Bouillaud concluded, "this proposition, so formulated, is a truth, I almost said a *physiological law,* henceforth acquired by science."[52]

Autopsies of dogs and horses in which air had spontaneously entered a vein revealed the presence of air in the form of frothy blood in the right heart and pulmonary artery. The commissioners rarely found air in the left heart or arteries of dogs opened immediately after the experiment. They did find, though, that dogs that survived from four to ten days generally had bubbles in the left heart and blood system. Horses almost always had air in the left heart and blood system regardless of time elapsed between introduction of the air and autopsy. From these observations, reported in the second article, the commission concluded that after a time air makes its way from the right heart via the pulmonary artery to the left heart and blood system.[53]

In a third article Bouillaud turned to the effects of introduction of air, in particular to those that often resulted in death. Approaching the experiments with the prior assertions of Amussat and other surgeons and physiologists in mind, the commission had expected to see sudden, instantaneous death. "What was our surprise," Bouillaud reported, "and if I dare say it, our *disappointment*, when we saw most dogs aspirate air in long draughts for several minutes, not only without dying but also without truly serious accidents." In place of this drama the commission found that in all dogs, within one to ten minutes respiration and circulation became difficult and more frequent, strength diminished, and signs of anxiety and agitation increased. If the experiment was stopped, some animals improved and recovered. If it was continued indefinitely these symptoms would intensify and the animal would die with a rapidity that varied with circumstances such as the size, species, and strength of the animal, the position in which it was placed, its previous state of health, the qualities and quantity of the introduced air, and the speed of introduction.

The commission concluded that, other things being equal, death occurred more promptly in dogs placed in a vertical position than in those placed in a horizontal position, perhaps because the former favored entry of air into the cerebral venous system. In both positions, the report added, death occurred more promptly in animals previously weakened or ill. Findings for horses were similar, with the important difference that time of death was much less variable. When the experimenter blew air into the blood vessels through a sound or tube, the animals died much more quickly than in cases of "spontaneous" introduction, a fact that Bouillaud tentatively attributed to the attenuated quality of expired air.[54]

Weighing its evidence, the commission settled on three principal causes of death. First in order and importance was the enormous distension of the right cavities of the heart by air dilated by the heat of the blood, which blocked the heart's regular function. Second was the presence of air in the pulmonary artery and its ramifications, which gave the blood a viscosity and spumescence that opposed its free movement in the pulmonary capillaries. Finally, the commission adopted Nysten's view that air reaching the veins of the brain would exert a compression, and perhaps other chemical or physical actions, that could contribute to death.[55]

On the point that Amussat had considered most important—namely, the means by which the introduction of air could be prevented, or remedied once it had taken place—Bouillaud had surprisingly little to report, and none of his findings was conclusive. Compression bandages on a dog's chest (Gerdy's suggestion) had not notably hindered the entry of air into the jugular vein, whether the dog was in a horizontal or a vertical position. The commission found that a sudden compression of the chest and abdomen could induce a certain quantity of blood mixed with air to leave an open vein, and that by using a syringe they could aspirate blood mixed with air. The experiments were inconclusive, however, because in these cases the subjects might have recovered anyway. Bouillaud had to end the brief fourth article by admitting that the prophylactics and therapeutics of the spontaneous introduction of air into the veins required new experiments.[56]

In the report's fifth and final article Bouillaud affirmed the applicability of the commission's experiments to man, and that there was no doubt that air could enter the veins during surgical operations. The same experiments showed, however, that the rapidity of death reported in clinical cases could not be solely a result of introduced air, given that animals typically survived for longer times or even indefinitely. Exhaustion, blood loss, and pain were among the possible contributing causes of death that Bouillaud thought might account for the difference.[57]

"Whether because of the results of the numerous experiments that he has done in the presence of the commission," Bouillaud concluded, "or because of the indefatigable zeal of which he has given evidence, our colleague M. Amussat appears to us very deserving of the gratitude of science and of the Academy, and we propose to this company to express to him, through its president, its thanks and high satisfaction." On this positive if vague note Bouillaud closed his report, noting also that the commission had done its best but wished that it had done better.[58]

Bouillaud's vagueness in praise of Amussat was well considered. For the discussion that followed the reading of the report revealed a surprising lack of consensus within the commission itself on the novelty, conclusiveness, and significance of Amussat's experiments and assertions. Velpeau and Barthélemy felt that Amussat's experiments were largely repetitive of earlier work. Velpeau and Gerdy conceded that the experiments made it very probable that surgical patients might die by the introduction of air, but neither believed that there was a single clinical case in which this had been positively proved. Gerdy listed thirteen ways in which the commissions's experiments were misleading or inconclusive for lack of rigor, exactitude, or precision, or because they were not properly interpreted. He even suspected that Amussat's presence in the commission had inhibited the reporter. Barthélemy rejected the commission's finding that a principal cause of death was distension of the right heart, and described his own experiments on horses in which he had measured the quantities of introduced air, a procedure the commission had neglected. Velpeau felt that although the whole debate lacked firm conclusions, it had served a very useful educative function in diffusing awareness of the problem and of the need for further research.[59]

Although annoyed by the revolt of his fellow commissioners, Bouillaud replied with calm and humor, defending the novelty of the commission's findings. He pointed out that even its critics had not directly attacked its fundamental conclusions, and that its report had been unanimously adopted. On 13 February 1838 the academy, having heard Bouillaud's last word, voted to adopt the commission's recommendation and to thank Amussat.[60]

IV

Together the two debates described here provide a window on the role and status of experimentalism in the Academy of Medicine. Most obviously they show that the academy embraced experimental science, gave it a respected role in the investigation of medical questions, and appealed to it on occasion as the authority of last resort. The academy saw itself as working within a tradition of physiological experiment that stretched from Harvey through Haller to Bichat, Nysten, Poiseuille, and Magendie. Although Magendie's primary institutional affiliations lay elsewhere and he did not participate directly in the academy's affairs, he was a member whose presence was felt even *in absentia,* and Academicians often referred to him as a model and authority.[61]

As Pariset had foreseen, the academy's adoption of animal experiment as method was reinforced and enhanced by its inclusion of veterinarians as medical professionals. Veterinarian members of the academy spoke with the same scientific and medical authority as their medical and surgical colleagues. Veterinary experience entered into the academy's debates with an ease and a naturalness that belie any sense of discomfort or condescension toward animal medicine on the academy's part. That experience took several forms. Veterinarians such as Dupuy, Barthélemy, or Jean Bouley reported observations from their own clinical practices that promised to illuminate human physiology or medicine. Amussat held up the veterinarians' use of animal experiment in professional training as a model for surgeons, and argued that the last step in surgical education should be practice on animals. In at least one instance, where he considered methods of hemostasis for small wounds in the skin, Amussat cited veterinary practice as a model for human practice. Most important in the present context, the domestic animals with which veterinarians were most familiar were also among the experimental animals most frequently used by the Academicians. Horses figure prominently in the experiments of the commission judging Amussat's work and in those reported by several of the veterinarians.[62]

The debates show that many of the principles of what Claude Bernard would later describe as experimental medicine were already in gestation within the academy in the 1830s, while Bernard was still a medical student. Most striking is the general—though not unanimous—acknowledgment by participants of what Bernard would later defend as the central tenet of experimental determinism: that biological processes are regular and consistent in their behavior, and that inconsistencies in results are to be traced to differences of experimental conditions or procedure. This view came closest to explicit formulation in the debate on the entry of air into the chest in the operation for empyema, when Cruveilhier had said that "facts are contradictory only when they comprise different elements not yet perceived," and "when two contradictory facts are advanced by different observers, there is necessarily an error on one side or the other; because nature cannot contradict itself."

Piorry, Cruveilhier's opponent, had also sought to resolve the apparent contradictions by fresh experiments, thinking that "there must be some cause of this difference in results that escaped us." The principle of experimental determinism was also implicit in the commission's report on Amussat, in which the language of "spontaneous" introduction of air into the veins was rejected in favor of a rigorous specification of the experimental conditions necessary and sufficient for the phenomenon to take place. When one of the commissioners, Gerdy, directly challenged the capacity of animal experiments to yield consistent results, he was answered by the commission's reporter, Bouillaud, who affirmed that apparent contradiction proved only that "the facts do not resemble one another, and that it is necessary to divide them into categories, otherwise we risk confusing everything and drawing false conclusions."[63]

Bernard's principles were approximated in other, subsidiary ways by the statements and actions of the academy's experimenters. They affirmed the need to repeat experiments and to systematically vary experimental conditions.[64] They adopted an empiricist posture that stressed observed fact as the starting point of investigation and the need to set aside preconceptions in the face of experimental findings.[65] They insisted on manual practice as an essential quality of the experimenter's art.[66] In the face of colleagues' persistent doubts, they repeatedly stated their belief in the applicability of the results of animal experiments to man.[67] They defended the morality of animal experiment in the name of the advancement of medical science and the conservation of human life.[68] They alluded to chemical findings, recognized the need to apply the quantitative spirit of chemistry in physiology and medicine, and generally held up as an ideal the qualities of rigor, exactness, and precision.[69]

For all that, the debates show with equal clarity that the academy— by intention or circumstance—placed material, organizational, and intellectual limits on experimentalism that were never transcended in the period under consideration. The material constraints were painfully obvious. Cramped quarters and a restricted budget precluded the allotment of space on the academy's premises for laboratories or experimental work. The commissioners judging Amussat's research complained of the lack of needed laboratory instruments. Amussat himself complained of the lack of an amphitheater for experiments at either the academy or the Faculty of Medicine. In lieu of such facilities Academicians turned to private laboratories, to the Faculty's École Pratique, or to the veterinary school at Alfort.[70]

Less obvious but also constraining was the lack of organizational maturity reflected in the academy's procedures for judging experimental investigations. Pariset had anticipated, and Academicians clearly recognized, the value of the academy as a forum. In the academy's debates medical questions—including those subject to experimental study—were clarified, might be resolved, and in any case might be imprinted on the consciousness of physicians. In practice the mechanisms did not always function so smoothly, a fact particularly evident in the second debate. Members quarreled over whether Amussat should be allowed to present new results before

the commission had reported on his initial claims, eventually decid-
ing that he should not. Despite the commission's attempt to follow a
rigorous and consistent format for reporting experiments, some of
its descriptions lack dates, times, or other particulars. Most seriously, the commission was unable to enforce discipline within its
own ranks, and the discussion that followed the initial report threatened to rob it of any force. After listening patiently but with growing
irritation to criticisms of his report by Gerdy, Blandin, and Velpeau—all fellow commissioners—Bouillaud finally rose to interrupt
yet another critique from Barthélemy, also a commissioner. Pointing
out that his report was based on the *procès-verbaux* of the commission
and had been prepared in the presence of the commissioners, Bouillaud maintained that it was not the place of members of the commission to attack it. Other Academicians objected to Bouillaud's interruption of free discussion, and the issue was resolved only by ad-
journment. At a subsequent meeting Dubois d'Amiens echoed Bouillaud's complaint and asked the majority who approved the report to
defend it and the minority who disapproved to withdraw from debate. In a lame effort to head off further conflict, Dubois d'Amiens
also suggested that the academy need not bring the report to a vote,
since a scientific investigator found his greatest reward in himself
and had no need of an academic decision. None of this was to any
avail, however, and the debate among the commissioners rumbled
on. A week after Dubois d'Amiens' remarks Rochoux protested in
vain that everyone was venting his own opinion as if the report did
not exist, which was a reversal of all academic usages.[71]

Least tangible but most significant were the methodological, conceptual, and programmatic limitations placed on experimentalism in
the Academy of Medicine. Despite their undoubted approach to
what Claude Bernard would later describe as the principles of experimental medicine, the academy's experimenters often fell woefully
short in practice. Not only were experiments not always repeated,
but often sweeping conclusions were drawn on the basis of one or a
handful of trials. Experiments that were done were not always well
described, as in Amussat's memoir on traumatic hemorrhage, where
the accounts were sparse and vague. Although the commission reporting on Amussat's work fully recognized the need for quantitative measurements of the air introduced into blood vessels, they had
to admit that the lack of such measurements was a major weakness
of their report. Academicians' formulations of the principles them-

selves were occasionally simplistic or confused, as when they failed
explicitly to recognize a role for hypothesis in investigation, or when
Amussat refused to recognize a constructive role for negative or
unexpected experimental results.[72]

Always in the background, and occasionally very much in the
foreground, were nagging doubts about the reliability of animal experiments and their applicability to man. In a passage comparable to
one in Niels Bohr's famous 1932 lecture entitled "Light and Life,"
Pariset had suggested that life itself imposed limits on experimental
investigation. "There are in the humors," he said, "conditions which
depend on life, and that undoubtedly the art of man will never be
able to grasp: because as soon as man intervenes, as soon as he puts
his hand on the object he wishes to know, the object dies; its interior
connections are broken, its intimate nature changes; henceforth it is
no more than a cadaver, that is, the contrary of what it was."[73]
Amussat noted that "prejudices of all kinds" still existed against
animal experiment as a research method, and the commissioners
judging his work conceded that "we are aware with what circum-
spection we must proceed when it is a matter in general of drawing
conclusions on what happens in man from what happens in animals."[74] The Academician Louis Castel voiced a reservation of a
different sort when, speaking as representative of a discursive
vitalism not yet deceased, he hoped that the commission's "conclu-
sioncules" or small conclusions based on observation and experiment might be replaced with reflection on "the highest regions of
physiology and the analysis of life."[75]

No one pushed his doubts about animal experiment further than
Gerdy, who was at once member and critic of the commission judging Amussat's work. Noting that the issues remained in part unresolved, Gerdy ventured that "experiments undertaken to confirm
the introduction of air into the veins have been and will always be
very variable in their results." Elsewhere he elevated this variability
into a general principle, stating that "vivisections do not always give
the same result to different experimenters." Behind these remarks
lay a vitalism that would pose a direct challenge to the notion of
experimental determinism, though Gerdy was not explicit on the
point in this context. Provoked by Amussat's reference to his
"known antipathy to experimentation," however, Gerdy did make
known his resentment of the dominance of experiment in contemporary physiology. Quoting his own textbook, he told his colleagues

that since around 1800 physiology had relied exclusively on experimentation. His own confidence in this method was, he said, limited:
"critical and not fanatical." He had therefore resolved to use experiment, but only when other means—which he did not specify—
proved inadequate. This methodological pluralism had, he admitted, drawn upon him the accusations of the intolerant. "And how
could it be otherwise," he lamented, when the Academy of Science,
"so rich in celebrated men of all kinds, but in which mathematicians,
physicists, chemists, etc., are much more numerous than physiologists, lends a considerable and almost exclusive support to the
method of vivisections?" In Gerdy's view it was now incumbent
upon the Academy of Medicine to reassert its proper authority. "It is
for you, gentlemen," he told his colleagues, "that it belongs to take
possession of physiology, because it is much more within your competence than in that of the Academy of Science. It is for you to
exercise a legitimate influence on the study of physiology and on the
methods destined to advance its progress." Since Amussat had
raised the subject, Gerdy concluded, "far from rejecting your jurisdiction, I make haste to recognize its legitimacy, and I ask that you
one day establish a discussion on the utility of vivisections or experiments on living animals in the study of the medical sciences."[76]

Gerdy got his discussion, and he did not have to wait long. In
January 1839 the academy began a debate on the status of recent
discoveries on the nervous system and on the methods used to
acquire them, an exchange of opinions that one of its participants
termed a "trial brought by M. Gerdy against experimental physiology."[77] Argument began in the context of the academy's consideration of a report by Bouillaud on a memoir by a Dr. Belhomme.
Belhomme's subject was vertigo (turnsick, or staggers, *le tournis*) in
animals and humans, which he compared to the affection resulting
from lesions of the cerebellum and its peduncles.[78] Belhomme reported several clinical cases in humans in which involuntary turning
behavior was associated with pathological alterations of the brain
observed at autopsy. He compared his findings with certain of
Magendie's experiments, concluding that his observations and Magendie's experiments agreed perfectly in their finding that disorders
of posture or position and of locomotion are under the influence of
the cerebellum and its peduncles. In a largely favorable report
Bouillaud emphasized the harmony of pathology and experiment
and commented that despite the great progress made recently in the

localization of functions in the great nervous centers, much remained unknown.

Here Gerdy saw—or made—his opportunity. He attacked both
Bouillaud's characterization of recent progress in the physiology of
the nervous system and his confidence in animal experiment as a
means to that end. In a debate extending over several months Gerdy
argued that little progress had yet been made in knowledge of functions of the nervous centers. Even the supposedly signal achievement
of the field—the differentiation of the spinal nerve roots into sensory
(posterior) and motor (anterior)—could not be cited as a firm result of
experiment because it was not clear what, if anything, had been established. Indeed, Gerdy doubted whether anything substantial had
been learned from experiments on the nervous system. He pointed to
frequent disagreements among experimenters, even when they ostensibly performed the same experiments. He claimed that during the
fifteen or twenty years that he had been "very seriously" engaged in
physiological research he had used animal experiment, but had been
disillusioned by the "inconstancy and obscurity of the results." He
had been embarrassed in his teaching of experimental physiology.
"Before beginning the experiment," he recalled, "I announced a result; I placed myself under obligation to produce it, and often enough
the animal made me a liar in the presence of my audience." Gerdy
denied total opposition to experimental method, citing toxicology as a
field that he considered to owe much of its recent progress to experiment. But in his view that method could not have the same weight in
physiology that it did in physics and chemistry. The recent excessive
preoccupation of physiologists with animal experiments and their
uncertain results was, Gerdy lamented, "not the history of nature, it
is the poetry of science." Neither could comparative anatomy and
physiology serve as reliable guides to human faculties and functions,
Gerdy maintained.[79]

By what means was physiology to be advanced, then? Gerdy
admitted that pathology and anatomy had their uses in the study of
normal function. He gave pride of place, however, to an alternative
method that he termed "complex, analytical, and logical." To judge
by the examples he used to illustrate it, this consisted mainly in
reflection on complex physiological phenomena accessible to observation in an effort mentally to resolve them into their components. It
did not involve intervention in or interrogation (Gerdy's word) of
the phenomena in the manner of animal experiment.[80]

In one sense at least, Gerdy got his way. Implicit in the whole debate on the distinction of motor and sensory nerves, and explicit in remarks by Gerdy and Blandin, was recognition of the authority of the Academy of Medicine to judge questions of physiology.[81]

In other ways Gerdy felt himself to be, and was, in a minority. Castel declared himself in Gerdy's camp but with a blanket and ill-informed condemnation of animal experiment that did little justice to his colleague's more nuanced arguments. Apart from this ally *manqué*, other participants in this debate, as in the two debates described earlier, did not hestitate to grant a privileged place to experimental findings. Bouillaud flatly affirmed animal experiment to be the primary authority in physiology. Not only had it "taught us almost everything that we know," he argued, but it had also provided useful guidance for practice. His examples came from studies of the nervous system.[82] While admitting that the experimental method could be abused, like any other, Rochoux pointed out that it was so far beyond attack that Gerdy himself had used it to criticize Charles Bell and Magendie.[83] Blandin conceded that animal experiments were laborious and their results often complex and difficult to analyze. In his view they had to be joined to clinical observation and anatomy in order to compel assent. Yet for Blandin the distinction of motor and sensory nerves was the result which "incomparably [had] been derived from the most numerous and ably executed experiments."[84]

In justifying the academy's authority to decide on the distinction of motor and sensory nerves, Blandin had said that "the practice of our art is almost as much interested in [the question] as is physiology." Indeed, the clinical dimension of the problem was never entirely set aside, and for these Academicians the importance of physiology was ultimately grounded in its promise of service to pathology and therapeutics.[85] What they shared with Gerdy and what placed limits on their experimentalism was a peculiarly medical vision of physiology that tended to subordinate knowledge of natural processes to therapeutic goals. The central problems of the debates on the operation for empyema and on the entry of air into the veins had a properly physiological dimension in that they sought to achieve objective knowledge of the behavior of the organism under specified conditions. On occasion participants explicitly recognized this goal—Bouillaud, for example, formulating a version of Amussat's assertions as a "physiological law."[86] Yet each investigation had its origins in a problem of medical practice, and the primary goal of each debate was to arrive at a result useful to therapeutics. Discussants repeatedly affirmed the clinical importance of the questions at issue and often called upon clinical experience for evidence or illustration.[87] The uses envisaged for experimental physiology tended to slide into the practical, as in Amussat's eloquent appeals for the use of animal experiment in the training of surgeons and in the improvement of surgical technique.[88] On the whole the debates reflect the academy's view that "practical medicine must occupy the first and largest place among the medical sciences."[89]

Erwin H. Ackerknecht has written that the founding of the Société de Biologie in 1848 "objectively ended the era of exclusive clinicism" in Parisian medicine.[90] The present study indicates that although hospital practice remained central to Parisian medicine through midcentury, there was never a time when clinical concerns held exclusive sway over Parisian doctors. At the heart of the Paris clinical school, among the membership of the Academy of Medicine, the professors of the Faculty of Medicine, and staff physicians of the hospitals, serious science was done and duly gained the recognition of the scientific community. The academy, the "Senate of Medicine" in Paul Ganière's phrase, embodied in its founding statutes, organization, stated goals, publications, and debates a commitment to the cultivation of the sciences related to medicine. Experimental physiology and pharmaceutical chemistry in particular gained respect and a significant role in medical discussion.

The Academy of Medicine, in a word, sought to incorporate experimental science. Incorporation was double-edged, however, because in bringing experimentalism into the academy its members tended to subordinate it to properly medical goals and sought to bring it within the intellectual and institutional jurisdiction of medicine. Implicit in Pariset's inaugural address, and explicit in Gerdy's remarks, is the view that physiology is not only a science that happens to be relevant to medicine but one that is rightly a part of medicine and in some sense subject to its corporate authority. If there was a failure in Parisian doctors' attitudes toward experimental science, then, it was not that they rejected it in favor of pathological anatomy or an ontological concept of disease but that they embraced it in such a way as to tie it too immediately and directly to clinical preoccupations.

In the 1830s and 1840s a few Academicians, among them Pierre Rayer and Charles Robin, began to evolve an ideal of a scientific medicine founded on biology. In so doing they reasserted the priority of scientific over immediately practical goals in medical science, and in this sense their program, which became that of the Société de Biologie, broke with the prevailing emphasis in the Academy of Medicine. Underlying this shift of emphasis, however, was a deeper continuity that linked the new society to more than two decades of thought and action in its parent institution. Far from being a sharp break with the past, the Société de Biologie gave separate institutional expression to a scientific tendency long present in Parisian medicine.

NOTES

Special thanks go to John Parascandola and the staff of the Historical Division of the National Library of Medicine, the Lane Medical Library of Stanford University, and the History Library of the University of California, San Francisco, for their assistance in the research for this chapter. I am also indebted to Paula Fass, Frederic L. Holmes, and three anonymous referees for the University of California Press for their comments on an earlier version.

1. Erwin H. Ackerknecht, *A Short History of Medicine*, rev. ed. (Baltimore and London: Johns Hopkins University Press, 1982), p. 70; Ludwig Edelstein, *Ancient Medicine* (Baltimore: Johns Hopkins University Press, 1967), pp. 173–191, 195–203.

2. Robert G. Frank, Jr., "The Image of Harvey in Commonwealth and Restoration England," *William Harvey and His Age*, ed. Jerome Bylebyl (Baltimore and London: Johns Hopkins University Press, 1979), pp. 103–143.

3. See, for example, Robert E. Kohler, "Medical Reform and Biomedical Science: Biochemistry—A Case Study" in *The Therapeutic Revolution: Essays in the Social History of American Medicine*, ed. Morris J. Vogel and Charles E. Rosenberg (Philadelphia: University of Pennsylvania Press, 1979), pp. 27–66; Gerald L. Geison, "Divided We Stand: Physiologists and Clinicians in the American Context" in ibid., pp. 67–90; and Russell C. Maulitz, " 'Physician versus Bacteriologist'; The Ideology of Science in Clinical Medicine" in ibid., pp. 91–107.

4. Erwin H. Ackerknecht, *Medicine at the Paris Hospital 1794–1848* (Baltimore: Johns Hopkins University Press, 1967), esp. pp. 121–127.

5. John E. Lesch, *Science and Medicine in France: The Emergence of Experimental Physiology, 1790–1855* (Cambridge, Mass., and London: Harvard University Press, 1984).

6. "Ordonnances relatives à l'Académie royale de médecine," Académie de Médecine, Paris *Mémoires* (hereafter *AMPM*) 1 (1828): 1–28; Paul Ganière, "Le baron Antoine Portal, Président perpétuel de l'Académie Royale de Médecine," Académie Nationale de Médecine *Bulletin* 150 (1966):

539–545. Portal had served as president of an earlier version of the Academy of Medicine that had failed because of limited membership and lack of official backing. See A. Corlieu, *Centenaire de la Faculté de médecine de Paris (1794–1894)* (Paris, 1896), pp. 552–553.

7. "Ordonnances," pp. 1–6; Etienne Pariset, "Discours prononcé par le secrétaire perpétuel, dans le séance inaugurale, le 6 mai 1824," *AMPM* 1 (1828): 57–106 (see pp. 65–69); Paul Ganière, "Les origines de l'Académie de Médecine," Académie Nationale de Médecine, Paris *Bulletin* 148 (1964): 44–49 (see p. 45). See also "Prospectus," Académie de Médecine, Paris *Bulletin* (hereafter *AMPB*) 1 (1836): 5–8.

8. Corlieu, *Centenaire*, p. 552; Paul Ganière, *L'Académie de médecine: ses origines et son historie* (Paris: Librairie Maloine, 1964), pp. 80–81; Ganière, "Les origines," p. 47. Pariset makes the political parallels explicit. See "Discours," pp. 67–69.

9. At its inception the academy was composed of sixty honorary members, eighty-five titular members, of which five were veterinarians, and three classes of associates: thirty *associés libres;* eighty *associés ordinaires,* of whom twenty lived in Paris; and thirty foreign associates. The 1829 ordinance reduced these numbers to sixty titular members, forty adjuncts, forty nonresident associates, ten *associés libres,* and twenty foreign associates. The reduction was effected by electing one new member for each three losses by death or resignation. "Ordonnances"; "Rapport au Roi sur l'Académie Royale de Médecine," *AMPM* 2 (1833): 61–75; Corlieu, *Centenaire,* pp. 553–554; Ganière, *L'Académie de médecine,* pp. 77–80, 84–85; Maurice Genty, *Index biographique des membres, des associés, et des correspondants de l'Académie de médecine de 1820 à 1970* (Paris: Doin, 1972), pp. vi–vii, x–xi.

10. Ackerknecht, *Medicine at the Paris Hospital pp. 26–27;* "Ordonnances," *pp. 1–4, 15, 26–27;* "Rapport au Roi," *pp. 73–74.*

11. "Rapport au Roi," p. 61; Corlieu, *Centenaire,* p. 554.

12. "Prospectus," *AMPB* 1 (1836); 5–8.

13. Ganière, *L'Académie de médecine,* pp. 83, 87–92, 94; idem, "Les origines," pp. 47–49; "Rapport au Roi," p. 62.

14. Ganière, *L'Académie de médecine,* pp. 82–85; idem, "Antoine Portal," p. 544; Ackerknecht, *Medicine at the Paris Hospital,* p. 116; Etienne Pariset, "Discours prononcé par le secrétaire perpétuel, dans le séance inaugurale, le 6 mai 1824," *AMPM* 1 (1828): 57–106. For a list of the functions of the permanant secretary, see "Rapport au Roi," pp. 66, 71–73.

15. Pariset, "Discours," pp. 57–69, 85–86.

16. Ibid., pp. 72–73.

17. Ibid.

18. Ibid., pp. 74–75. On the connections between therapeutic skepticism, pharmacy, and chemistry, see Lesch, *Science and Medicine in France,* pp. 125–165.

19. Pariset, "Discours," pp. 89–93, 95. On the nervous system and pathological physiology in the 1820s, see Lesch, *Science and Medicine in France,* pp. 166–196.

20. Pariset, "Discours," pp. 72–73, 89–93.

21. Ibid., pp. 86–89, 101–102.

22. For purposes of this study original members of the Academy of Medicine are those listed as honorary or titular members of the sections of medicine, surgery, or pharmacy; resident associates; resident adjuncts of the sections of medicine, surgery, or pharmacy; and deceased members who fell into one of the preceding categories before their deaths. Not included are *associés libres, associés ordinaires non résidents, associés étrangers,* or *adjoints correspondants.* Note that dates of nomination for these original members range from 27 December 1820 (when the king named the first members) to 31 January 1826. *AMPM* 1 (1828): 29–56.

Membership in the Academy of Science was determined by consulting the Institut de France, *Index biographique des membres et correspondants de l'Académie des sciences de 1666 à 1939* (Paris: Gauthier-Villars, 1939); Maurice Genty, *Index biographique;* and Corlieu, *Centenaire,* pp. 576–595.

After 1835 all members of the Academy of Medicine were assigned the same rank. Before that date promotion could occur—for example, from resident associate to titular member of a section. Therefore some of those found in the aforementioned figures for original members also appear in the figures for promotions. Promotions and new members for this period are listed in Genty, *Index biographique,* pp. 197–221.

For a list of members of the Academy of Medicine in 1849, see *AMPM* 14 (1849): v–vii.

23. Corlieu, *Centenaire,* pp. 224–225, 235, 246, 261, 269, 278, 285, 293, 299, 308, 323, 331, 345, 349, 355, 364, 369, 374, 393–394, 439–440, 454–455, 575–595; Genty, *Index biographique;* Institut de France, *Index biographique; AMPM* 14 (1849): v–vii.

24. On the founding of specialized societies, see Ackerknecht, *Medicine at the Paris Hospital,* p. 116. On the program and original membership of the Société de Biologie, see Lesch, *Science and Medicine in France,* pp. 222–224; and Frederic Lawrence Holmes, *Claude Bernard and Animal Chemistry* (Cambridge, Mass.: Harvard University Press, 1974), pp. 401–402. Sources for the figures given here are Société de Biologie, Paris, *Comptes rendus des séances et mémoires* 2 (1850): ix–xi; *AMPM* 14 (1849): v–vii; Genty, *Index biographique;* Institut de France, *Index biographique;* and Corlieu, *Centenaire,* pp. 576–595.

25. *AMPM* 1 (1828): 27–28.

26. *AMPB* 9 (1843–1844): 268–292.

27. *AMPM* 3 (1833): 44.

28. *AMPM* 5 (1836): 84.

29. *AMPB* 12 (1846–1847): 187.

30. Categories were defined by me but in every case would have been recognizable to contemporary physicians. As would be the case with any categorization, they involve some overlap. Pathology, as used here, includes pathological anatomy, reports of clinical observations, and, in general, any description of disease. Some disease descriptions, however, are grouped here under psychiatry or public health. Therapeutics comprises articles mainly devoted to treatment, but memoirs including discussion of treatment are also grouped under pathology, surgery, or pharmacy. Both

definition of categories and assignment of memoirs to them could be slightly different, but I do not believe that these differences would have a significant effect on the overall results.

31. René Prus, "Mémoire sur les deux maladies connus sous le nom d'apoplexie méningée," *AMPM* 11 (1845): 18–81; and Hippolyte Larrey, "Mémoire sur les plaies pénétrantes de l'abdomen compliquées d'issue de l'epiploon," ibid., pp. 664–682.

32. See *AMPM* 1 (1828): 259–316, 371–393, 417–439, 440–449; 3 (1833): 1–13, 46–62, 63–68, 340–349; 4 (1835): 298–307, 308–323; 5 (1836): 41–63, 68–90, 212–220; 6 (1837): 605–624; 8 (1840): 375–567, 676–696; 9 (1841): 1–56, 57–71, 234–275; 10 (1843): 206–222, 722–745; 11 (1845): 608–663; 12 (1846): 1–151, 604–648; 13 (1847): 36–486; 14 (1849): 408–500.

33. "Exposé sommaire d'expériences faites sur les animaux dans le but de constater si la sécrétion urinaire est suprimée dans l'empoisonnement par l'acide arsénieux," *AMPM* 11 (1845): 608–663.

34. "Rechercher les cas dans lesquels on observe les abcesses multiples et comparer ces cas sous leurs différents rapports," *AMPM* 12 (1846): 1–151.

35. *AMPB* 1 (1836–1837): 62–67, 120–126, 138–148, 159–160.

36. Ibid., pp. 138–148, 164–169, 180–191.

37. Ibid. pp. 183–186.

38. Ibid., pp. 280–284, 397–400.

39. J. Z. Amussat, "Nouvelles recherches expérimentales sur les hemorrhagies traumatiques, suivies de quelques considerations sur l'importance des vivisections pour former les chirurgiens operateurs," *AMPM* 5 (1836): 68–90.

40. *AMPB* 1 (1836–1837): 894–897.

41. Ibid.

42. Ibid.

43. Ibid., pp. 899–901.

44. Ibid., pp. 901–909.

45. *AMPB* 2 (1837–1838): 182–254.

46. Ibid., pp. 182–183.

47. Ibid., pp. 183–204.

48. Ibid., pp. 205–206.

49. Ibid., pp. 206–207.

50. Ibid., pp. 208–239.

51. Bouillaud here inadvertently substitutes "inspiration" for "expiration." See his comment on Poiseuille's findings, discussed earlier in this chapter, and note 32.

52. *AMPB* 2 (1837–1838): 239–241. Bouillaud's emphasis.

53. Ibid., pp. 242–244.

54. Ibid., pp. 244–248.

55. Ibid., pp. 249–250.

56. Ibid., pp. 250–251.

57. Ibid., pp. 251–253.

58. Ibid., pp. 253–254.

59. Ibid., pp. 280–294, 305–314, 363–382, 418–430, 454–481.

60. Ibid., p. 481. The debate continued sporadically at long intervals for several years, without reaching more definitive conclusions. See, e.g., *AMPB* 3 (1838–1839): 465–471, 934–942; 6 (1840–1841): 178–186; 9 (1843–1844): 416–417.

61. For references to Magendie, see, e.g., *AMPM* 5 (1836): 68–69, 81–82; *AMPB* 1 (1836–1837): 894–897, 899–901; *AMPB* 2 (1837–1838): 197–199, 270.

62. See descriptions of the debates cited earlier and *AMPM* 5 (1836): 78, 86–90; *AMPB* 1 (1836–1837): 894–897, 903–904, 922–923; *AMPB* 2 (1837–1838): 182–254 passim, 269, 278–280, 368–382, 457; *AMPB* 3 (1838–1839): 465–471; *AMPB* 6 (1840–1841): 178–186, 1029–1030.

63. *AMPB* 1 (1836–1837): 168, 180–181, 185–186, 280–284; *AMPB* 2 (1837–1838): 182–254 passim; *AMPB* 3 (1838–1839): 471. Compare Frédéric Dubois d'Amiens' remarks on experimental method in a subsequent debate on the motor and sensory nerves, in *AMPB* 3 (1838–1839): 793, 823–830.

64. See, e.g., *AMPB* 2 (1837–1839): 206–207.

65. See, ibid., pp. 206–207, 249–250, 466 (note 1).

66. *AMPM* 5 (1836): 83, 86–90; *AMPB* 2 (1837–1838): 278–279.

67. *AMPM* 5 (1836): 68–69; *AMPB* 2 (1837–1838): 251–253, 422, 425–430.

68. *AMPM* 5 (1836): 69–70, 86–90. See also Pariset's remarks in his "Discours" of 1824, pp. 89–93.

69. See, e.g., *AMPB* 2 (1837–1838): 184, 239–241, 280–294, 377–381.

70. See earlier in this chapter and *AMPB* 1 (1836–1837): 899–901; 2 (1837–1838): 245 (note 1), 457, 469.

71. *AMPB* 2 (1837–1838): 35, 42–43, 55, 182–254 passim, 371, 404–410, 425, 461–481.

72. *AMPM* 5 (1836): 72–73, 78, 81–82; *AMPB* 2 (1837–1838): 245 (note 1), 249–250, 253 (note 1), 295–296, 466 (note 1).

73. Pariset, "Discours," p. 87. For an English text of Bohr's lecture, see *Nature* 131 (1933): 421–423, 457–459.

74. *AMPM* 5 (1836): 68–69; *AMPB* 2 (1837 1838): 251–253.

75. *AMPB* 2 (1837–1838): 412, 414–415.

76. *AMPB* 2 (1837–1838): 458–460; 3 (1838–1839): 470; 6 (1840–1841): 185–186.

77. *AMPB* 3 (1838–1839): 392–403, 413–421, 426, 691–693, 739–759, 770–786, 789–798, 802–810, 820–832, 853–881. The quotation, from the Academician Charles Londe, occurs on page 868.

78. Discussion of Belhomme, "Considérations sur le tournis chez les animaux et chez l'homme, comparé à l'affection provenant de la lésion du cervelet et de ses pédoncules" *AMPB* 3 (1838–1839): 392–403.

79. *AMPB* 3 (1838–1839): 401–402, 414–415, 739–759.

80. *AMPB* 3 (1838–1839): 401–402, 739–759.

81. For Blandin's remarks, see *AMPB* 3 (1838–1839): 691–693, 774. On Gerdy see previous discussion and note 76.

82. *AMPB* 3 (1838–1839): 403, 420–421, 791–792.

83. *AMPB* 3 (1838 1839): 417.

84. Ibid., pp. 417–420.

85. See, e.g., Bouillaud's remarks in *AMPB* 3 (1838–1839): 420–421; and Blandin's in ibid., pp. 691–693, 778.

86. *AMPB* 2 (1837–1838): 239–241. See also ibid., pp. 182–183, 186.

87. On the clinical significance of the problems, see, e.g., *AMPM* 5 (1837): 81–82; *AMPB* 1 (1836–1837): 280–284, 894–897, 899–902, 905–912; *AMPB* 2 (1837–1838): 182–183, 185–186, 239, 250–251, 278–280. For examples of the appeal to clinical experience, see *AMPB* 1 (1836–1837): 397–400, 903; 2 (1837–1838): 20–23, 146–147, 199–204, 244–245, 251–253, 305–314, 418–425; 3 (1838–1839): 934–942.

88. *AMPM* 5 (1836): 83, 86–90; *AMPB* 2 (1837–1838): 278–279.

89. "Avertissement de l'Editeur," *AMPM* 2 (1833): vii–viii.

90. Ackerknecht, *Medicine at the Paris Hospital,* p. 116.

CHAPTER FOUR

Science for the Clinic: Science Policy and the Formation of Carl Ludwig's Institute in Leipzig

Timothy Lenoir

INTRODUCTION; THE INSTITUTIONAL REVOLUTION IN GERMAN SCIENCE

In 1877 Emil du Bois-Reymond welcomed a throng of state dignitaries, professors, and students to his sumptuous new institute for physiology. In characteristically baroque style, this seasoned ideologue of Bismarck's *Kulturkampf* and high priest of German nationalism told his audience,

> You are looking at the regal lodgings that have been prepared for physiology, the queen of the natural sciences. This is one of the state institutions which are a symbol of the present age, institutions which neither the highest culture of Antiquity with its temples and amphitheaters nor that of the Renaissance with its domes and palaces had even dreamed of in the least.[1]

To be accurate du Bois-Reymond should have added Prussia to the list of those countries which, until recently, had been unable to imagine that institutes of natural science would furnish the temples of the new Kaiserreich. For in spite of its reputation as the *"Staat der Wissenschaft,"* prior to the late 1860s support of the natural sciences in Prussia had been meager. Du Bois-Reymond could easily have recounted his own experiences as evidence for this fact. In 1860, for example, the budget for the physiological laboratory he headed was 750 thaler, and before 1871 it did not increase above 1,140 thaler.[2] The operating budget of the institute for physiology du Bois-Reymond was christening in 1877, however, was a stately 40,220 marks, and the building in which it was housed had cost well over 200,000 marks. In contrast to the special grant of 975 thaler received in 1859 for an assortment of instruments, including three microscopes, a kymograph, ophthalometer, and heliostat, du Bois-Reymond was authorized to spend 32,400 marks to equip the laboratories of the new institute.[3] Du Bois-Reymond's experiences were by no means singular. Ample evidence supports the claim that during the same period the fortunes of other scientific disciplines, particularly chemistry and physics, had also changed.[4]

In discussing the reasons behind the massive funding of these new temples of science, du Bois-Reymond made explicit reference to the science policy of the Kultusministerium. At the base of the bright future lying before the young imperial German state was the conviction "that in medicine no less than in industry even the most apparently insignificant fact discovered in the pursuit of purely theoretical interests and abstract concerns can suddenly receive an immeasurable practical importance."[5] Du Bois-Reymond was giving expression to the attitude widespread among German industrialists, academics, and state ministers that leadership in the production of scientific knowledge was essential to the economic and political strength of the Kaiserreich. Modern scholarship has confirmed this view and demonstrated furthermore that its investment in scientific and technical education was one of the most significant factors in the meteoric rise of imperial Germany to the first rank among world powers at the end of the nineteenth century.

According to present interpretations, it was possible for science to play such a critical role in the modernization of Germany because it was not necessary to create *de novo* the entire framework of scientific institutions needed for these explosive developments. Rather it was possible to adapt structures that had been nurtured within the German academic system since the late 1830s, particularly in the Prussian universities. The key elements of this system were the research imperative, the support of pure science for its own sake independent of practical application, and intense competition within the decentralized German universities. This institutional framework permitted the growth of abstract research-oriented disciplines that only later became the basis for Germany's industrial and military strength; so that when the industrial demand for academic science began during the 1870s, Germany already possessed facilities for organized research and training in laboratory techniques which could be expanded to meet the new demand.[6] According to this point of view, the creation of the new scientific institutes was a continuation and expansion of existing structures rather than the effects of an institutional revolution in German science, as du Bois-Reymond's rhetoric would lead us to believe.

There is, however, much to recommend the view that radical changes had taken place in the institutional structure of German science since the late 1860s. A comparison between du Bois-Reymond's new institute and his earlier physiological laboratory reveals something of the nature and magnitude of these changes. Most striking is the number of students the institute was designed to serve. Its main lecture hall seated 217 with space for additional removable folding chairs which could enlarge its capacity to 259. There was in addition a small lecture hall, designed primarily for lectures of the institute's *ausserordentliche Professoren* and *Assistenten*, which seated sixty-five students.

The institute contained several departments, each with its own director; a section for physical physiology, another for chemical physiology, and a third for histology. The sections for chemical physiology and histology each had laboratory space to accommodate seventy students. These laboratories were intended particularly for the medical students, for whom practical laboratory exercises in chemistry and microscopic anatomy were required. A much smaller laboratory cluster including a main laboratory for vivisectional experiments and special physiological experiments and two adjoining labs for precision instrument work was reserved for the small number of the "more talented and especially diligent students" who intended to go on in physiological research.[7]

The organization of the institute bore little resemblance to du Bois-Reymond's previous physiological laboratory. Founded in 1851, for many years the laboratory was located on the second floor of the main building of the university. It consisted of two rooms, one of which was a partitioned-off section of the main corridor of the building. Before 1858 the laboratory had no regular students, and, in no small part a result of the cramped conditions, its student clientele never numbered more than seven. The primary and in fact exclusive subject of study in this laboratory was muscle and nerve physiology. Yet in spite of the severe limitations in space and equipment, major physiological discoveries were made and a significant number of the leading physiologists of the nineteenth century were trained in this laboratory.[8]

At least two aspects of this comparison call into question the assumption that the institutional transformation of the late 1860s and 1870s was based on the simple continuation of a previous science policy and the expansion of structures already in place. First is that, irrespective of the level of its financial support, in the period preceding the Gründerzeit laboratory science was supported primarily for the cultivation of elite scientists. Furthermore, when we consider the number of important advances made within this institutional framework, limited as it was, the conclusion is inescapable that the earlier system was adequate to produce a core of productive, elite scientists in most fields. Du Bois-Reymond was explicit about the fact that the primary objective behind the new institutes was not to make up for past inadequacies in support of individual scientific achievement.

> Adequate space, good apparatus, material support of all sorts are clearly essential today in order to insure further advances in physiology. But they are not responsible alone. . . . In the rule it is talent that makes discoveries, and while circumstances are responsible for bringing talent to light, its influx is dependent upon chance. In any case the opening of our institute will only increase the present possibilities by a small fraction. It would be beyond our expectations if in the average a single talent were always to emerge at each institute; for in the final analysis the production of young physiologists is limited by the saturation of the market, which temporarily diverts talent into other paths. Therefore, it would not be impossible that, while from the dismal "holes-in-the-wall" of our previous laboratories wave after wave of teachers of physiology came forth, the shining new institutes could for some time remain relatively unfruitful. . . . [But] it is not on account of the geniuses (may there be many among you) that this institute is here; geniuses have always succeeded in making their way even without such institutes. Rather to impart sound physiological intuition and rigorous inductive training as light and armour in the insecure half-darkness of medicine to the person of average intelligence, indeed to the person of lesser ability; that is the reason for the existence of this institute, and if it achieves this purpose, the sacrifices for it will not have been too great."[9]

The construction of the new scientific institutes, therefore, was predicated on a major shift in the orientation of science policy. Once regarded as the proper mental equipment for the elite intellectual leadership of the nation, natural science and rigorous methodical thinking was now regarded as essential for the rank-and-file professional, the "*Durchschnittsköpfe*," as du Bois-Reymond referred to them. The new institutes with their well-provisioned laboratories were the places where the catechism of the scientific age was to be transmitted to the faithful.

A second feature differentiating the new physiological institute from its predecessor was its disciplinary organization. Although du Bois-Reymond's earlier physiological laboratory was specialized for "physical physiology," the institute housed under a single roof the various subdisciplines of physiological research, including histology, physiological chemistry, and experimental physiology. At first glance it might appear that this was the result of the natural evolution of the conceptual structure of the discipline. It might be argued, for example, as William Coleman has argued in a recent paper,[10] that by the 1870s the cognitive structure of physiology had evolved to a level that *demanded* the organizational structure represented in du Bois-Reymond's institute. In keeping with this argument, it could be maintained that limited funding prevented du Bois-Reymond from pursuing a more expansive disciplinary perspective in his earlier physiological laboratory and that when circumstances permitted, he gave full institutional expression to the cognitive structure of his discipline. Indeed, as I too shall argue, the evolution of cognitive structure in physiology was intimately related to the form of its mature disciplinary organization. But my investigation into the formation of physiological institutes in Germany suggests an interactional perspective in which the institutional form of the disciplinary landscape was shaped not only by the cognitive interests of scientists but equally by the interests of the state and by a variety of local factors best captured by the term "institutional momentum." It is in investigating these aspects of disciplinary formation that we come to appreciate the magnitude of the institutional revolution that occurred in German science during the Gründerzeit.

Once again the situation of du Bois-Reymond is suggestive of the role of noncognitive factors in the institutionalization of physiology. Mention has already been made of the specialized orientation of research in du Bois-Reymond's physiological laboratory. This orientation was not exclusively the result of lack of funds for expanding the type of physiology done in the laboratory. Du Bois-Reymond simply did not pursue research problems unconnected with electrophysiology. The few examples of vivisectional work done by him or the students in his laboratory were all in connection with nerve and muscle physiology. Similarly, the few instances in which chemical methods were employed in his research were all directed at issues related to electrophysiology.

This narrow focus was in part responsible for difficulties du Bois-Reymond encountered in the early advancement of his career, in spite of the reputation he had attained as one of Europe's leading young physiologists. Du Bois-Reymond acknowledged in a letter to Ludwig in 1854 that his hopes for advancement in Berlin hinged on incorporating vivisectional demonstrations into his lectures, techniques that he had not mastered. In order to improve his prospects du Bois-Reymond learned several vivisectional experiments, such as Ludwig's experiment on the electrical stimulation of the salivary gland of the dog, which would soon become fare in the large lecture classes on physiology. In his letter to the Kultusministerium recommending du Bois-Reymond for promotion to the position of extraordinary professor several months later, Johann Lucas Schönlein observed that both he and Müller were now in agreement that du Bois-Reymond had sufficiently expanded his repertoire of lectures so that no further obstacle stood in the way of his promotion.

But this experience did not lead du Bois-Reymond to broaden his vision of the discipline. The several proposals he submitted to the Kultusministerium for a physiological laboratory beginning in 1858 and his various requests for equipment in the 1860s were all aimed at building a larger and better-equipped laboratory for physical physiology. He was not motivated to erect an integrated approach to physiology. Factors other than his own convictions about the cognitive structure of the discipline intervened to bring about the integrated physiological institute du Bois-Reymond opened in 1877.

The fact that other physiologists, such as Ludwig and Helmholtz, exhibited a more diverse range of research interests should not lead us to think that du Bois-Reymond was singular in not aiming at an integrated physiology as his disciplinary goal. In the period from the late 1840s through the late 1860s physiology in Germany was not dominated by a single approach. At least three self-conscious competing "schools" can be identified, each of which had its own vision of physiology. As the self-appointed leader of the physical reductionist school, du Bois-Reymond represented its vision of physiology rather more dogmatically than its other members. But in opposition to this approach was the school of Liebig, Voit, Pettenkofer, and Bischoff in

Munich. These men all treated the experimental work of the physical school as secondary to work on metabolism and relied on chemistry rather than physics to provide the principal explanatory framework for physiology. A third contender on the disciplinary horizon during this period was the older morphological tradition, the senior members of which included Johannes Müller and Rudolph Wagner. Their approach, which emphasized the priority of structure in understanding function, was manifested, among others, in the microscopical and histological work of Henle in Heidelberg and later Göttingen and by Reichert in Berlin.

I can find no evidence that prior to 1865 either of these schools defended an integrated conception of physiology resembling what afterward became the norm and that was institutionalized in the many institutes that have served ever since as the organizational locus of the discipline. The prototype for the new physiological institutes was Carl Ludwig's institute in Leipzig. Rich archival sources in Leipzig today permit an examination of the events leading to the establishment of that institute, and they illuminate the forces structuring the institutional revolution in German science. In particular, these sources suggest that the transition in physiology from a disciplinary landscape populated by competing schools to an approach integrated in its concepts, methods, and institutional structures resulted from the emergence of new interests and the formulation of new priorities by the German states in the period between the Revolution of 1848 and the Gründerzeit. Although the need for an "integrated" approach to physiology was emerging in Ludwig's work prior to his move to Leipzig, particular local circumstances and a shift in the science policy of the Saxon Kultusministerium provided a context in which his disciplinary program received both its concrete formulation and its institutional structure. In Leipzig, where the new priorities of industrializing states in Germany came to bear on physiology for the first time, economic constraints and the local institutional context gave Carl Ludwig's institute and the discipline of physiology its specific institutional form.

THE RESEARCH IMPERATIVE: SHIFTING PERSPECTIVES

In order to understand the factors restructuring the role of laboratory training in scientific and medical education from the late 1860s onward, it is useful to consider laboratory training in the earlier decades. Such an analysis reveals that although laboratory research was already considered essential to the production of knowledge, laboratory training played an insignificant role for the practitioner. Only those preparing for a career as academic scientists acquired extensive laboratory experience. Moreover even these advanced students do not seem to have acquired "laboratory training" systematically. Rather they were permitted to work in the laboratory of a major professor, where they picked up the skills of laboratory science by following his example. The paradigmatic case of this informal approach to laboratory science was the famous physiological laboratory of Johannes Müller.

Friedrich Bidder, who was himself a student in Müller's lab in 1834, provides a vivid description of the activities there in his *"Lebenserinnerungen."*[11] Müller's exercises in dissection, offered every winter semester, were attended normally by about 150–200 medical students. The students were divided into groups working on twenty different corpses.

> After the group assignments had been made, the students were left completely to their own designs. Müller appeared at most for a half-hour in the hall to cast a quick glance here or there; a rigorous introduction to anatomical preparation was out of the question.
>
> . . . Most of the students had not the slightest idea what the parts were they were supposed to prepare. A few of them had a handbook for anatomical preparation.[12]

Bidder, who had already completed a course of medical study in Dorpat with Heinrich Rathke, where the only human dissection he had ever done was on the day of his state medical qualifying exam, attracted Müller's attention on one of his dashes through the anatomical theater. His skilled hand in dissection earned Müller's praise and the "electrifying invitation: Herr Doktor, why don't you join me upstairs in my *Kabinet*. You will be able to work much better there away from all this confusion."[13] In the two-room private laboratory of Johannes Müller, Bidder joined Henle, Schwann, and Reichert. He learned the art of anatomical preparation and was initiated into physiological research at the side of these future scions of Müller's school. Perhaps most revealing of the level of anatomical instruction at that date was the presence of no more than a single microscope in Müller's lab.

The lectures on physiology held every summer term were equally disappointing. Bidder had expected that

> the man who was so deeply concerned to give the doctrines of physiology empirical foundations would have made every effort to give his auditors such experiences and to demonstrate the methods by which they are acquired. That was, however, not the case at all. The students and other auditors had to be satisfied with theoretical discussions. In his lectures encompassing the entire domain of physiology Müller only twice offered the students an occasion to observe something.[14]

At the root of the problem described in these passages by Bidder was a particular conception of the objectives of physiology as a discipline. Physiology for Müller was *Wissenschaft;* and he understood that term precisely in the sense of the Prussian educational reformers. What he sought was a unified science of life, the pillars of which were comparative anatomy, particularly embryological investigations, and experiment. Both in his inaugural address as a professor in Bonn and in the introduction to his monumental *Handbuch der Physiologie des Menschen,* Müller, declaring himself to be the heir and continuator of the biological tradition of Kant and Goethe, stated that observation and experiment were instruments leading to a synthetic philosophical understanding of the nature of life. To construct this *verständige Physiologie* was Müller's announced purpose. Operative control over nature was not necessarily an end consonant with this disciplinary objective.

In his dealings with the Kultusministerium Müller always stressed his program for a unified science of life. It was a program that appealed to ministers for whom the support of *Wissenschaft um sich selber willen* was part of a plan for providing for the spiritual elite the values they would then disseminate to the youth of the nation. Such thinking was behind not only the call of Müller to Berlin but also his appointment in *both* the philosophical and medical faculties.[15] Through Müller's activities they hoped to enrich the empirical, technician-like orientation of the medical curriculum with the spirit emanating from the research seminars of the reformed philosophical faculty, the spiritual bulwark of the nation.

The attitudes I have attributed to Müller were not unique among the natural scientists in the Prussian professoriate. R. Steven Turner has recently shown similar attitudes in the memoranda prepared by chemists for the Kultusministerium in response to Liebig's scathing critique of the condition of the natural sciences in Prussia in 1840.[16] They regarded Liebig's laboratory as a factory in which young men worked from morning until late evening and as much too utilitarian in its orientation. Prussia had technical schools and *Realschulen* to attend to the practical needs of the state. The medical faculty in particular rejected Liebig's claims for chemistry as not growing out of an appreciation of the unity of learning. Moreover Liebig's laboratory exploited a set of techniques and apparatus he had developed for performing organic analysis. Though valuable, such methods, which could be taught even to ordinary minds, did not yet qualify as *Wissenschaft*. Chemistry of the kind taught by Liebig had not progressed beyond the stage of describing and classifying. It was not yet a theoretical science seeking the causes of phenomena.

Institutes designed in light of the principle of *"Wissenschaft um sich selber Willen"* were extremely individualistic in their orientation toward research. This was in keeping with one of the fundamental concepts behind the Humboldt reforms; namely, to produce creative minds freed from the oppressive regimentation of the Frederician state. The effects of this science policy are illustrated once again in the work of Johannes Müller. In contrast to Liebig, for example, Müller did not pursue a single objective in his research. He moved from work in experimental physiology utilizing vivisectional techniques in the early 1830s to work in sensory physiology. Next came a period of work on digestion (with Schwann) utilizing chemical methods in the mid-1830s. This was followed by research on cellular development (particularly in its application to pathology). Interspersed throughout these researches was extensive work in comparative anatomy, embryology, and, finally, work on the alternation of generations.

As Müller's research interests shifted, so did the orientation and fields of research of the inner circle of his research assistants and students. The result was successive student clusters entering the academic market with different research objectives and frequently different disciplinary aims. Through the orientations he gave his students Müller has correctly been credited with contributing to the foundation in Germany of several different research fields in the biological and medical sciences, including experimental physiology, cellular pathology, embryology, and zoology.

This approach was not conducive to the sustained development of research skills, techniques, and instrumentation in a particular area such as physiology and of refining them so that through laboratory training they would enter the repertoire of standard practice. Indeed between 1835 and 1858 the average amount spent in Müller's institute on materials and experimental animals for instruction in physiology was 18 thaler.[17] This was hardly the sort of investment needed to transform the practice of medicine by infusing it with results obtained at the research front. But this, of course, was precisely the genius of Liebig's institutional reform proposals. In 1840 they went strongly against the grain of the reigning ideology of *Wissenschaft*.

A new wind began to stir during the 1840s, however. Its direction was being determined by developments in the clinic. In 1840 Johann Lukas Schönlein accepted a call to Berlin. Schönlein aimed to reform clinical medicine by linking diagnostic procedures to causal theories based in physiology and pathology.[18] In this goal he was not alone. At exactly the same time in Tübingen Carl Wunderlich was calling for the construction of a rational medicine. They were soon to be joined by others in this endeavor, most notably Virchow, Henle, and Pfeuffer. The programs of these individuals differed in their emphasis on key elements of the reform package, and while these differences were not without consequence for the theory and organization of clinical practice, there was essential agreement on the core of their proposed scientific medicine. For my purposes Wunderlich's "physiological medicine" is most significant because it largely shaped the local institutional context in Leipzig that prepared the call of Ludwig.

Wunderlich's physiological medicine was based on the notion that illness and disease result from a disturbance in the normal functioning of an organ or system of organs. In his journal, the *Archiv für physiologische Heilkunde,* Wunderlich waged war against the defenders of specific disease entities. He also opposed the view that pathological anatomy provided the sole source of scientific medicine. Rather he advocated the investigation through experimental physiology of the laws of normal organ function. Grounded in physiology, scientific medicine would investigate the causes of pathological lesions and the relationship between lesions and symptoms of disease. Wunderlich's central objective was to trace changes in organ function back to chemical and physical changes transpiring at their anatomical locus. In his program, therefore, pathology was only a tool to be employed in tracing the pathways of disturbed organ function. Similarly he argued that scientific medicine must use the microscope and chemical investigations both as a research tool and as diagnostic aids. But their relevance as diagnostic tools was dependent upon establishing a causal relationship to the physical and chemical basis of normal organ function.[19]

This interest in medical reform was reflected in gradual changes in the course offerings in medical faculties. The University of Berlin, which had the largest number of medical students during the period, is representative of the difficulties encountered by the reformers. The first of the new generation of courses that offered laboratory training to the general medical student was Henle's two-hour course in general microscopic anatomy in the summer semester of 1839.[20] Considering that Müller's cabinet possessed only one microscope, Henle's course could not have accommodated large numbers of students. Interested students had to share Henle's microscope or supply their own, a possibility realizable for the first time in the late 1830s with the introduction of the inexpensive achromatic microscopes produced by Plössel in Vienna and by Pista and Scheick in Berlin.[21] That there was indeed growing student interest in the new scientific medicine and the microscope as a potential diagnostic tool is indicated by the fact that after Henle's departure Ehrenberg began to offer exercises in the use of the microscope for physiology.[22]

Following the arrival of Schönlein in 1840 one small private course began to be offered on the new diagnostic techniques of auscultation and percussion. By 1843 the interest in diagnostic methods had expanded to include offerings on the chemical analysis of blood, urine, and other secretions. In the winter semester of 1843 Simons, a future cofounding member of the Berliner physikalische Gesellschaft, offered two courses in pathological and physiological chemistry accompanied by demonstrations with chemical and microscopic experiments.[23]

The turning point in the perceived importance of such practical courses emphasizing training in the use of the microscope and in the new diagnostic methods seems to have occurred in Berlin about 1845. In the summer semester of that year Brücke offered a course on the theory of the microscope and its use in the examination of healthy and diseased tissues. This course, along with Ehrenberg's exercises in the use of the microscope for physiology, Simon's (now four-hour) course on pathology and therapeutics with demonstrations with the microscope, Heintz's course on physiological chemistry with experimental demonstrations, and Ebert's practical exercises in auscultation and percussion, made at least five course offerings in which medical students were being initiated into the technical methods of the emerging scientific medicine. From 1847 onward the number of such courses offering practical experience in microscopy, experiment, and the use of chemical and physical diagnostic methods increased to seven; in 1848, eight such courses were offered; fifteen in the revolutionary summer semester of 1849; and by 1856 there was an average of eleven courses offering practical exercises in experimental technique and diagnostic procedures to medical students. By the late 1850s science-based medicine was fully recognized as the organizing principle of the medical faculty. That victory was finally attained in 1861 when Virchow, du Bois-Reymond, and Langenbeck engineered the demise of the old *Tentamen philosophicum* and its replacement with the *Tentamen physicum*. Where technical subjects had previously been absent from the exams, the *physicum* examined over six areas related to experimental physiology, pathological anatomy, and physiological chemistry.[24]

CARL LUDWIG AND THE INTEGRATED APPROACH TO PHYSIOLOGY

At the same time interest in rational medicine was growing among students and the younger *Dozenten*, new developments in physiology were pointing to the need for an integrated approach to the discipline. Carl Ludwig was at the forefront of these disciplinary developments. In this section we shall follow the cognitive developments that led Ludwig to his integrated approach to physiology, developments that are best illustrated through his work on kidney function. Ludwig's work on kidney function spanned his entire career. The further he pressed on in understanding urinary physiology, the more he was forced to resort to methods and techniques that expanded his original conception of the field.

Ludwig first took up the problem of kidney function in his doctoral dissertation, completed in 1842.[25] Kidney function was one of the primary examples employed by the older generation in its defense of teleological forms of explanation in physiology. The apparent ability of the kidneys selectively to remove harmful substances from the blood was regarded as evidence that forces irreducible to physics and chemistry guide organ function. According to the commonly accepted model, urine was produced through a process of secretion in the kidneys. Ludwig's dissertation and the much expanded version of the thesis published in Rudolph Wagner's *Handwörterbuch der Physiologie* two years later (1844) attempted to demonstrate that the kidneys do not secrete urine at all but serve rather as a hydraulic device for mechanically filtering the blood.[26]

Ludwig's model was based on the observation that whereas in normal capillaries the increase in cross-sectional areas in the passage from artery to capillary significantly lowers the pressure, in the glomerulus, because the afferent arterioles are larger than the efferent arterioles, an increase in pressure results. This pressure differential is the mechanism driving the expulsion of urine from the blood.

In order to account for the selectivity of the filtration process, Ludwig drew upon experiments by Ernst Brücke and on recent work on osmotic pressures. Brücke had shown that certain organic membranes, such as the amniotic membranes in birds, are pervious to water and crystalloid solutions but impervious to proteins.[27] Ludwig coupled to this finding the results of work on diffusion gradients to explain how the concentration of urea and other crystalloids in the blood could be less than their corresponding concentrations in the urine and why the entire water content of the plasma is not eliminated through the kidneys. According to Ludwig's model, because of the permeability of the glomular membranes to water, an increased concentration of water occurs in the lumen of the surrounding Bowman's capsule. The concentration gradient across the membrane creates a reverse current reabsorbing water into the blood plasma.

This explanation, ingenious though it was, could not completely account for the mechanism of kidney function. Karl Valentin pointed out that Ludwig's hypothesis implied that the urine should be a more concentrated solution of all the substances present in the blood minus the proteins impermeable to the membrane. Chemical analysis of the urine, however, exhibited differences from the composition of blood plasma. Instead of concluding that an active function of the kidney restoring certain substances from the filtrate back into the blood plasma could not be excluded, Valentin completely rejected Ludwig's explanation in favor of the older vitalistic models.

In the following years Ludwig attempted repeatedly to shore up his filtration theory of kidney function. Together with his students Friedrich Goll and Max Hermann he performed a variety of experiments demonstrating the dependence of urine production on blood pressure. By stimulating the vagus nerve or by removing a sufficient quantity of blood to reduce blood pressure to 40–50 mmHg in the aorta, Ludwig and Hermann found that under such conditions urine production ceases altogether. Reversing the procedure restored urine production to normal. In a further experiment Ludwig and Hermann inserted a manometer into the ureter of a dog and measured the maximal secretion pressure of the kidney. They showed that at 40 mmHg in the ureter urine production ceased and increased levels of urea began to appear in the blood.[28]

Ludwig's work on kidney function depended upon a variety of techniques and results from different disciplines. In revealing the difference in cross-sectional area between the afferent and efferent arterioles, microscopic anatomy provided the entrée for his application of hydrostatic principles drawn from mechanics. Vivisection techniques in combination with instrumentation for registering pressure, which Ludwig pioneered in developing, enabled him and his students to provide convincing evidence for the role of filtration in the formation of urine. But as he pressed further in understanding organ function, the importance not only of utilizing the results and methods of these different areas but, more significantly, of integrating and refining them in a manner specifically suitable for addressing strictly physiological questions became ever more imperative.

In responding to Valentin's criticism, for example, Ludwig succeeded in providing conclusive evidence for his filtration theory. But he had not removed the objection that some additional process must be involved in regulating the concentration of various substances in the plasma. Concentration gradients were clearly not a sufficient mechanism. This problem was a constant source of concern, and though he never resolved it, he seems to have searched long and hard for the answer. One solution he contemplated was a chemical-physical model for the regulation of membrane permeability. Thus in 1849, responding to Valentin's criticisms, Ludwig gave as a dissertation topic to his student Carl Loebell the task of performing a variety of experiments on the permeability of arterial membranes to various solutions.[29] With Ludwig's assistance Loebell showed that if an arterial membrane is placed between blood serum and a two percent saline solution, no proteins penetrate the membrane, just as Brücke had shown in experiments in which he used amniotic membranes. But if instead of saline solution distilled water were used, the membrane suddenly became permeable to protein molecules. If, furthermore, the membrane had been soaked in distilled water *before* placing it between a saline solution and the blood serum, protein molecules penetrated the membrane into the saline solution. Bathing the membrane in distilled water had rendered it permeable to protein molecules. Reflecting on these experiments in a letter to Jacob Henle, Ludwig speculated that perhaps each molecule of the membrane became surrounded by a layer of water molecules which altered the normal chemical affinities of the membrane. The resulting change in chemical affinity of the membrane might have rendered it permeable to specific components of the blood serum.[30] This was not a particularly enlightening solution to the problem, and as far as I can determine, Ludwig nowhere published it.

Ludwig continued his search for a chemical-physical model to explain membrane permeability to specific substances. In 1855, shortly after his arrival in Vienna, he began working seriously with Brücke on a new model for secretion. They attempted to determine whether an electric current might impart different velocities to particles in a mixture, perhaps through inducing differential charges on the particles, and thereby providing a mechanism for differentially separating the components of the mixture. Ludwig's hopes for this model, however, were disappointed by a series of experiments conducted by Brücke.[31]

But Ludwig maintained his belief in the need for investigating physical mechanisms for active transport. On one occasion he even did so in an area where his earlier strictly mechanical model ultimately prevailed. Thus commenting in 1860 on the results of blood, milk, and urine analyses done by one of his students, Alexander von Schäffer, Ludwig noted that much more CO_2 appears to be transferred between the alveoli and pulmonary capillary blood than is transferred in the formation of urine. This finding led him to conclude that some specific active transport mechanism must be involved in the expulsion of CO_2.[32]

Ludwig's work in urinary and respiratory physiology continually impressed upon him the need for more detailed knowledge of processes involving physiological chemistry. The further he penetrated into organ function, the more essential it became to him to be able to unravel each step in a physiological transformation. Some of these steps could be revealed with the aid of methods drawn from physics, but increasingly he began to perceive that the simple application of mechanics could not account for the complex interrelations between physiological functions. Ludwig's letters to Henle from the mid-1850s contain persistent references to the need for more and improved chemical knowledge. At issue was not merely improved methods of analyzing organic compounds. Rather for the kinds of questions Ludwig was confronting a new sort of chemistry that went beyond the techniques of the "blood and urine analysts" was needed, one that addressed the chemical transformations in a functioning physiological context. Thus in 1853 he wrote that nothing significant had been added to the understanding of chemical transformations in the blood since the work of Prevost and Dumas in the 1820s.[33] Ludwig's awareness of the need for breaking new ground in physiological chemistry led him to encourage his students during the 1850s and early 1860s to visit various German universities in order to learn more advanced methods in mathematics, physics, and, above all, organic chemistry.[34] "I hope that you are in agreement with me," Ludwig wrote Henle, "that in our field chemistry in the true sense of the word provides the prospects for the most significant advances. No doubt you are no less sensitive to the present need of true physiological chemists than I am."[35]

An equally important condition for progress in physiology was the continued refinement and improvement of microscopic anatomy. Each stage in the extension of Ludwig's program of experimental physiology required a deeper understanding of the intimate connection between structure and function. Nothing demonstrated this more clearly than his work in urinary physiology. His filtration theory successfully accounted for one of the central components in the production of urine, but Ludwig was all too aware that it provided only part of the picture. In 1863 Jacob Henle opened the prospect of enlarging the explanatory domain through his discovery of the hairpinlike loops in the nephronic tubules that have ever since born his name, the Henle loops.

Two features of Henle's discovery are of present interest. The first is that after Henle announced the discovery, it took Ludwig three months of careful work to duplicate Henle's observations for himself. To make progress in microscopic anatomy, it was not enough simply to look through the microscope. Each new discovery demanded improvements in existing techniques or the development of new ones. By the early 1860s even an experienced microscopist such as Ludwig could duplicate the work of his specialist colleagues only through an enormous investment of effort. "From all of this," he confided to Henle, "it is clear that insofar as one takes it seriously microscopic anatomy is one of the most difficult observational sciences."[36] Ludwig later admitted that had it not been for the rough impressions he had obtained from Henle's descriptions of what to look for, he would never have found the loops by himself.[37]

The second aspect of this episode relevant to our story is the extent to which it reinforced in Ludwig's mind the close interdependent working relationship that must exist between microscopic anatomy and physiology. "That your kidney structures are of great functional importance is evident even if one only considers the necessary effects of the mechanical characteristics of the tube. Even the comparative anatomy of animals with and without renal medullae as well as those that produce dry and fluid urine will now become significant, for they are now more capable of being investigated."[38] Ludwig saw in these thin, hairpin-loop sections of the nephron tubules the structure needed to overcome the deficiencies in his earlier filtration theory. Following the hydrostatic model once again, he thought that the restriction of flow of the glomular filtrate as it passed through the narrow confines of the Henle loop might lead to further filtration. The enveloping peritubular capillary network might furnish the pathway for reabsorption of materials from the glomular filtrate into the plasma.[39]

Ludwig had come to appreciate the value of integrating microscopic anatomy and physiological chemistry into experimental physiology long before the early 1860s. In response to the first volume of Henle's *Handbuch der rationallen Pathologie* (1846) Ludwig had stated that "it is clear to me that we quantitative and experimental heads could not live without a man like you, and I could wish for nothing more than to see you collect the fruits of my efforts together with those of all others into a single edifice."[40] But when the time came to construct that edifice Ludwig changed his mind about who should be its rightful architect. That person necessarily had to be a physiologist. Ludwig adopted this view not as a strategy for defending his professional turf from rivals. Rather it developed out of his own perception of the cognitive demands of physiology as a discipline. Ludwig provided a remarkable statement of those cognitive demands in a letter written in 1854 responding to Henle's reservations concerning Ludwig's *Lehrbuch der Physiologie des Menschen*.

Henle had criticized the *Lehrbuch* for excluding all discussion of morphological questions. No comparative anatomy, not a single sentence concerning embryology, and only those aspects of the cell theory relating to function are to be found in Ludwig's text. In Henle's view this had been a one-sided treatment of the subject, emphasizing only the experimental viewpoint while completely neglecting the morphological approach. To this Ludwig responded that it was not a matter of preference whether one emphasized physics over anatomy in a textbook on physiology. "All physiological processes consist of motions of larger or smaller masses in the animal body which are dependent either upon the transmission of motion or the transformation of tensional forces into vis viva."[41] Given that the motions referred to could be conceived only as movements of complicated chemical atoms in accordance with the principles of chemical combination, the conclusion was inescapable that "physiology is nothing other than applied physics."[42]

From these considerations Ludwig drew the further and, to a man from Henle's discipline, far more alarming conclusion that anatomy does not stand in conflict with physiology, "because the results of [anatomical] research—namely the determination of the properties of structure—*are included as an element in the physicalist point of view.*"[43] Ludwig explained that from his perspective the anatomical structure is the means for inhibiting or channeling motions in particular directions. Anatomical structures produce physiological effects not in virtue of their shape or structure but rather because particular conditions are determined by the organization of the matter contained in them. "If this is correct," Ludwig concluded, "then anatomy is by no means sufficient in order to obtain any sort of insight into physiological processes; because the object studied by anatomy only acquires significance under the condition that some movement is present."[44]

This statement implied that research in microscopic anatomy should receive its guidance from physiology. To be sure, Ludwig acknowledged a deep interdependence of the two disciplines. As our examination of his own work in urinary physiology has shown, each stage in the progress of Ludwig's explanatory model was aimed at unraveling the deep interdependence of form and function. But the leading edge of that research program was defined by the functional constraints of particular anatomical structures as revealed by the principles of mechanics and organic chemistry. When available models proved incapable of providing a complete explanation, as in the case of Ludwig's model of glomular filtration, attention needed to be shifted to the search for additional structures that would provide the conditions for a refined description of function. The functional perspective thus provided the framework for orienting research, and the microscopic anatomist had to take the search for structural solutions to problems defined by the physiologist's perspective as the focus of his research. The fact that Henle, Leuckart, Rudolph Wagner, and others interpreted this as a rationalization for the imperialistic disciplinary aims of the Berlin "physical" school did not deflect Ludwig in the least. In that optimistic, boyish naiveté that seems to have characterized his style, Ludwig in a later communication attempted to smooth over the obvious points of potential confrontation at the institutional level. "In what concerns form and content," he wrote Henle, "our efforts are directed toward the same end. That we work on different ends of the building should not hinder us from exchanging a friendly greeting during working hours."[45]

The problem was, of course, that not everyone had been convinced of the correctness of Ludwig's disciplinary perspective. In an era when *Wissenschaft um sich selber Willen* implied the equality of all abstract knowledge, few scientists were willing to take on employment in Ludwig's laboratory as first-class technicians, tailoring their research to the needs of his disciplinary program. This was a persistent problem Ludwig faced, even in Leipzig, where, as we shall see, local circumstances had offered a means for resolving it. Thus when Ludwig went to Leipzig a primary consideration was to acquire a microscopic anatomist as an assistant in the institute.

To find such a person proved to be no easy task. For while there were able enough microscopists, few were imbued with the appropriate perspective needed to work well with a physiologist. Schweiger-Seidel, a histologist who became Ludwig's associate in all his early research endeavors in Leipzig, turned out to be a rare species among microscopic anatomists at that time. The features of Schweiger-Seidel's professional profile that rendered his breed increasingly indispensable for Ludwig's program are spelled out in letters to Henle during the late 1860s:

> That I am extremely fortunate in having won Schweiger-Seidel for
> Leipzig and have been able to keep him here, you can well appreciate.
> Considering the present refinements in the development of micros
> copy it would be inefficient [*untunlich*] to press on alone. Together
> with Schweiger-Seidel I have already seen many things that I would

never have seen by myself; and this is not simply because I would not have had the time or interest in making the necessary preparations.[46]

Just how scarce microscopists of this stamp were was driven home to Ludwig in 1870 following Schweiger-Seidel's untimely death. He was ultimately replaced by an assistant named Merkel. Though an extremely talented and accomplished microscopic anatomist, Merkel proved to be an ineffective assistant for a physiological institute: "My desire," wrote Ludwig, "that the anatomist also take the functioning organ into consideration, that whenever possible he make measurements on the active organ, has simply made no impression on him."[47]

Ludwig and his colleagues in the "physicalist school" faced a dilemma. In order to advance their own disciplinary goals, they were dependent upon work of the microscopists and organic chemists. Allowed to pursue disciplinary goals of their own definition, however, practitioners in these research fields could not be counted upon to provide the results required by the physiologists when they were needed. On the other hand, Ludwig knew well from personal experience that the techniques of both microscopic anatomy and organic chemistry had become advanced enough so that it was neither efficient nor in many cases possible for the physiologist to provide the anatomical and chemical discoveries required for progress in his own house. Some more efficient working arrangement between the various biomedical research areas had to be established if physiology were to achieve its disciplinary aims. The solution to that problem was not cognitive; it was institutional.

KNOWLEDGE IN CONTEXT: CARL LUDWIG AND THE INSTITUTIONALIZATION OF SCIENCE-BASED MEDICINE IN LEIPZIG

Throughout the 1850s and early 1860s developments were under way in Leipzig which provided a context for the institutional solution to the problems confronting Ludwig's vision of physiology as a discipline. The creation of the institutional form in which Ludwig's integrated approach to physiology was realized can be viewed on the one hand as the culmination of these earlier institutional patterns in Leipzig. On the other hand, the call of Ludwig to Leipzig and the creation of his institute should be seen from the perspective of its role in resolving certain concrete institutional obstacles to the larger goals of the science policy of the state of Saxony. Ludwig created the science that Leipzig needed for its program of modernization.

Institutional developments during the 1850s in the Leipzig medical and science faculties must be interpreted in the context of three closely interrelated aspects of the Revolution of 1848. Foremost, in my view, is the widespread interest in medical reform that surfaced everywhere during the revolution. The leader in this movement was Rudolf Virchow. In the popular press and in journals such as his *Medizinisches Reform,* Virchow and others who joined his cause were able to focus many of the criticisms of old regime, *ständisch* German society in a concrete issue directly affecting large numbers of persons. It was not the support for his radical democratic politics that Virchow hoped to generate from his analysis of sanitation and public health that are of interest for our story, however. At the heart of his demands for reform were the notions that good health is a right of each citizen and that the state has the responsibility to provide it. Virchow was the self-appointed spokesperson of those who believed that support of science-based medicine would enable the state to meet its responsibility. Increasing numbers of people shared his view. At nearly every German university during the revolutionary period petitions were made to reform the medical faculties and abolish the old system of state exams. Frequently these petitions were coupled with proposals for increasing the role of the natural sciences in the curriculum.[48]

Closely allied with these reform efforts was a concern, particularly among younger physicians, for upgrading professional standards.[49] Therapeutic nihilism was gradually falling into disfavor among academically trained physicians. In part they were inspired by general humanistic concerns and a growing confidence in the ability of scientifically trained physicians to make a difference in the battle against disease. No less significant, however, were the genuine concerns about the inroads being made into their practice by homeopathic medicine and the *Anthroposophen.* Academically trained physicians wanted to enhance the image of their profession and improve their status in society. Scientific medicine offered them a tool for achieving their ends.

Another important factor was the general fear aroused by the cholera epidemic of 1848–1849.[50] By the summer of 1849 papers in major cities such as Berlin, for example, were reporting weekly death rates

in the hundreds attributable to cholera. In an age increasingly dominated by the belief that men can shape their own destinies, active
control of epidemic disease emerged as the moral imperative of a
progressive society.

Motivated by concerns to reform medicine as well as by an interest in appointing a popular teacher who would improve their slump-
ing medical student enrollments, the University of Leipzig called
Carl Wunderlich as the director of the Jakobshospital in 1850. Leipzig seemed to offer everything Wunderlich desired in order to establish his program of "physiological medicine." As colleagues he had
Ernst Heinrich and Eduard Weber, the early fathers of the
physicalist school of physiology. Moreover in Carl Lehmann he
found one of the leading physiological chemists of the day. With his
path-breaking *Handbuch der Pathologie und Therapie* (1850–1852), begun shortly after his arrival in Leipzig, Wunderlich wasted no time
in announcing that Leipzig was a center of the new medical reform
movement.

The difficulties in shaping a program according to one's own plan
and the role of local circumstances in determining the final outcome
are emphasized by the situation Wunderlich found in Leipzig on his
arrival. One of the principal difficulties he would face over the next
decade had been created by a faculty and administrative decision
made on a proposal by his new colleague, Lehmann, shortly before
his arrival. In July 1849, seizing upon the opportune circumstances
of the revolution and the readiness of most regimes to accede to
reforms, Lehmann had made a bold and imaginative proposal for
creating a new institute for physiological chemistry.

In his memorandum, seventeen folio pages in length, Lehmann
criticized the role of laboratory training in chemistry within the medical curriculum.[51] Although every serious medical program was beginning to emphasize chemical diagnostic procedures to be performed
by the practicing physician at the bedside, in no German university,
with the notable exception of Würzburg, were medical students required to have advanced practical laboratory training in quantitative
chemistry. The medical student was presented with an occasional
demonstration of some important aspect of prevailing views on metabolism, respiration, and the chemical compositions of blood and
urine, but he was not expected to become a master of the chemical
techniques he observed in operation. Students were also shown a
variety of simple tests for analyzing the composition of urine, blood,

and feces. The working assumption, however, was not that as physicians they would ever perform such tests themselves, but simply that the normal practicing physician should be aware that such tests existed and what they indicated.

Lehmann made a two-front assault on this conception of laboratory science. On the one hand he argued that the number and sophistication of the chemical tests and diagnostic techniques being developed daily and already capable of entering the standard repertoire of the practicing physician justified an expanded role for laboratory training in the medical curriculum. But his main assault centered on the need to rethink the relation between the theoretical and practical disciplines. At present laboratory training functioned as an uninspired transmission of technical expertise rather than an embodiment of the notion essential to a university education; namely, that theoretical knowledge should inform practice. Lehmann advocated a curriculum incorporating serious laboratory training that treated scientific knowledge not as window dressing but rather as the heart and soul of the thought processes of the practicing physician.

With the means at the disposal of the one-room laboratories typically present in teaching clinics it was possible, for example, for students to determine certain components of the urine, such as urea, uric acid, and a variety of salts and gases. But if the student were asked to determine whether fats are present in the urine, the laboratory exercise would fail. To be sure, fats could be identified with the aid of the microscope; but if, as in most cases, they were present only in small quantities in solution, it was impossible to distinguish them from a variety of other similar substances also present in the urine without the aid of precise elementary analysis and the determination of atomic weights. Lehmann provided other examples of blood analyses and analyses of various pathological secretions of interest to the practicing physician, all requiring mastery of advanced quantitative techniques.[52] The point he wanted to make with these examples was that if it was in the interest of the state and the medical profession to infuse medical practice with methodical scientific thinking and procedures, then it was essential to inculcate this frame of mind in the medical students through the appropriate laboratory training. In describing the objectives of that laboratory training Lehmann stressed the importance of having students perform difficult, lengthy elementary analyses that worked every time they were performed correctly. By assigning problems in physiological chemistry that could be solved but only after mastering rigorous, precise techniques, students would leave their medical study not only with an understanding and appreciation of the basis of scientific medicine and the powerful results to which it could lead but, more important, with a deep confidence in the scientific method and the readiness to apply it to whatever problem they encountered in their medical practice.[53]

The objective of Lehmann's proposal was not to turn crude technicians into more sophisticated ones. He stated that in his view medical education should prepare the physician to associate outward signs with causal processes going on at the level of organs, tissues, and cells. When the physician performs an examination, he should have a clear conception of the relationship between those outward signs and the internal mechanisms to which they are ultimately causally connected. In order to achieve these ends, Lehmann advocated an eclectic program for providing the medical student with a fundamental understanding of basic organic and physiological processes. Study of the basic processes and reactions of the animal body would be preparatory to studying the locations and manner in which they transpire in the fluids and tissues of the body. In this he was advocating a program far more ambitious than contemporary efforts to draw up a statistical-chemical balance sheet of inputs and outputs. Lehmann wanted to pursue the problem of metabolism to the dynamic level of the step-by-step modification of substances as they pass through the organism. In order to follow organic transformations throughout their entire course, chemical knowledge had to be coupled with microscopic technique and vivisectional experimentation. Training in the use of the microscope as well as in staining techniques would provide tools for teaching students to think in terms of causal models.

The small but significant number of foreign students who came to Leipzig to study with Lehmann in his private laboratory already received the kind of training he outlined. But his proposal to bring it to the average medical student required a commitment of resources and facilities far beyond the damp, poorly ventilated, and dimly lit one-room laboratory in the basement of the Jakobshospital then allotted to physiological chemistry. Lehmann required not only space for training between fifteen to twenty students; he needed space for experimental animals, as well as equipment and space for advanced chemical analysis and experimentation. In order to ensure its relevance to medical practice, Lehmann saw great advantage in attaching the laboratory to the hospital, where it could provide chemical analyses for the clinicians and benefit from access to pathological material. But his preferred solution was the construction of a separate institute for physiological chemistry, where advanced quantitative research could be conducted in addition to providing medical students with the requisite knowledge and skills to perform sophisticated diagnostic procedures.

Lehmann's vision of the relation between the theoretical and practical domains of biomedical science was clearly in accord with Wunderlich's prescriptions for physiological medicine. Indeed, before his departure from Tübingen, Wunderlich had made some small beginnings toward the establishment of a laboratory similar to the one described by Lehmann. But Lehmann's proposal was ultimately rejected by the Kultusministerium. The minutes of the medical faculty reveal that the faculty supported Lehmann's proposal but that they favored more enthusiastically another proposal for a chemical laboratory submitted at the same time by the locally powerful professor of organic and pharmaceutical chemistry, Otto Kühne. The medical faculty emphasized the diversity of Kühne's clientele, in contrast to the small number of students who would benefit from Lehmann's laboratory. Kühne's course in inorganic chemistry averaged thirty-three students per semester; organic chemistry, twenty-five students per semester; pharmaceutical chemistry, nine students per semester; general chemistry for medical students, thirty per semester. The concluding statement of the report provided the clinching argument: Kühne's discipline was

> no longer, as was once the case, of interest only to physicians, pharmacists, students of mining and metallurgy. Rather, since the recent discoveries made by several famous men, chemistry is widely held to be essential, and its valuable influence is being felt in agriculture and industry. Furthermore, since engineers, students of economics and businessmen have begun to introduce scientific principles into their activities, chemistry, whether in its most general form or in one of its specialized fields, has come to be regarded as a fundamental requirement. It is essential, therefore, to build laboratories in which theory and practice in all branches of chemistry will be taught and in which the students will receive practical training.[54]

Lehmann had made the fatal mistake of proposing that his laboratory specialize in *advanced* chemical analysis. The faculty minutes point out that Lehmann's course of study presupposed previous training in laboratories of the kind proposed by Kühne. Although the institute proposed by Kühne was not funded, the warm endorsement of the faculty did succeed in persuading the Saxon Kultusministerium to provide additional support for improvements to the chemical laboratory. In the years following this decision Lehmann resubmitted his proposal. He did ultimately receive funding for the minimal laboratory he had described as suitable for the limited teaching of diagnostic procedures in the Jakobshospital, but he was never able to convince the faculty or the ministry to fund a separate institute for advanced quantitative work in physiological chemistry. Disillusioned, Lehmann accepted a call to Jena in 1856. Though unsuccessful, his memorandum had nonetheless planted the seed for important future developments.

A "new era" in scientific and medical education began with the appointment of Johann Paul Freiherr von Falkenstein as director of the Saxon Kultusministerium in 1853. Falkenstein was already experienced in state administration. In 1830, then twenty-nine years of age, he entered state service as a member of the Landesregierung. Having received promotion to Geheimer Regierungsrath in 1834, he became superintendent of the district of Leipzig. In this position Falkenstein was to Saxony what Beuth and Rother were to Prussia. He was an ardent proponent of the need to build railroads to stimulate industrialization; he advocated the removal of barriers to trade through the creation of a customs union; and in his ministerial role it was Falkenstein who mediated the conflict between Harkort and Friedrich List which threatened to bring the Leipzig-Dresden railroad to collapse. Once the line was completed Falkenstein personally negotiated on behalf of the company to build a further line linking Munich, Nürnberg, Bamberg, and Hof.

Falkenstein was no less enlightened when it came to matters of public health. In response to the outbreak of cholera in 1831, he went to Halle and then to Prague, where he consulted with Purkyně on the appropriate countermeasures to be taken. In 1844 Falkenstein was appointed minister of the interior, a post he held until the Revolution of 1848.[55] When he returned to power as Kultusminister in 1853, Falkenstein was determined to continue his policies of bureaucratic liberalism. Two concrete concerns directed his attention toward the natural sciences. On the one hand, as Kultusminister his task was to make the university competitive in the market for students, particularly by attracting students from other German and foreign states. Leipzig had not done particularly well in student enrollment during the 1840s and early 1850s; new matriculations for that period in Leipzig averaged 357. The standard antedote of all educational ministers in this enterprise was to appoint faculty with the most outstanding reputations. A further strategy for improving enrollment, particularly in the period immediately after the revolution, was to build up the medical faculty, for these were the faculties with the largest matriculation.

But Falkenstein had another pressing concern which exerted an equal if not greater influence on his policies. Like several other states in the postrevolutionary period, Saxony was confronted with the need to improve its agricultural production. The causes behind the crisis in agriculture and its relation to increased support for the natural sciences in the universities has been best documented by Peter Borscheid's brilliant study of the Baden chemical industry.[56] As Borscheid has shown, the regime in Baden harbored no illusions about the fact that the immediate cause of the Revolution of 1848 was not unrequited demands for freedom of the press or concerns about differing slogans for national unity. It was hunger that had driven the people into the streets. The leading government officials were clear about the fact that the revolution would reerupt unless serious measures were taken to eradicate increasing hunger and poverty among the small farmers and farming proletariate. Industrialization alone could not solve the economic problems of Germany. Rather, German industrialization depended on the simultaneous expansion of agricultural production. In the face of the ever declining crop yields that resulted from soil exhaustion and the ineffectiveness of traditional farming methods, the Baden regime began to take seriously the arguments made by numerous persons before the revolution in the Baden assembly to the effect that the only solution seemed to be that offered by harnessing chemistry to the needs of agriculture. This was the program that Justus Liebig had been vigorously promoting since 1840.

Immediately after the revolution the Baden ministry of the interior set forth determined to make Heidelberg a center for chemical instruction in Germany. Over the decade from 1850 to 1860 an unprecedented 97 percent of all new expenditures at the university were devoted to expanding faculty and providing laboratories and the various support facilities for carrying through the full set of measures required to introduce the system of chemical education as conceived and promoted by Liebig.[57] Liebig's program, which was carried through in Heidelberg by Robert Bunsen, benefited not only chemistry but physiology and physics as well. Both Liebig and Bunsen were convinced that chemical instruction linking theory and practice in a manner capable of obtaining useful results for industry, agriculture, and medicine could not be achieved simply by investing in chemical laboratories. Crucial to the entire program of improving chemical education was the simultaneous development of disciplines regarded as auxiliary to chemistry. These were above all physics and physiology. Bunsen made it clear to the Baden ministry that the greatest possible cooperation had to be established between chemistry, physics, and physiology if they were to succeed in their goal.[58]

A parallel set of concerns was operative in Saxony after the revolution. Indeed, in 1851 the state educational ministry constructed an agricultural experiment station in Möckern on the outskirts of Leipzig.[59] But it was not until the 1860s, under the ministry of Falkenstein, that deliberate steps were taken to focus chemical instruction at the university on the needs of agriculture and industry.

Concerned to increase the enrollment of the university in an academic market in which it was necessary to compete with other great universities such as Heidelberg and Berlin, and conscious of the pressing economic needs of his state, Falkenstein turned his attention toward improving the Leipzig natural science faculties in 1861.[60] He seems to have been no less impressed by the Liebig model than other state ministers, but local circumstances and existing institutions dictated a different course in Leipzig. The matrix within which Falkenstein's plans for the university were worked out received its concrete shape in 1863 with the unexpected death of Otto Kühne, the professor of chemistry. In the deliberations over Kühne's successor the issues concerning both physiological chemistry and the expansion of laboratories for organic chemistry and pharmacy, neither of which had received a satisfactory resolution during the 1850s, came once again to the fore. By 1863 the ever increasing numbers of pharmacy students far exceeded the capacity of existing facilities to meet the demand. This problem could no longer be handled by a patchwork solution. In addition, the needs of the medical faculty for

a physiological chemist were now more pressing than a decade earlier.[61] Wunderlich in particular had already begun calling attention
to these needs in 1860.

In the years following Lehmann's departure the laboratory in the
Jakobshospital had fallen into total disuse. Wunderlich had come to
miss sorely the services of that laboratory, and in a lengthy memorandum he emphasized the increasing importance of physiological
chemistry and microscopic anatomy for his program of physiological
medicine.[62] For an increasing number of diseases, he observed, diagnosis without the use of the microscope and a battery of chemical
tests was unthinkable; moreover no medical school could remain
among institutions of the first rank without following the lead of
Virchow in Berlin, who had introduced advanced training in pathological chemistry. In his memorandum of 1860 Wunderlich demanded, and Falkenstein provided, a new position for an assistant
in physiological chemistry to head the laboratory in the Jakobshospital. Determined to satisfy his own immediate needs for a technician,
Wunderlich was concerned that the person filling this position
would pursue an independent research agenda with the facilities
placed at his disposal.[63] He therefore specified that the laboratory in
the hospital be directed completely by the hospital administration
and work only on problems approved by the hospital directorship.[64]
Wunderlich did not, however, dismiss the importance of contributing to the advancement of knowledge in physiological chemistry
through support of research facilities.[65] On the contrary, he suggested that in the future provision be made for advanced research in
physiological chemistry and microscopic anatomy.

In 1860 Wunderlich did not specify whether the solution he had in
mind involved separate institutes for these fields. But his suggestion
stands clearly in the background of the memorandum composed in
1863 by Falkenstein outlining the interests of the state in the matter of
Kühne's successor.[66] A primary concern of the state, he noted, was
the improvement of agriculture through the expansion of courses in
agricultural chemistry.[67] The person they chose for Kühne's replacement, therefore, should be interested in developing agricultural chemistry. The second point Falkenstein emphasized was that Leipzig was
a small university. It could not compete with larger universities such
as the University of Berlin. The state educational budget, furthermore, was limited. Under such conditions the best strategy was to
develop first-class competence in a few select areas. Falkenstein was

committed to the research ideal, but he made it clear that the expansion of research facilities, the appointment of faculty, and the support of particular disciplines were to be guided by the economic interests of the state rather than by the principle of *Wissenschaft um sich selber Willen*.

Debates in the faculty over the person to be appointed and whether the position should be in the philosophical or medical faculty dragged on for several months. Finally, in an angry memorandum dated 28 April 1865, Falkenstein urged the faculty to make the appointment as soon as possible, and he queried whether in their deliberations the faculty had come across the name of Hermann Kolbe (he knew full well they had not considered him).[68] Kolbe had been Bunsen's successor in Marburg, and he was one of the leading figures in the synthesis of organic compounds upon which the new science-based dyestuffs and pharmaceutical industries were being erected. Within a fortnight the faculty had a recommendation for the vacated chair of chemistry: it was Hermann Kolbe, who joined the faculty in the summer semester of 1865.

The circumstances surrounding Kühne's successor had highlighted certain glaring inefficiencies in the system for making appointments. If the state were going to formulate and pursue its interests in the expansion of research facilities and the hiring of personnel, then it should not allow itself to be caught unaware by the death of a professor and be forced into a makeshift policy dictated by circumstances. Furthermore, given the enormous costs of creating new facilities, it was imperative for a small university such as Leipzig to look for inventive means to fulfil a variety of needs with a single appointment. Both of these considerations played a role in the appointment of Carl Ludwig.

CONCLUSION; CLINICAL MEDICINE IN LEIPZIG AND THE "INTEGRATED APPROACH" TO PHYSIOLOGY

The script for a typical sequence of events leading up to the establishment of institutes in Germany would have the state minister, Falkenstein in our drama, seeking star talents in order to polish the reputation of his university. The star talent, Ludwig in our tale, would exploit his momentary advantage in the marketplace by demanding as a condition for recruitment the facilities and resources necessary to achieve his disciplinary goals. The real world does not always follow the script, however. In any case, the archival material concerning Carl Ludwig's call to Leipzig suggests a script altered to fit the local circumstances.

On 28 December 1864 Falkenstein sent a memorandum to the medical faculty informing them of the status of his plans for expansion.[69] Falkenstein was planning to build an institute for pathology and a separate institute for physiology. He had already laid his plans before the Saxon Ständesversammlung in its meeting the previous spring. The idea was to build the most up-to-date facilities possible, which meant that physiology had to be separated from anatomy. Falkenstein stated that he was guided by the view that in the current academic market the only way an outstanding physiologist could be won was to build such an institute. He proposed that the physiologist to be appointed also be consulted in the organization of the institute.

A second consideration guiding Falkenstein was the need to avoid a situation similar to that occasioned by the death of Kühne. Without demeaning the many services of the current ordinarius for anatomy and physiology, Ernst Heinrich Weber, Falkenstein observed that Weber's energies had diminished and that, with the rapid growth of these two fields in the last decades, it was impossible for one man to represent both. Considering the central place of physiology among the medical disciplines, Falkenstein suggested that the best course of action in preparing for the day when Weber would step down was to appoint a young but first-rank physiologist and for Weber to confine his future teaching exclusively to anatomy.

Falkenstein concluded his memorandum by stating that in his view, the man best fitting the criteria he had outlined was Carl Ludwig. It was not at all clear that he could win Ludwig for Leipzig, however, for he knew that Ludwig received a substantial salary in Vienna, and it might be difficult to offer him better conditions. Falkenstein asked the faculty to consider his proposal and comment upon it so that he could proceed. Dutifully acquiescing to a foregone conclusion, the faculty offered no opposition. Weber agreed to give up physiology, and the faculty unanimously supported the recruitment of Ludwig. Falkenstein contacted Ludwig concerning the position in the first week of January 1865.[70]

Several aspects of the events leading to Ludwig's call to Leipzig deserve critical examination. First, if his call is taken in isolation from the circumstances and limiting factors in which it developed, then the standard script based on the market model and the commitment to the research ideal provides a reasonable and satisfactory account. But as I have indicated, a broader analysis reveals the primary determinants in the decision to have been the immediate needs of the state as perceived and executed by the Kultusminister, Falkenstein. The ministerial archives indicate that prior to calling Ludwig, Falkenstein had embarked on a full-scale renovation of the science and medical faculties at Leipzig. Prompted by the need for a successor to Kühne, he determined to create a new and expanded chemical laboratory to serve agricultural students and pharmacists. But in an era when the medical faculty was the "bread and butter" of the universities, Falkenstein was equally concerned to concentrate his resources in the area of his existing strength: clinical medicine. It is no accident, in my view, that we find him in 1863 laying plans for an institute for pathological anatomy, a gynecological clinic, and an institute for physiology. At the center of these plans was the construction of the full complement of scientific institutes needed to support Carl Wunderlich's program of physiological medicine.

Since the late 1850s Wunderlich's program had continued to gain strength. By the early 1860s Wunderlich was deeply involved in his studies on thermometry. Both these studies and continued work in pathological anatomy strengthened the conviction he had repeatedly expressed over the years that the closest cooperation ought to develop among experimental physiology, pathological anatomy, and the development of diagnostic techniques for the clinic. Not only experimental physiology but also microscopic anatomy and physiological chemistry were essential components of Wunderlich's disciplinary program. For the variety of reasons that surfaced during the debate over Lehmann's proposal, and in light of the additional constraints now dictated by the institutional needs of chemistry, the preferred solution to the needs of the medical faculty was the construction of institutes for physiology and pathology, each with positions for assistants in physiological chemistry and microscopic anatomy. Before negotiations were ever commenced with a physiologist, therefore, the disciplinary objectives of the Leipzig school of clinical medicine, the fiscal restrictions within which the Saxon educational ministry was forced to operate, and existing institutional constraints had structured a field in which an integrated approach to physiology was a precondition of appointment.

In light of these considerations it is not surprising that Carl Ludwig was the only name on the list of candidates for the directorship of the physiological institute. In all the discussions concerning the institute for physiology only one name was ever mentioned. The reason, I urge, is that except for Ernst Brücke, Carl Ludwig was the only German physiologist who fit the requirements of both the disciplinary and institutional needs in Leipzig. Other outstanding physiologists—Helmholtz and du Bois-Reymond, for example— were openly interested in offers to move, but neither shared the integrated view of physiology that was growing prominent in Ludwig's work. Moreover neither of these men had Ludwig's commitment to place physiology in the service of medicine.

A more harmonious fit than that between Ludwig's perspective on physiology and Wunderlich's program for physiological medicine could scarcely be imagined. In a letter to Henle written during his years in Zürich, for example, Ludwig stated:

> It is my hope someday to work with a capable clinician or pathological anatomist at a university with a medium-sized hospital and together with him experimentally reproduce the conditions of disease. By proceeding with sufficient care, it ought to be possible to generate innumerable illnesses similar to those found in man; and were this to be accomplished, a field of investigation would be opened which would quickly pay dividends in excess of the statistical method.[71]

That Ludwig's perspective was compatible with his own was certainly not lost on Wunderlich, whose advice was crucial to Falkenstein in his plans for the university. Indeed, Ludwig's years in Vienna and the increasing number of students who were coming to study experimental physiology with him seem to have led him to the conviction that a more practical turn must be given to the discipline. Thus in the fall of 1864 as the air was filled with rumors of an impending call to Leipzig, Ludwig's thoughts turned once again to the prospects of working more closely with clinicians:

> It is a propitious sign for the future of German science that there is never a shortage of independent young researchers. But their numbers are larger than they ought to be. The number of truly inventive minds must certainly be much smaller. Why is it that so few turn their talents to practical medicine? Much more is to be accomplished at present in that domain than in ours. . . . Circumstances lie hidden

here for which either the teachers of physiology or those in the clinic are responsible.[72]

To train persons of average talent—du Bois-Reymond's "*Durch-schnittsköpfe*"—that was the mission physiology had to set for itself if it were to continue to grow and prosper as a discipline. In an era when state ministries were harnessing science to the needs of agriculture, industry, and the military, Ludwig had come to realize that in order to secure the funding for experimental apparatus and personnel essential to extending the boundaries of his discipline, it was necessary to render his science and its methods serviceable to the practical needs of clinical medicine.[73] This did not imply giving up the disinterested pursuit of knowledge. Rather, it meant coordinating scientific research with the material interests of the state. The realization of Ludwig's disciplinary aims implied that his science must become an integral part of the new system then in the process of formation, a system composed of distinct but coordinated elements: government, universities, and industry.

A few months later, on 1 May 1865, as he addressed his students and colleagues in Leipzig for the first time, Ludwig set forth the importance of the theoretical and experimental disciplines for the training of physicians. At the end of that lecture he alluded to the circumstances surrounding the establishment of the physiological institute, the clientele it was intended to serve, and the concept that had guided the state officials in the plan of its construction:

> We hope that the connection established between them [the physiological institute and the clinic] today will remain a victorious one. And if the work becomes too great for either of us, either for the physiologist or the clinician, we can be sure that the insightful directors of our university will not be sparing in providing the forces required to establish helpful, binding links between the physiological laboratory and the clinic. In this sense it is with glad thanks that I greet the decision taken by our highest administrators to establish simultaneously with the founding of the physiological institute another dedicated to experimental pathology.[74]

Ludwig was bearing witness to the intersection of the interests of modern industrializing states in supporting clinical medicine and the special constellation of institutional factors in Leipzig that brought his own recently formulated disciplinary goals to fruition.

NOTES

1. Du Bois-Reymond, "Der physiologische Unterricht sonst und jetzt," *Reden* (Leipzig, 1912), 1:645.

2. From records in the Zentrales Staatsarchiv Merseburg, Historische Abteilung II, Generalia Universitäts-Sachen, Acta betreffend "Die ordentlichen jährlichen Ausgaben für die naturwissenschaftlichen und medizinischen Institute der deutschen und österreichischen Universitäten," Rep. 76 V a Sekt. 1, Tit. XV, Nr. 17, Vol. I. Quoted from Axel Genz, *Die Emanzipation der naturwissenschaftlichen Physiologie in Berlin* (Dipl. med. diss., Magdeburg, 1976) p. 33.

3. Albert Guttstadt, *Die naturwissenschaftlichen und medicinischen Staatsanstalten Berlins* (Berlin, 1886), p. 286. The ratio of Reichsmarks to the old Prussian taler was 3:1. See Frank R. Pfetsch, *Zur Entwicklung der Wissenschaftspolitik in Deutschland 1750–1914* (Berlin: Duncker & Humblot, 1974), 93n.

4. See especially David Cahan, "The Institutional Revolution in German Physics, 1865–1914," *Historical Studies in the Physical Sciences*, 15 pt. 2 (1984); 1–65; R. Steven Turner, "Justus Liebig versus Prussian Chemistry: Reflections on Early Institute-Building in Germany," *Historical Studies in the Physical Sciences* 13 (1982): 129–162.

5. Du Bois-Reymond, "Der physiologische," p. 648.

6. This position is developed most forcefully in the writings of Joseph Ben-David, Awraham Zloczower, and R. Steven Turner.See in particular Awraham Zloczower, "Career Opportunities and the Growth of Scientific Discovery in Nineteenth-Century Germany, with Special Reference to Physiology" (Ph.D. diss., Hebrew University, Jerusalem, 1960); Joseph Ben-David and Awraham Zloczower, "Universities and Academic Systems in Modern Societies," *European Journal of Sociology* 3 (1962): 45–84; Joseph Ben-David, "Scientific Growth: A Sociological View," *Minerva* 2 (1963): 455–476; R. Steven Turner, "The Growth of Professorial Research in Prussia, 1818 to 1848—Causes and Context," *Historical Studies in the Physical Sciences* 3 (1971): 137–182; and Steven Turner, Edward Kerwin, and David Woolwine, "Careers and Creativity in Nineteenth-Century Physiology: Zloczower Redux," *Isis* 75 (1984): 523–529.

7. Guttstadt, *Der naturwissenschaftlichen*, pp. 273–274.

8. See Karl E. Rothschuh, *Physiologie. Der Wandel ihrer Konzepte, Probleme und Methoden vom 16. bis 20. Jahrhundert* (Freiburg/Munich: Alber Verlag, 1968); Ilse Jahn, Rolf Löther, and Konrad Senglaub, *Geschichte der Biologie: Theorien, Methoden, Institutionen und Kurzbiographieen* (Jena: Gustav Fischer Verlag, 1982).

9. Du Bois-Reymond, "Der physiologische," pp. 647–648, 651.

10. William Coleman, "The Cognitive Basis of the Discipline: Claude Bernard on Physiology," *Isis* 76 (1985): 49–70.

11. Excerpted and published by P. Morawitz in an article entitled "Vor Hundert Jahren im Laboratorium Johannes Müllers, von weil. Prof. Dr.

Friedrich Bidder, Dorpat," *Münchener medizinischer Wochenschrift* 81 (1934): 60–64.

12. Ibid., p. 62.

13. Ibid.

14. Ibid., p. 63.

15. See Manfred Stürzbecher, "Zur Berufung Johannes Müllers an die Berliner Universität," *Jahrbuch für die Geschichte Mittel- und Ostdeutschlands* 21 (1972): 184–226, esp. 192.

16. See Turner, "Justus Liebig versus Prussian Chemistry," esp. pp. 133–139.

17. Genz, *Emanzipation der naturwissenschaften*, p. 7.

18. Johanna Bleker, *Die naturhistorische Schule 1825–1845. Ein Beitrag zur Geschichte der klinischen Medizin in Deutschland* (Stuttgart: Gustav Fischer Verlag, 1981).

19. Carl Wunderlich, "Das Verhältniss der physiologischen Medicin zur ärtzlichen Praxis," *Archiv für physiologische Heilkunde* 4 (1845): 1–13. The various programs for scientific medicine that proliferated during the 1840s are discussed in Bleker, *Die naturhistorische Schule* pp. 114–126.

20. Vorlesungsverzeichniss of the University of Berlin, 1839.

21. See chapter 2 of the present volume, by Arleen Tuchman.

22. This course appears in the *Verzeichniss* for the first time in the summer semester of 1842. Ehrenberg continued to offer it every year thereafter.

23. These courses were announced in the listings under the natural sciences in the philosophical faculty.

24. See Theodor Billroth, *Über das Lehren und Lernen der medicinischen Wissenschaften an den Universitäten der deutschen Nation nebst allgemeinen Bemerkungen über Universitäten. Eine culturhistorische Studie* (Vienna, 1876), pp. 208–213.

25. Carl Ludwig, *De viribus physicis secretionem urinae adjuvantibus* (Marburg, 1842).

26. Carl Ludwig, "Nieren und Harnbereitung," in *Handwörterbuch der Physiologie*, ed. Rudolph Wagner (Göttingen, 1844), 2: 628 ff.

27. Ernst Brücke, "Beiträge zur Lehre von der Diffusion tropfbarer flüssiger Körper durch porose Scheidewände," *Poggendorff's Annalen der Physik* 58 (1843): 77–94.

28. Friedrich Goll, "Über den Einfluss des Blutdrucks auf die Harnabsonderung," *Henle und Pfeuffers Zeitschrift für rationale Medizin* IV, new series (1854): 78 ff.; Max Hermann, "Über den Einfluss des Blutdrucks auf die Sekretion des Harnes," *Sitzungsberichte der Kaiserlichen Akademie der Wissenschaften zu Wien* 45 (1862): 317 ff. These results are summarized in Ludwig, "Einige neue Beziehungen zwischen dem Bau und der Funktion der Niere," *Sitzungsberichte der Kaiserlichen Akademie der Wissenschaften zu Wien* 49 (1863): 725 ff.

29. Carl Eduard Loebell, *De conditionibus quibus secretiones in glandulis perficiuntur* (med. diss., Marburg, 1849).

30. Ludwig to Henle, 23 March 1849, in Astrid Dreher, ed.,*Briefe von Carl

Ludwig an Jacob Henle aus den Jahren 1846–1872 (med. diss., Heidelberg, 1980), pp. 68–70.

31. Ibid., 6 December 1855, in Dreher, *Briefe*, pp. 149–150.

32. Ibid., 11 July 1860, in ibid., p. 172.

33. Ibid., 30 May 1853, in ibid., pp. 118–119.

34. Ibid., 18 October 1857, in ibid., pp. 156–157.

35. Ibid., p. 157.

36. Ibid., 3 June 1863, in ibid., p. 184.

37. Ibid., 18 August 1863, in ibid., p. 186.

38. Ibid., p. 187.

39. See Ludwig, "Einige neue Beziehungen zwischen dem Bau und der Funktion der Niere," *Sitzungsberichte der Kaiserlichen Akademie der Wissenschaften zu Wien* 49 (1863): 725 ff.

40. Ludwig to Henle, 19 July 1846 in Dreher, *Briefe*, p. 44.

41. Ibid., 14 April 1854, in ibid., p. 122.

42. Ibid., p. 122.

43. Ibid., pp. 122–123. My emphasis.

44. Ibid., p. 123.

45. Ibid., 7 December 1857, in ibid., p. 160.

46. Ibid., 17 April 1867, in ibid., pp. 214–215.

47. Ibid. (n.d.), March 1870, in ibid., p. 225.

48. See the discussion in Max Lenz, *Geschichte der königlichen Friedrich-Wilhelms-Universität zu Berlin*, 4 vols. (Halle, 1910–1918), vol. 2. An outstanding example of this reform literature is provided by the pamphlet written by Gustav Karsten but published anonymously, *Von der Stellung der Naturwissenschaften, besonders der physikalischen, an unseren Universitäten* (Kiel, 1849). Carl Ludwig also participated in efforts to reform science education in Marburg during 1849. His role in university reform politics was responsible for his departure from Germany.

49. Discussed by Theodor Billroth, *Über das Lehren und Lernen der medicinischen Wissenschaften an den Universitäten der deutschen Nation nebst allgemeinen Bemerkungen über Universitäten* (Wien, 1876), pp. 169–175. This point has been emphasized more recently by Thomas Nipperdey, *Deutsche Geschichte 1800–1866. Bürgerwelt und starker Staat* (Munich: Beck, 1984), pp. 142–143. The role of increased standards as a strategy employed by professionalizing physicians during the 1840s in Baden is explored by Arleen Tuchman in her dissertation *Science, Medicine and the State: The Institutionalization of Scientific Medicine at the University of Heidelberg* (Ph.D. diss., University of Wisconsin, 1985).

I have emphasized the importance of technical competence and experimental control as a professionalization strategy employed among competitors for academic positions in medical faculties during the 1840s in "Social Interests and the Organic Physics of 1847," to appear in Yehuda Elkana, ed., *Israel-Boston Colloquium Series in the History and Philosophy of Science*, in press.

50. This factor is credited by Billroth for an increased interest in scientific medicine. See Billroth, *Über des Lehren*, p. 246. The effects of the cholera epidemics in reshaping attitudes of German physicians toward scientific

medicine has not, to my knowledge, been explored. It is a topic much in need of further attention.

51. Universitätsarchiv Leipzig, Med. Fak. B III, Nr. 2b, Bd. I: Acta das Lehrstuhl für physiologische Chemie betreffend, Bl. 1–16. (Henceforth cited as Lehmann, *Denkschrift*).

52. Lehmann, *Denkschrift*, Bl. 4–6.

53. Lehmann, *Denkschrift*, Bl. 9R–11R.

54. Universitätsarchiv Leipzig, UAL, Med. Fak. B III, 2b, Bd. I: Bl. 19–22, quoted from Bl. 22.

55. See "Falkenstein," in the *Allgemeine deutsche Biographie*, vol. 48, pp. 489–494. His departure from office in 1848 prevented Falkenstein from introducing the plans he had formulated for introducing freedom of the press and a revision of the chambers along English lines.

56. Peter Borscheid, *Naturwissenschaft, Staat und Industrie in Baden (1818–1914)*, (Stuttgart: Klett Verlag, 1976).

57. Ibid., p. 80.

58. Ibid., pp. 76–78.

59. Ibid., p. 107. Also see *Verein Deutscher Dünger-Fabrikanten 1880–1930. Die Geschichte des Vereins in den letzten 25 Jahren 1905–1930* (Hamburg, 1930), p. 358.

60. Falkenstein's efforts to increase enrollment through his policy of attracting the most outstanding faculty and expanding the science facilities of the university are described by Friedrich Zarncke in the annual address he delivered as rector of the university in October 1871. See *Reden der Universität Leipzig beim Rektoratswechsel*, pp. 7 ff.

Zarncke noted the following new matriculations (in hundreds) as a result of Falkenstein's efforts:

1862	400 +
1865	500 +
1867	700 +
1869	800 +
1870	900 +
1871	1100 +

61. See UAL, Med. Fak. B III, 2b, Bd. II, Acta physiologisch-chemische Lehrstelle betreffend, 1863. This supports the claim of R. Steven Turner that expanding facilities for pharmacy students was a major desideratum in the post 1848 period. See Turner, "Justus Liebig versus Prussian Chemistry."

62. UAL, Med. Fak. B III, 2b, Bd. I: Bl. 62–68R (Memorandum of Wunderlich to the medical faculty, April 1860. Henceforth cited as Wunderlich, *Denkschrift*).

63. Ibid., Bl. 66–67.

64. Ibid., Bl. 63–63R.

65. Ibid., Bl. 68.

66. UAL, Med. Fak. B III, 2b, Bd. II: Bl. 26–28R (Memorandum of Falkenstein to the faculty, 9 December 1864. Henceforth cited as Falkenstein, *Memorandum*).

67. Ibid., Bl. 27R–28.
68. UAL, Med. Fak. B III, 2b, Bd. II: Bl. 62–68 (Falkenstein, *Memorandum*, 28 April 1865).
69. Universitätsarchiv Leipzig, Med. Fak. Bd. V 1864: UAL, PA 2243, Acta Prof. Ludwig betreffend: Bl. 1–13.
70. Although a newspaper report of the meeting of the Saxon Standesversammlung in which Falkenstein's plans were debated indicated that Ludwig would receive a call to Leipzig, in letters to Henle and du Bois-Reymond Ludwig insisted that the first and only contact he had with Leipzig was in the first week of January. See Ludwig to Henle, 26 January 1865, in Dreher, *Briefe*, p. 197.

Ludwig to du Bois-Reymond, 30 October 1864, *Zwei grosse Naturforscher des 19. Jahrhunderts. Ein Briefwechsel zwischen Emil du Bois-Reymond und Carl Ludwig*, ed. Estelle du Bois-Reymond and Paul Diepgen (Leipzig, 1927), pp. 156–157.

For his own part Falkenstein was adamant about the "leak" of his plan to recruit Ludwig before formal contact had been made. A connoisseur of the entrepreneurial spirit, Falkenstein pointed out that telegraphing his moves could only result in driving Ludwig's price up, perhaps beyond the limits his budget could bear. See Falkenstein's memorandum, Universitätsarchiv Leipzig, Med. Fak. Bd. V 1864.

71. Ludwig to Henle, 5 September 1852, in Dreher, *Briefe*, p. 112.
72. Ibid., 27 October 1864, in ibid., pp. 195–196.
73. In a letter to Helmholtz dated 6 February 1865, Ludwig intimated that persistent difficulties in convincing the Austrian government to provide better facilities for his research at the Josepheneum was a major factor in his decision to leave Vienna. See Ludwig to Helmholtz, 6 February 1865, Nachlass Helmholtz, Akademie der Wissenschaften der DDR, Berlin.
74. Carl Ludwig, *Die physiologischen Leistungen des Blutdrucks* (Leipzig, 1865) p. 24.

CHAPTER FIVE

The Formation of the Munich School of Metabolism

Frederic L. Holmes

The relations between scientific investigations and the institutions within which they take place are complex. These connections cannot be captured in simple formulas, such as that local institutional settings "shape" research programs; nor, in the converse, that the state of development of the scientific disciplines determines the forms of the institutions that will house them. Local factors interact at multiple levels with larger-scale configurations, both spatial and temporal. Intensive studies of events within localized settings can nevertheless reveal to advantage the nature of those developments that occur along the intersections between intellectual and institutional history. As the essays in the present volume suggest, the relations between the science that is pursued in a particular place and the contextual framework within which it is pursued vary widely from case to case. We should therefore avoid premature generalization. Only through numerous detailed studies of specific historical situations can we come to understand "the ways in which natural knowledge is . . . enveloped by material conditions and institutional restrictions."[1]

In order to elucidate the dynamics of scientific activity within localized settings, historians have recently begun to focus on scientific "schools" and "research groups." Often, although not invariably, such units function within physically bounded institutions, such as academic departments or research institutes. There is therefore considerable overlap in the identities of schools, research groups, and institutional structures. Frequently these terms appear to define different perspectives on the same activities. A research group or a school is often synonymous with a "laboratory." A scientific school may be viewed as a forceful research group, commonly operating within an institutional structure. A research group may be said to attain the level of a school if it displays a distinctive style of work or a prominent research program in which its members participate, and it exerts some influence upon the practice of science in its field beyond its immediate setting. Frequently, but not inevitably, a research school coalesces around the strong leadership of a single founder. Research schools tend to be concentrated in local institutions because personal influences and styles have the most powerful effects on people working in physical proximity to one another. A scientific school, even if it is characterized as a "research school," ordinarily includes an educational dimension, since participation of the younger members in the research activity serves simultaneously as training for future independent work. Gerald Geison has recently given a definition of a research school that incorporates all of these criteria. By "research schools," he writes, "I mean small groups of mature scientists pursuing a reasonably coherent program of research side-by-side with advanced students in the same institutional context and engaging in direct, continuous social and intellectual interaction."[2]

Geison's definition may be taken to represent an "ideal type," which any given research school resembles to some degree but from which each particular school is likely to deviate somewhat in one or more of its features. An important recent article by Joseph S. Fruton points out that styles of scientific leadership in research groups vary widely, reflecting divergent individual personalities as well as disciplinary or institutional conditions. At one extreme, the director of such a group may bind the efforts of all of its members tightly to his personal research agenda. At the other end of the spectrum, he may subordinate his own research interests in order to nurture the diverse interests and strengths of the younger members of his group.[3] Kathryn Olesko's study of Franz Neumann's pioneering physics seminar at Königsberg shows that a scientific school may owe its coherence mainly to a training program stressing the acquisition of skills, rather than to a research program aimed at specific unsolved problems.[4] Moreover, considering that the influence of an important scientific leader normally spreads beyond his local group, research at some other institutions in his field may come to resemble his own sufficiently to appear as extensions of his school. When those trained within one school move to positions in other institutions, some of them may implant "colonies" of the research groups from which they have come, so that the school ceases to be identified exclusively with its original home. These, and further modifying influences that we might readily add, suggest that the research school is a pliable entity and that it will be fruitful to examine the formation and growth of numerous such entities in depth in order to grasp the range of variations compatible with the generalized concept.

The Munich School of Metabolism provides a rich case for examining the interplay of scientific, personal, and institutional factors that condition the formation of a research school. In its mature stage it exhibited the hallmark features of a scientific school that was at once a local research group working within a formally structured institute and also an influence diffused across an international field of activity. For four decades the Munich school dominated the investigation of metabolism. Its leader, Carl Voit, directed an overarching research program that could be sustained indefinitely while generating numerous subproblems that members of his group could solve in reasonable lengths of time. Voit's own early successes, and his forceful leadership, had such impact that his student and successor, Otto Frank, could realistically assert after his death "that all laboratories in which exact metabolic investigations are now being carried out have been, in their way of working, directly or indirectly influenced by the methods of the Munich Institute."[5]

As Frank's statement indicates, the Munich school was identified with a particular institution, the Munich Physiological Institute, which was housed in a well-defined physical structure. Within its walls Voit gathered a circle of younger investigators, who were both research assistants and advanced students being prepared for future scientific careers of their own. Voit was known not only as the leader of this research group but as a dedicated, inspiring teacher.[6] At its peak the Munich Institute must have appeared a highly coherent integration of research activity, institutional form, and social utility. Its director, its physical facilities, much of its teaching, its experimental work, and its extensive consulting functions on practical problems of nutrition must have projected a harmonious composite image, reflecting a unified nexus of concerns.

The subject of the present chapter is not the character of the Munich school in its fully developed state but its origins. Unlike the institutes described in some other essays in this volume, the Munich

Physiological Institute was not the realization of a design clearly planned from the beginning. The eventual state of affairs was the unforeseen outcome of interactions between various personal aspirations and responses to opportunities and restrictions not controlled by any single vision or authority. The Munich Institute emerged from negotiations, partnerships, and compromises between individuals with diverse personal purposes and views and differing perspectives on the educational and research objectives that this institution might serve.

The research program that became so closely associated with the Munich Physiological Institute did not originate there. It was created by a combination of the ideas of Justus Liebig at the University of Giessen and the decision of Theodor Bischoff to join Liebig in Giessen in order to test Liebig's ideas experimentally. Before these two could get under way, however, a research program strongly influenced by Liebig's views emerged at the distant University of Dorpat. Liebig and Bischoff were, in turn, influenced by the results attained in Dorpat. When Liebig and Bischoff were successively called to Munich as part of the plan of King Maximilian II to make his capital a major center for *Wissenschaft,* their research program migrated with them. There it was grafted onto an institute that had recently been founded with a scientific orientation unrelated to Liebig and Bischoff's research aims. The history of the formation of the Munich School of Metabolism is therefore not coextensive with the local history of the Munich Physiological Institute, even though the research program and the institution that came to house it eventually became nearly synonymous.

I

The moving spirit behind the research program that ultimately shaped the Munich School was Liebig. The views Liebig published in 1842 in his influential book *Animal Chemistry* provided the conceptual inspiration from which the program emerged. Moreover Liebig's command of research facilities in the laboratory at Giessen, which he had established as the leading center in Europe for chemical experimentation and teaching, and his immense personal stature in Germany enabled him to direct extensive attention and resources toward solution of the problems he posed. Because these problems required investigations in domains outside his own fields of professional competence, however, he could not personally implement the full program of experimental testing that his formulation of animal chemistry invited. The success of his endeavor depended, therefore, as much upon his ability to attract others to take up the problems he defined as upon his ability to pursue them himself.

The point of departure for Liebig's *Animal Chemistry* was the theory of respiration developed by Antoine Lavoisier half a century earlier. Lavoisier had viewed respiration as a form of combustion in which carbon and hydrogen are combined with oxygen to form carbonic acid and water, releasing animal heat.[7] Liebig restated Lavoisier's theory in a form that incorporated the knowledge of organic compounds that had accumulated during the five intervening decades. The carbon and hydrogen he could now describe as constituents of the two classes of nonnitrogenous nutrient compounds, carbohydrates and fats, which he designated *respiratory aliments*.[8]

To the nitrogenous foodstuffs Liebig assigned a quite different role. They were the *plastic aliments,* for only they became assimilated into the organized tissue of the body. Liebig reached this conclusion from recent elementary analyses carried out by the Dutch chemist G. J. Mulder, and extended in his own laboratory, which appeared to indicate that the proportions of carbon, hydrogen, oxygen, and nitrogen were identical in the major recognized classes of nitrogenous animal substances—albumin, fibrin, and casein—and that for each of these substances there were corresponding substances in plants. Whether an animal were a carnivore or an herbivore, therefore, no extensive changes in chemical composition seemed to be required to convert nitrogenous food substances into blood and blood into organized tissue, and Liebig assumed that none took place.[9]

In the course of producing the vital actions that tissues carry out, Liebig argued, some of its substance must be broken down. In particular, the mechanical effects that muscles produce cause part of the muscle substance to be degraded, losing its functional properties, and it was this particular process that he designated the *Stoffwechsel*. The breakdown products are swept into the circulation. The nitrogenous portion is excreted through the kidneys in the form of urea or uric acid, whereas the nonnitrogenous residue is carried to the liver, secreted as bile, and reabsorbed into the blood until it is gradually consumed by respiratory oxidation.[10]

Liebig's account of what goes on inside the animal was highly speculative. He derived it by combining his own deep knowledge of the chemical properties of the substances then regarded as the main constituents of plant and animal matter with a superficial knowledge of physiology gleaned from standard textbooks and a few journal articles. Nevertheless his analysis was brilliant and revealing. No one since Lavoisier had so fully perceived that the balance of matter consumed in respiration and supplied in nutrition, and the connection between these processes and the production of heat and motion, were the principles around which the entire complex of internal chemical changes could be understood. No one before him had ever attempted to integrate within this framework all of the current knowledge of the substances involved, to construct a broad picture of how these internal processes might be organized. In his *Animal Chemistry* Liebig displayed the fresh illumination that an imaginative scientist can provide when he crosses disciplines to bring the experience he has acquired in his own field to bear on unsolved problems in an adjacent field. His approach also exhibited, however, the drawbacks of being a novice in the field he entered.

Liebig's teaching laboratory was organized in such a way that the students made a gradual transition from elementary analytical exercises to assigned research projects that reflected Liebig's own experimental interests. When his interests changed, therefore, he was able to change the direction not only of his own personal research but that of an entire group of advanced students. During the 1840s he and his students concentrated much of their effort upon the chemistry of substances that were significant to his physiological views. Because the nature of muscle substance had been fundamental to his conception of the chemical processes within animals, he gave special priority to reinvestigating experimentally what was known about the organic compounds contained in this tissue. In 1847 he published a monograph summarizing the results he and his students had attained. They confirmed that muscle is composed largely of albumin and muscle fiber. They verified also that it contains lactic acid, and they found in addition two highly nitrogenous compounds: creatine and creatinine.[11]

Such results were essential to an eventually more refined understanding of the conversion of nutrients to tissue and of tissue to breakdown products, but they did not bear directly on the most salient and controversial physiological claims Liebig had made. One claim was that bile is reabsorbed in large enough quantities to account for the passage into the blood of the nonnitrogenous residues of the *Stoffwechsel* consumed in respiration; another was that all nitrogenous aliments must become part of organized tissue before decomposing to give the nitrogenous end products; still another claim was that "the quantity of the tissue substance decomposed in a given time is measurable through the nitrogen content of the urine."[12] Such views could be tested only by experiments on living animals and humans. Liebig's laboratory was not equipped for such experiments, however, nor did his personal scientific experience prepare him to undertake them. Liebig himself soon came to appreciate some of his limitations. Harsh criticisms of his book[13] led him to realize, by 1843, that the chemist who ventures alone into animal chemistry "makes too many physiological errors, through which the impression made even by the best work is weakened, often entirely destroyed." The two sciences of chemistry and physiology, he predicted, would have to be joined if more progress was to be made, eventually by training people "who know the organism precisely and who are at the same time confident with chemical work." In the meantime the gap could be filled if the chemist were to collaborate with someone able to compensate for his lack of anatomical and physiological expertise.[14]

Some physiologists rejected Liebig's *Animal Chemistry* for reasons similar to those to which he alluded in the earlier passage. Some of his protégés accepted it uncritically and began enthusiastically to promote it. More significant than either of these extremes was the response of a number of well-established physiologists, including Johannes Müller. Instead of dismissing it for the naiveté of its description of certain anatomical and physiological details, they appreciated that Liebig brought to their subject a perspective from which they could greatly benefit. Younger physiologists were especially attracted to Liebig. Some of them saw in his *Animal Chemistry*, and in the investigations in his laboratory which had led up to it, the dawn of a new era, and they tried to associate their work with his leadership.[15]

II

Soon after the appearance of *Animal Chemistry*, Liebig himself acquired the potential collaborator who could supply his need for deeper physiological and anatomical knowledge. Theodor Bischoff, who taught those subjects at Heidelberg, had reviewed Liebig's book very favorably in Müller's *Archiv* in 1842, emphasizing that the conclusions Liebig had reached were of the greatest importance, even though they called for further proofs, and perhaps even some corrections, by anatomists and physiologists. Liebig wrote Bischoff in 1843, asking him to bring to his attention any weak points in the book. Bischoff replied with a meticulous critique that both praised its main ideas and pointed out significant flaws that resulted from Liebig's anatomical and physiological misconceptions. Soon afterward Bischoff accepted an offer to come to Giessen as professor of physiology. After his arrival he and Liebig began almost daily exchanges of views on subjects related to Liebig's views on animal chemistry. For a long time, however, they did not make any investigative progress. The main obstacle to such research was probably the heavy load of other responsibilities Bischoff took on with his new position. In 1844 he became in addition professor of descriptive and comparative anatomy. In Giessen he found no organizational structure or anatomical materials for his teaching. During the next six years he established an anatomical and physiological institute, oversaw the construction of a building to house it, and built up an anatomical collection. He also devoted much time to his lectures, and continued his investigations in mammalian embryology. There was no close link between Bischoff's primary teaching and research fields and the kind of experimental program that Liebig's views on animal chemistry invited.[16]

While Liebig and Bischoff delayed, the first collaborative team of the type Liebig had envisioned entered the investigative field, not in Giessen but in the German-speaking University of Dorpat in far-off Latvia. Carl Schmidt, trained in chemistry in Liebig's own laboratory, became *Privatdozent* in physiological chemistry at Dorpat in 1846 and there encountered Friedrich Bidder, professor of Pathology, who had been trained in anatomy by Johannes Müller. Schmidt and Bidder decided to undertake a joint research endeavor that would include studies both of the rate of flow of the digestive fluids within the organism and of the exchange of materials between the organism and the environment. Beginning in 1847 they carried out a long series of experiments that culminated in 1852 in their landmark monograph, *The Digestive Fluids and the Stoffwechsel*. The portion of their investigation concerned with the *Stoffwechsel* included numerous measurements of the food intake of cats and their excretions in the form of urine and feces, under a variety of dietary conditions, as

well as measurements over short periods of their respiratory gaseous exchanges.[17]

From each of these experiments Bidder and Schmidt calculated a
complete balance sheet of the quantities of carbon, hydrogen, nitrogen, and oxygen consumed by the animal in its food, drink, and
inspired air, and the quantities of each of these elements excreted in
the urine, feces, and expired gases. In order to do this they first had
to analyze samples of the meat fed to the animals to determine how
much water, fat, and muscle fiber plus collagen it contained, and
then to establish the elementary composition of these substances.
They could then express the matter consumed in terms of the total
quantities of each of the elements. If the animal gained weight, they
counted the gain as meat assimilated to its tissues and deducted that
amount from the quantity of meat they treated as consumed. In
most of their experiments the nitrogen contained in the alimentary
meat and the muscle substance consumed (when the animal lost
weight) was very nearly accounted for by the quantity of nitrogen
excreted.[18]

Although Bidder and Schmidt did not explicitly describe their investigation as an application of Liebig's views, they clearly thought
about the problems of nutrition and respiration from within the framework that he had provided. Implicitly they treated his ideas not as a
rigid doctrine but as the outline for a research program. They did not
hesitate to modify specific aspects of his physiological system, as
when they found that the quantity of bile reabsorbed was far too small
to account for a significant proportion of the respiratory oxidations.
Finding a large difference between the rate of formation of urea when
the animal was fed the minimum diet required to maintain its weight
and the rate when it was fed a rich nitrogen diet, they designated the
latter condition a *"Luxusconsumtion."*[19]

In 1850, when Bidder and Schmidt were nearing the end of their
Stoffwechsel investigation in Dorpat, Liebig and Bischoff were finally
getting under way on their own collaborative venture in Giessen.
Bischoff, who was to carry out the animal experiments, intended to
concentrate on the relation of the formation of urea to the *Stoffwechsel*, a project that would require numerous measurements of the
urea content of urine. Believing that the difficulty of carrying out so
many analyses with the tedious methods currently available was the
largest obstacle he faced, he pressed Liebig to find a simpler, more
rapid method. After working on the problem intently for a long time

and devising method after method that proved inadequate to Bischoff's purpose, Liebig finally came up with a procedure, based on titration with mercurous nitrate, that could be carried out with great ease. When he reported on the method in 1851, Liebig stressed how important it had been to work it out in cooperation with a physiologist. It was, he claimed, only because Bischoff could test the application of each method that many difficulties came to light and that they were able to arrive at a chemical method fully suitable "to solve a physiological problem." Liebig thus appeared to be aware that he was now beginning the collaboration he had foreseen a decade earlier as the first step toward bringing together the sciences of chemistry and physiology.[20]

Bischoff began the physiological experiments on 1 January 1852. Keeping a large dog in a cage arranged so that he could collect all of its urine and feces, he measured its daily urea output for a period of eight months. During that time he fed the dog different types of diets, ranging from fasting to pure meat, pure fat, bread, combinations of meat and fat and of meat and carbohydrate. For each type of diet he varied systematically the daily quantities of the aliments.[21]

Not long after Bischoff had begun this work, Bidder and Schmidt's book appeared. The publication of their *Stoffwechsel* investigation made a strong impact on the nascent Giessen effort. The most visible effect was negative. Bischoff vehemently rejected their concept of *Luxusconsumtion* as deadly to Liebig's views on animal chemistry. A major motivation in his subsequent course was to disprove their assertion. He also thought that they had tried to include too many factors in their complicated experiments and inferences. Nevertheless from the changes in procedures that he began to make in his own experiments, and from the form in which he presented his results, it is evident that Bischoff adopted some of the methods and standards that Bidder and Schmidt had introduced into this emerging research field.[22]

No sooner had the investigative link between chemistry and physiology been forged at Giessen than it was broken again by Liebig's departure from the institution at which he had established his career, his school, and his reputation. During the summer of 1852 he accepted a call from Munich to become professor of chemistry. The Bavarian king, Maximilian II, personally intervened to bring Liebig to his capital as part of his strong commitment to use his own resources to advance all areas of *Wissenschaft* in Bavaria. Maximilian wished particularly to support those fields, such as physics, chemistry, and technology, which were most suited to favor the solution of practical problems because he hoped to bring science and industry into closer touch. His aims were typical of an era in which the growing power of science to foster economic and social progress was becoming ever more visible. Maximilian pursued such policies with special fervor because of his own deep respect for all forms of learning and his concern that in an age in which the monarchical principle had been severely shaken he must demonstrate that he could further the material interests as well as the spiritual needs of Bavarian citizens.[23]

As part of his plan Maximilian hoped to establish new institutions to stimulate research and teaching in science and technology; but he and his advisers soon came to appreciate that if they were to make Munich a leading center for *Wissenschaft*, they had to attract outstanding leaders in various fields to migrate there. Liebig was a prime target for such aims. Not only was his scientific prestige enormous, but he himself had become increasingly preoccupied with the practical applications of chemistry to agriculture, industry, and medicine. With the new views on agricultural chemistry that he had been promulgating since 1840 he was attempting to transform the ways in which farmers grew crops. His animal chemistry, too, acquired a practical orientation as he focused in his popular writings on his theories of nutrition as the essential basis for utilizing available food resources in the most efficient manner to provide for the nutritional requirements of the people.[24]

In order to entice Liebig to Munich, Maximilian provided him with a new laboratory, generous budgets, and freedom from all responsibilities that did not interest him. Liebig accepted the offer in part because he had long grown weary of the arduous teaching burdens he carried in Giessen, in part because he believed that in the future only universities in the larger German states would have the resources necessary to meet the growing needs of the burgeoning sciences, and in part because Munich was a more lustrous setting than Giessen in which to play the part of a scientific statesman.[25]

For Theodor Bischoff, Munich's gain was a devastating loss. The little provincial town of Giessen suddenly ceased to have the attraction for him that it had held when scientific exchanges with Liebig were central to his daily professional life. For a time he was too dispirited to continue the experimental investigation they had begun together. Worse still, when he began to reduce the data from the experiments already completed, he ran into difficulties for which he sorely missed Liebig's presence and help. He began writing Liebig frequently for advice about the many pitfalls he was encountering, and he lamented that his own chemical experience was inadequate to resolve the analytical discrepancies he found. The problem that most tormented him was that when he compared the quantity of nitrogen excreted in the urine with that supplied in the food or from the animal's own flesh, one third or more of the nitrogen consumed was regularly "missing." Bischoff could find no persuasive explanation for this deficit. A second vexation for him was that the addition of fat to a meat diet in some circumstances increased the quantity of urea excreted, in contradiction to Liebig's theory that nonnitrogenous aliments protect some of the nitrogenous tissue substance from decomposition. Early in 1853 Bischoff began a second series of experiments on another dog, hoping to obtain more satisfactory results, but the same problems continued to plague him.[26]

In spite of these unresolved dilemmas and his deep private doubts about the validity of his results, Bischoff proceeded to incorporate them into a lengthy monograph entitled "Urea as a Measure of the *Stoffwechsel*," which appeared during the spring of 1853. Putting the best light he could on the experimental difficulties, he interpreted the experiments as a confirmation of Liebig's views on animal chemistry. In particular he believed that he had been able to lay to rest a threat to Liebig's theories that Theodor Frerichs had posed five years earlier. Finding that a fasting dog excreted only a small fraction of the urea that it did on a mixed diet of meat and vegetables, Frerichs had inferred in 1848 that the nitrogenous aliments in excess of the minimum nutritional requirement must be oxidized directly in the blood. Bidder and Schmidt's concept of *Luxusconsumtion* was, in Bischoff's view, a second expression of the same idea. In refuting these claims Bischoff believed he had successfully defended Liebig's conception that all of the nitrogen excreted represented the products of the *Stoffwechsel* as Liebig defined it.[27]

III

In 1852 Maximilian's plans to attract distinguished scientists and to provide them with ample facilities resulted in the foundation of the Munich Physiological Institute. Carl von Siebold, the successor to Purkyně as director of the Physiological Institute in Breslau,[28] accepted an offer to come to Munich as professor of comparative anatomy and physiology and to establish a physiological institute to complement the existing Anatomical Institute. When he arrived, in April 1853, one of Siebold's first tasks was to supervise construction of the building that would house the new institute.[29]

The choice of Siebold indicates that the Physiological Institute was not envisioned as a home for the type of experimental physiology that was emerging in France around Claude Bernard and in Germany around the group that included Carl Ludwig and Emil du Bois-Reymond, whose practitioners were seeking autonomy from anatomy. Rather, it was conceived from the viewpoint of an older generation, exemplified by Johannes Müller, for whom anatomy and physiology were intimately connected. Siebold's own original research had been in the fields of zoology and comparative anatomy. His special field of interest was the invertebrates. He had elucidated the life cycles of parasitic worms, established the definition of protozoa as single-celled organisms, and produced a comprehensive handbook of comparative anatomy based largely on his own observations. Beyond constructing the institute itself, Siebold's most urgent priority in his new position was to build up the comparative anatomy collections.[30]

After he accepted the offer, Siebold found that in addition to the two fields for which he was officially responsible, he would be required to give lectures in human anatomy. It was recognized that he would be overburdened, and even before his arrival plans were under way to appoint a second professor of physiology. The first person approached for the post was Jacob Henle, who had revitalized the teaching of anatomy and physiology in Heidelberg after his arrival there in 1843[31] and had just moved to Göttingen. The acquisition of Henle would have reinforced the anatomical orientation of the Physiological Institute, for Henle was one of the leading investigators of the microscopic anatomy of tissues oriented around the cell theory of Theodor Schwann. Negotiations with Henle broke down, however, and rumors began to circulate that Johannes Müller would receive the next offer.[32]

During the course of this search Liebig began to exert an influence on its direction. On 18 April 1853 he wrote to Bischoff to inquire if Bischoff himself would be interested in the position.[33] For Liebig's interests Bischoff would be an ideal choice. His background in anatomy and embryology would make him very suitable for an institution featuring the anatomical aspects of physiology. In his teaching Bischoff would emphasize conventional gross anatomical dissections and microscopical observations, just as Henle would have done. Bischoff's presence, however, would also provide Liebig with an opening to revive within that institution his own research program for physiological chemistry. For Bischoff such a move would enable him to rejoin that person whose company he so missed and to revitalize the joint experimental enterprise that he was now on the point of abandoning in his isolation.

Nevertheless Bischoff did not leap at the chance to regain in Munich what he had lost in Giessen. He was reluctant to leave the place where his family had close personal ties. He resisted abandoning the fine anatomical collection and facilities he had built up, in order to start over where nothing comparable existed. He distrusted the political and bureaucratic system in Bavaria and believed that academics were not accorded the same legal protection and other benefits there that they enjoyed elsewhere in Germany. Although he respected Maximilian's objectives and integrity, he felt that the situation depended too heavily on that monarch's uncertain health. Within the organization of the Physiological Institute itself he saw major problems. There were questions about Siebold's attitude toward him, about how the teaching responsibilities and authority over the resources of the institute would be divided between them. Learning that there were two adjunct professors of anatomy whom he regarded as incompetent and as creatures of the "ultra-Montanes," who were hostile to academics recruited from other parts of Germany, he refused to consider coming unless these impediments were removed. He made it clear to Liebig that his only motivation for coming to Munich at all would be so that the two could work together again.[34]

Liebig was as persistent as Bischoff was recalcitrant. Acting as intermediary, Liebig pursued negotiations between Bischoff and the Bavarian Ministry of Education for more than a year and a half. Each time the matter appeared settled, Bischoff found reason to draw back. Not until the beginning of 1855 was he ready to give his final acceptance. In April of that year he finally made the move.[35]

The institution that Bischoff joined had become a patchwork, stitched together out of the diverse interests of those who found places in it. Bischoff and Siebold worked out mutually satisfactory arrangements for sharing responsibilities and resources. Siebold became conservator of the anatomical collection and retained the teaching of zoology and comparative anatomy, while Bischoff took over the lectures in physiology and human anatomy. Siebold shared with him the budget for instruments in the Physiological Institute, but Bischoff also had available a budget of his own for physiological research and an assistant in physiology. He held out and was able to obtain funds for improvements to the building.

The Physiological Institute also housed two other professors. Max Pettenkofer, who had been in on Maximilian's plans for science from the start and had been the principal intermediary in Liebig's *Berufung*, was rewarded with a chemical laboratory in the institute where he could pursue his various projects in applied chemistry and public health. Emil Harless, who had been on the scene as extraordinary professor of physiology for several years before the institute was founded, retained his position and brought his physiological collection into the new building. The institute itself belonged to the Bavarian Academy of Sciences rather than to the university, but Pettenkofer and Harless were university professors. Siebold and Bischoff were appointed to the institute itself.[36]

The Munich Physiological Institute was neither the manifestation of a single vision nor the institutional setting for a unified research program. It was the product of multiple influences, negotiations, confrontations, and accommodations. It existed in part because Maximilian wanted to make this political capital a scientific capital as well. Its institutional outlines were shaped initially around the anatomical-physiological tradition that its first director represented. Had the second professorship been filled by Henle or by Müller, this general orientation would have been solidified, although undoubtedly with a different emphasis reflecting the distinctive research program that either of these well-established investigators would have brought with him. With Bischoff, however, the institute took on a second dimension because Liebig had perceived in Bischoff's dual interest the opportunity to implant within it a foothold for his own combination of physiology and chemistry. Space was found as well for the still different personal aims of Max Pettenkofer. The previous era of physiology in Munich was also accommodated; Emil Harless moved into the institute. What remained to be seen was whether there was room under one roof for interests, programs, and ambitions as diverse as those of the four professors who came together there.

IV

Soon after establishing himself in Munich, Bischoff hired a "very industrious" young man, Carl Voit, as his physiological assistant. Voit had begun studying medicine in 1848 in Munich and had gone to Würzburg in 1851 to continue his studies. In 1852 he returned to Munich and completed his medical training there in 1854. Then he began attending lectures in physics, anatomy, zoology, and chemistry. For the latter he followed the course taught by Liebig. He did laboratory work under Pettenkofer, for whom he carried out determinations of the urea content of the muscles of victims of cholera. Liebig's writings on animal chemistry made so deep an impression on Voit that he decided he wanted to investigate the laws of nutrition and of the *Stoffwechsel*. He attracted the interest of Liebig, who advised him first to study more chemistry with Friedrich Wöhler in Göttingen. Voit spent the year 1855 there, completing a study of certain benzene compounds with what were by then classical methods of organic chemistry. Excited by the work of Bidder and Schmidt, Voit planned next to study with them in Dorpat but was diverted from this intention when Bischoff offered him the assistantship in Munich.[37]

During his last year in Giessen, Bischoff had attempted to investigate the effects of a bile fistula, which would divert the flow of bile from the intestine to the outside, upon the nutrition of an animal. Several of the animals died from the effects of the operation. In the one that survived long enough to carry out nutritional measurements, the results were only puzzling. From Liebig's theory that the bile is reabsorbed and oxidized in the blood, one would predict that the loss of this respiratory material would severely alter the nutritional condition of the animal. Instead the dog maintained its weight and health on diets very near to what it had required before the operation.[38] In Munich Bischoff continued these experiments on bile fistula animals and assigned Voit to assist with them. Soon, however, Voit encountered the more general technical difficulties that Bischoff had not yet overcome and decided to try to resolve them. The central problem remained the large proportion of the nitrogen consumed that was missing from the urea. Voit turned his attention, therefore, to experiments with normal dogs in order to improve the overall procedures, while Bischoff carried on with the bile fistula experiments.[39]

The division of labor established between Bischoff and his assistant was in keeping with their respective technical skills. Bischoff was apparently not known for great expertise in vivisection experiments,[40] his major research contributions having been in the realm of microscopical observations. As an anatomist, however, he was able to carry out with reasonable facility the rather difficult operation required to create the bile fistulas. Voit had already acquired much more experience in chemical methods of investigation than Bischoff possessed; consequently he was better equipped than Bischoff to detect and eliminate pitfalls in the analytical procedures so central to the quantitative measurements of the material exchanges of an animal with the exterior.

At first Voit looked for forms other than urea in which the missing nitrogen in Bischoff's experiment might be excreted, but he found none. He could not check the possibility that nitrogen is eliminated through the lungs or skin because he had no apparatus for conducting respiration experiments. As he refined the various procedures for measuring the nitrogen intake in the food, for establishing a uniform composition of the food, and for collecting the excretions, however, he found that the difficulty he had set out to explain had somehow disappeared. In five sets of experiments carried out between September 1856 and May 1857, Voit found that in each case the quantity of nitrogen consumed was very nearly equal to that found in the urea. Confidently he declared, "We can now with full justification designate the urea as a measure of the *Stoffwechsel*."[41] The way was clear for extended investigations of nitrogenous nutrition according to the principles set forth by Liebig.

Between October 1857 and June 1859 Bischoff and Voit carried out a long series of nutritional experiments on dogs, repeating much of what Bischoff had done in 1853 but more systematically and thoroughly, and with results that now consistently fulfilled their expectations. Now, for example, they were able to show in every case that an addition of fat to a given meat diet reduced the quantity of urea formed. From the outcome of several series of experiments in which they gradually raised or lowered the daily meat ration of their dogs, they came to realize that what was an adequate diet when the animal was in one physiological state might not be adequate in another state, for the rate of formation of urea depended not only upon the nutritional intake but upon the weight of the animal.[42]

In 1860 Bischoff and Voit published their massive quantity of accumulated results in a book whose title, *The Laws of the Nutrition of Carnivorous Animals, Established through New Investigations,* succinctly summarized what they believed they had achieved. In practical terms, they thought, they had established the methods through which one could determine the most economical quantitative combination of nitrogenous and nonnitrogenous foods that would maintain a given animal in a stable condition. Theoretically they affirmed, as Bischoff had already done in 1853, the validity of Liebig's distinction between respiratory and plastic aliments and his claim that all nitrogenous substances must be assimilated into the tissues before they can be converted into urea. Once more they rejected the view that excess nitrogenous aliment can be directly oxidized. Elaborating on Liebig's ideas, they proposed a general and notably vague theory to account for the variations they observed in the rate of nitrogen consumption of an animal. The rate of the *Stoffwechsel,* they asserted, is a product of the actions of three factors upon one another: the mass of the organs, the mass of the nutrient fluids delivering nitrogenous aliments to the organs, and the mass of oxygen present.[43]

In making their results public Bischoff and Voit claimed for themselves the authority to set the standards by which future research in animal nutrition must be judged. Only investigations in which, as in their own, "all of the metamorphosed nitrogen re-appears in the excretions," they asserted, will be worthy of attention.[44] They were just as confident that they had fully confirmed Liebig's conception of the *Stoffwechsel.* For the unprecedented range of nutritional conditions they had tested, and for the meticulous care devoted to the analyses, their work was quickly accorded a leading position in the field. Neither their results nor their conclusions, however, were accepted as definitive. The treatment of their work in the second edition of the *Lehrbuch der Physiologie des Menschen* by Carl Ludwig, head of the most influential school of physiology in Germany at the time, was representative of the more cautious contemporary judgments. Ludwig admired their "comprehensive" research sufficiently to devote more than one third of his section on the "comparison of losses and gains of weighable substances" in nutrition to a summary and analysis of Bischoff and Voit's results. He interpreted their significance, however, in quite different ways than the authors of the work had done, and he tactfully dismissed the theories concerning internal nutritional processes that Bischoff and Voit had drawn from their experiments by remarking, without explicit reference to them, that one cannot derive theories concerning the mechanism of the *Stoff-wechsel* by means of investigations of the "income and output of the animal body" alone.[45]

During the course of the investigations that led to their joint publication, the roles of Bischoff and Voit in the research that Voit had entered as Bischoff's assistant gradually shifted. In the main line of investigation they carried out between 1857 and 1859, both men shared in planning and interpreting the experiments. Bischoff, however, was largely occupied with his anatomy and physiology courses and his administrative responsibilities, and he left all of the actual operations to Voit. As late as 1859 Bischoff himself carried out one more set of experiments on a dog with a bile fistula, but after that he retired to the background in the enterprise that he had brought from Giessen to Munich. The publication of Charles Darwin's *Origin of Species* attracted Bischoff's attention to evolutionary questions, diverting him ultimately to the study of anthropology.[46] Voit meanwhile became a *Privatdozent*, and Bischoff made the resources of the institute's laboratory available to him to carry out independent experiments in animal nutrition. In 1860 Voit received an offer from Tübingen, which he declined in return for promotion to extraordinary professor in the Faculty of Medicine at Munich, with a modest budget for his research activity.[47] By this time Voit had clearly become the driving force in the research program that Bischoff and Liebig had initiated. Unlike Bischoff, who had carried on this work as a digression from his own main fields of interest, undertaken through his admiration for Liebig's views and his conviction that Liebig's ideas required testing by a physiologist, who had had misgivings about his competence in the type of analytical operations the investigation required, and who probably viewed his involvement all along as a limited one, Voit devoted himself single-mindedly to this field of investigation. Soon he came to regard it as his life work, and he pursued it relentlessly.

For his own research project, in 1859 Voit took up a study of the effects of three conditions upon the quantity of urea formed by a dog. Two of these were the addition to the normal diets of coffee and salt, substances whose nutritive roles had long been matters of controversy. Voit found that neither additive altered the nitrogenous consumption.[48] During these investigations, however, he learned something about his methods that proved to be of far broader significance than the specific questions he had set out to answer. Only if an animal is in a state of nutritive equilibrium can one determine the effects on its nutrition of an added factor, because if the constituents of the animal's body are changing, its nutritive requirements are concurrently altered. More specifically, Voit established that the animal must be placed in nitrogen equilibrium—that is, that the nitrogen excreted in the urea must be brought into balance with that assimilated from the food—before one could proceed to test the action of the specific factor in question.[49] This procedure became a basic criterion for future nutritional research.

The third factor that Voit studied was the effect of muscular activity on nitrogen consumption. In order to measure that effect, Voit constructed a treadmill on which his dog ran for ten minutes at a time, six times per day. In keeping with Liebig's view that the breakdown of the nitrogenous tissue constituents is the source of mechanical work, Voit expected that the dog would excrete considerably more urea on days that it ran than on days of rest. To his great surprise, he found no significant difference. This unexpected result did not induce Voit to give up Liebig's view, for, like Bischoff, he believed that Liebig's distinction between plastic and respiratory aliments was one of the basic foundations for the whole science of nutrition. Instead he constructed a secondary hypothesis according to which the decomposition of nitrogenous substance proceeds at a steady rate determined by the nitrogenous mass of the body and the nitrogenous nourishment. When the animal does not do mechanical work, the energy released by this *Stoffwechsel* is stored as electrical energy, which can be converted rapidly to mechanical work when the animal requires it.[50]

V

When Bischoff and Voit presented the results of their general nutritional experiments, they not only determined the quantities of nitrogen ingested and excreted but, through calculations based on the quantities of carbon, hydrogen, and oxygen in the food and excretions, they estimated indirectly the quantities of fat and water gained or lost by the animal, the oxygen absorbed, and the carbonic acid exhaled. In so doing they followed the precedent set eight years earlier by Bidder and Schmidt. Bischoff and Voit were very aware that these calculations involved multiple uncertain assumptions and that a rigorous balance sheet of the input and output of the elements involved in nutrition could be attained only by expanding their procedures to include direct measurements of the respiratory gaseous exchanges.[51] To combine such measurements with the type of measurements of the food intake and excretions that they were already carrying out was, however, a very difficult task. Respiratory measurements had to be made in chambers enclosing the experimental subject, with provision for renewing the oxygen consumed and removing the carbonic acid and water produced while accurately measuring the quantities involved. In 1849 the French investigators Victor Regnault and Jules Reiset had greatly improved the methods for carrying out such experiments. Their apparatus enabled them to maintain an animal in the respiration chamber for two to three days while maintaining a nearly normal atmosphere.[52] The size of their chamber, however, restricted them to experiments on small animals, and they did not attempt to measure the food or excretions of their animals. Bischoff and Voit required circumstances that would enable them to do not only the latter but to utilize large animals and, if they were to extend their results to practical nutritional problems, to accommodate humans as well.

In order to resolve these problems Bischoff and Voit decided, in 1859, to embark on the audacious project of constructing a respiration chamber in which a large dog or a person could live comfortably for a day or more. To do so they enlisted the aid of their colleague Max Pettenkofer. Although occupying four rooms in the Physiological Institute, Pettenkofer had until then devoted himself entirely to problems in applied chemistry and in public health that were unrelated to the work of the other members of the institute. His ongoing study of the air in dwellings, however, which included devising a method for carbon dioxide determinations and methods for exchanging the air in buildings, provided him with technical expertise relevant to the design of a large-scale respiration apparatus.

Pettenkofer's apparatus was as complex as it was grandiose. Although derived from Regnault and Reiset's apparatus, it was far more elaborate and much larger. The chamber was the size of a small room. Air passed continuously through the chamber in quantities as large as six hundred cubic meters per day. The total volumes of entering and outgoing air were measured, and samples of both, as well as of the air remaining in the chamber at the end of the experiment, were collected in order to determine the content of carbonic acid and water. Pettenkofer went to great lengths to assure the accuracy of the system by eliminating potential sources of leaks and by means of control experiments. The average error for the carbonic acid measured in the apparatus was only three-tenths of a percent.[53]

Pettenkofer's respiration apparatus was far more than the largest specimen of its kind; it introduced experimentation on a physical scale unprecedented in physiology. One awed observer likened its operation not to a scientific experiment but to a factory, which nevertheless had to function with the precision of a watch. The apparatus also represented a new level of financial investment in physiological experimentation. The project could be funded only because, with the aid of Liebig's influence, Pettenkofer and Voit were able to obtain from Maximilian a special subsidy of 10,000 fl. to build the apparatus. When Pettenkofer reluctantly concluded that it would be necessary to incorporate a steam engine, housed in a special wooden building, to drive the equipment, the cost went up by another 1,300 fl. Maximilian supported the project with his habitual generosity. He undoubtedly foresaw that it could lead to practical nutritional knowledge; but he also took a special personal interest in it, so much so that he himself once spent an hour in the respiration chamber.[54]

By February 1861 the apparatus was ready for Pettenkofer and Voit to try on feeding-respiration experiments.[55] For two years they encountered anomalous results and other experimental obstacles that forced them repeatedly to refine the apparatus and their procedures. Finally, early in 1863, they were able to carry out with notable success an experiment on a dog in which they attained a complete balance of the incoming and outgoing elements, with the animal in equilibrium on a pure meat diet. After establishing a nutritive balance, they measured the food intake and the excretions for fourteen days. They measured the respiratory exchanges for twenty-four-hour periods during five of these days. When all of the inputs and outputs were added up, the totals agreed to within less than one percent of the total mass of the material exchanged. In reporting their results they claimed with justifiable pride that

> every single value is ascertained by experiment. All *Stoffwechsel* balances put forward up to now have suffered from the serious defect that for certain factors, partly of the intake, partly of the output, they assumed hypothetical values instead of values actually determined during 24 hours, and consequently left a rather open field for arbitrary interpretations.

> The equation which we now [have established] . . . for the *Stoff-wechsel* over 24 hours rests on values which are all actually determined over this time and is, indeed, the first which has ever been established without any recourse to hypotheses.[56]

This was an experimental triumph of great magnitude, a fitting climax to an endeavor on which Liebig, Bischoff, Voit, and Pettenkofer collectively had toiled for more than a decade. They had now laid the groundwork for many further years of investigations of the quantitative metabolic exchanges of humans and animals under varied conditions of nourishment, health, and disease. They had also established the dominance, in this field of inquiry, of the Munich school of physiology.

As he moved toward a commanding position within the field of metabolism, Voit moved also toward a dominant role in the Munich Physiological Institute. Bischoff remained a staunch defender of the research program he had initiated and a benevolent observer of its further development.[57] Liebig stood even farther in the background. Meanwhile that program was preempting more and more of the institute's resources. Siebold's working space in the institute began to contract as soon as he turned physiology over to Bischoff. Eventually the anatomical collections that Siebold had established there were transferred to the buildings of the Bavarian Academy of Sciences, and Siebold's domain within the Physiological Institute was reduced to two small rooms crowded with books and specimens.[58] In 1862 Emil Harless died, and Voit applied for Harless's professorship, as well as for the research budget of 600 fl. that Harless had enjoyed. At first Voit was denied the promotion, but he received the research funds. In 1863, however, he succeeded to Harless's position as ordinary professor of physiology.[59] By then he had established effective control over the institute, except for the activities in hygiene that Pettenkofer continued to carry on there. With Harless gone, Siebold and Bischoff working in other fields, and Pettenkofer partly coopted into his own program, Voit was essentially setting the direction for a thriving investigative activity that increasingly came to identify the institute as a whole. In 1855 the institute had provided a home for independent research activities of the four scientists who were incorporated into it. By 1863 one of these lines of investigation had all but crowded the others out. From this time onward the institutional contours of the Munich Institute of Physiology became more and more congruent with the needs of this research program and of its single-minded director.

VI

Some historians of science have recently attributed to local institutional and social contexts the primary role in shaping scientific research programs.[60] The story of the Munich school of physiology illustrates the significance of this point of view but also its incompleteness. At every stage the institutional, social, and political surroundings conditioned the development of the particular line of investigation that eventually became the hallmark of the Munich school. Liebig was able to formulate the problems of animal chemistry in the way he did in 1842 partly because he stood at the center of an organized field of organic chemistry that had attained a certain degree of maturity. The experimental and training facilities he had earlier built up at Giessen were essential to his position in that field. His ideas about animal chemistry were influential in part because of his general power and influence within the German scientific community. He was able to move rapidly into the chemical problems most relevant to his physiological concerns after 1842 because he commanded a large group of students and associates whose central research efforts he could shift to the questions that most interested him. Theodor Bischoff was able to join him in Giessen to undertake a collaborative experimental program because of the mobility that well-established German scientists then enjoyed, in an era in which German universities were competing to attract leading figures to build up their local teaching and research activities. In Dorpat Bidder and Schmidt were able to sustain an intensive, prolonged research program partly because German-speaking universities had become generally supportive of such research and had created conditions under which determined professors and *Privatdozenten* could carry them out, with the aid of students whom they were at the same time training. Liebig and Bischoff were able to move their program from Giessen to Munich, and to assemble there the costly resources necessary to succeed with it again, among other reasons, because of the competition for outstanding talent among German universities,[61] enhanced by the special vision of a monarch who connected the well-being of his state with the advancement of science. Liebig and his followers were further able to increase the support for this particular program by promoting effectively, in a time of acute food shortages in Germany, the idea that it was necessary in order to utilize agricultural resources efficiently.

If such exterior factors created the general opportunities in which a research program demanding much time, assistance, and material support could thrive, they were nevertheless not the principal factors that gave the program of the Munich school its distinctive shape. The contours of that program are traceable most directly to the ideas of its founder and to a tradition that he drew upon reaching back to the ideas and investigations of Lavoisier. At no time during its formative period did this program arise from the organizational contours of an existing institution. Rather, it evolved within institutional frameworks that had been established for other purposes. It was Liebig's forceful vision and restless personality that diverted the research focus of his laboratory at Giessen from inorganic and organic chemistry to agricultural and physiological chemistry. It was the magnetic attraction of Liebig's vision for Bischoff that caused him to uproot himself twice from his existing institutional positions and to devote himself to a research endeavor having little connection with his previous areas of interest, his teaching responsibilities, or the microscopes and anatomical collections that represented institutional investments in his own scientific specialty. Throughout their collaborative enterprise Liebig and Bischoff had to improvise in order to adapt to their purpose institutional settings that were not primarily designed for the type of investigation they had in mind. Even when he went to Munich on terms that he was largely able to set, Bischoff occupied an institution shaped mainly by the needs of other occupants with different scientific orientations. Most of his own demands were dictated by his responsibility for teaching anatomy, an activity unrelated to the joint research plan. The Physiological Institute had to accommodate the very different field of interest of its initial director Siebold, and to make room for holdovers from a past era such as Harless and for intermediaries such as Pettenkofer who had their own ambitions, as well as for the goal that Bischoff came there to pursue.

Not until after the research program that Liebig and Bischoff undertook had already achieved auspicious success did the Physiological Institute in Munich come, in its organizational structure and its physical resources, to reflect mainly the needs of that program.

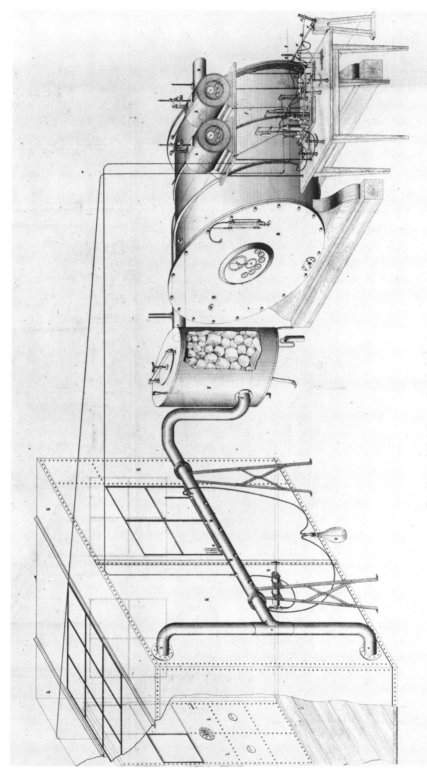

Portion of the Pettenkofer Respiration Apparatus

When the huge respiration apparatus was in place, when Carl Voit finally succeeded to a professorship and began to attract students to learn the methods of metabolic investigation that had made him the leader of the field, then the shape of a research program and of the institute that housed it came to be more and more congruent. The driving, shaping force, however, was not the institute, not the state in which it was built, not the monarch who backed it, but the ideas and determination of the scientists who imposed their research plans across preexisting institutional forms until those forms were finally forced into line with their aims.

The present case is relevant also to current discussions of the way in which disciplinary boundaries define research programs. It is sometimes suggested that existing specialty areas divide up the intellectual horizon in such a way, and so socialize those who enter these areas into their practices, as to channel research into problems that fit within each specialty boundary.[62] In this instance, however, the problem preceded the discipline, for physiological chemistry did not yet exist as a field when those whose story we have followed decided to devote their investigative efforts to it. Practitioners of two adjacent fields moved toward it from opposite directions. Some of them contested for jurisdictional control from within their own disciplines. In France, for example, Claude Bernard maintained that physiology must set the problems and that chemistry could provide only the tools.[63] Liebig at first seemed to believe the opposite: that chemists could solve the problems that physiologists could not even define clearly. He soon learned, however, that he needed help. He recognized that animal chemistry was not a part of chemistry, nor yet a scientific field at all, but a borderland between two existing fields. Until a generation trained in both of the relevant disciplines could emerge, it would be necessary for chemists and physiologists to work together. When the interdisciplinary research program thus put together, by Bidder and Schmidt as well as by Bischoff and Liebig, had become visible enough to attract disciples into it, then a new generation, which included particularly Carl Voit, emerged with the requisite combination of skills to create a subdiscipline oriented around the problem. It was, therefore, not the existing disciplines that shaped the problem but a problem arising athwart them that reshaped the disciplines.

The Munich Physiological Institute was both a teaching and a research institution. Bischoff was appointed to teach physiology and anatomy. The most crucial arrangements that had to be worked out between him and Siebold pertained to the division of their respective teaching areas, not their research domains. His physiology courses probably occupied Bischoff's time in Munich more than his experimentation did. As a research assistant Voit could at first spend all his time on experimental work, but when he became a *Privatdozent* he also began to teach. When he applied for Harless's position in 1862, Voit stressed as his qualifications "my prior success as a teacher at this university in all branches of physiology, as well as my scientific activity."[64] We may well ask what interactions there were between the teaching functions of the institute and the research programs present there. A preliminary assessment might suggest that in the institute's formative stages neither of these activities strongly shaped the other. Professors were required to teach a standard array of comprehensive courses in anatomy, zoology, and physiology, while a very specialized research program in the interdisciplinary zone that would eventually become physiological chemistry arose from the joint enterprise of Liebig and Bischoff. In the Munich Institute of Physiology, during the period in which it was still taking shape, teaching and research appear to have been loosely complementary activities of the same professors rather than tightly coordinated aspects of the same activity.

Research and teaching eventually grew closer in the Munich Institute as advanced students were drawn there to learn the investigative methods that had come to mark it as a scientific school. Justus Liebig, Theodor Bischoff, and Carl Voit had been able to found a research school within an institution whose educational role had been designed for other ends. That school could be sustained, however, only by the formation of another educational layer, through which were trained the generations of investigators who would carry on their research program. By then only Voit remained as the active leader of that program, and so it was he who became renowned as the grand old master and head of the Munich school of physiology.

NOTES

1. The orientation of this paragraph is influenced in part by a prospectus written by Kathryn M. Olesko for a proposed volume of essays to be entitled *Science in Germany: Problems at the Intersection of Institutional and*

Intellectual History. The quoted passage is from a letter by Olesko to the author (11 September 1984) outlining the themes for that volume, which will be complementary to the themes of the present volume.

2. Gerald L. Geison, "Scientific Change, Emerging Specialties, and Research Schools," *History of Science* 19 (1981): 21. For a thoughtful application of Geison's criteria, see Leo J. Klosterman, "A Research School of Chemistry in the Nineteenth Century: Jean–Baptiste Dumas and his Research Students," *Annals of Science* 42 (1985): 1–80.

3. Joseph S. Fruton, "Contrasts in Scientific Style: Emil Fischer and Franz Hofmeister: Their Research Groups and Their Theory of Protein Structure," *Proceedings of the American Philosophical Society* 129 (1985): 313–370.

4. Kathryn M. Olesko, *Physics as a Calling: Discipline and Profession in the Königsberg Seminar for Physics* (in press).

5. Otto Frank, *Carl von Voit, Gedächtnisrede* (Munich: Akademie der Wissenschaften, 1910), p. 10.

6. Graham Lusk, "Carl von Voit, Master and Friend," *Annals of Medical History* 3 (1931): 583–594.

7. See Frederic L. Holmes, *Lavoisier and the Chemistry of Life: An Exploration of Scientific Creativity* (Madison: University of Wisconsin Press, 1985), pp. 91–128, 237–259, 440–468.

8. Justus Liebig, *Die Thier-Chemie, oder die organische Chemie in ihrer Anwendung auf Physiologie und Pathologie*, 2d ed. (Braunschweig: Vieweg, 1843), pp. 3–36.

9. Ibid., pp. 37–53, 88.

10. Ibid., pp. 51–61, 220.

11. Justus Liebig, *Chemische Untersuchung über das Fleisch und seine Zubereitung zum Nahrungsmittel* (Heidelberg: C. F. Winter, 1847).

12. Liebig, *Thier-Chemie*, pp. 57, 222.

13. See F. L. Holmes, "Introduction," in Justus Liebig *Animal Chemistry: or Organic Chemistry in Its Application to Physiology and Pathology*, (New York: Johnson Reprint Corp., 1964), pp. lviii–lxv.

14. Mauritz Dittrich, "Motive und Hintergrunde des Greifswalder Anatomie-Baues," *Medizinhistorisches Journal* 4 (1969): 285. William Coleman has drawn my attention to this source.

15. Holmes, "Introduction," pp. lviii–lxxiii; Johannes Müller to Liebig, 1 August 1842, Liebigiana, Staatsbibliothek, Munich; Carl Vierordt to Liebig, 9 December 1846, *ibid.*; Hermann Nasse to Liebig, 17 January 1842, ibid.; C. G. Lehmann to Liebig, 3 September 1841, ibid.

16. K. E. Rothschuh, "Bischoff, Theodor Ludwig Wilhelm," in *Dictionary of Scientific Biography*, ed. C. C. Gillispie (New York: Charles Scribner's Sons, 1970–1980), 2: 160–162; Th. L. W. Bischoff, *Entwicklungsgeschichte der Saugethiere und des Menschen* (Leipzig: Boss, 1842); Bischoff, "Bericht über die Fortschritte der Physiologie in Jahre 1841," *Archiv für Anatomie, Physiologie und Wissenschaftliche Medizin* (1842): LXVI–LXXII; Bischoff to Liebig, 15 January 1843, 10 April 1843, Liebigiana 58, Staatsbibliothek, Munich; Bischoff to Liebig, 4 June 1843, Darmstaedter Coll., Staatsbibliothek, Berlin; Bischoff, *Der Harnstoff als Maass des Stoffwechsels* (Giessen: Ricker, 1853), p. vi; Carl

Kupffer, *Gedächtnissrede auf Theodor L. W. von Bischoff* (Munich: Verlag der b. Akademie, 1884), pp. 25–31.

17. J. C. Poggendorff, *Biographisch-Literarsches Handwörterbuch zur Geschichte der Exacten Wissenschaften*, vol. 2 (Leipzig: Barth, 1863), pp. 818–819; Charles Culotta, "Bidder, Friedrich H.," in *Dictionary of Scientific Biography*, ed. C. C. Gillispie (New York: Charles Scribner's Sons, 1970–1980), 2: 123–125; F. Bidder and C. Schmidt, *Die Verdauungssaefte und der Stoffwechsel* (Mitau: G. A. Reyher, 1852).

18. See, for example, Bidder and Schmidt, *Verdauungssaefte*, pp. 333–337.

19. Ibid., pp. 292, 354–355.

20. Bischoff, *Der Harnstoff*, pp. 8–18; Richard Blunck, *Justus von Liebig* (Hamburg: Hammerich and Lesser, 1946), p. 193; Justus Liebig, "Ueber einige Harnstoffverbindungen und eine neue Methode zur Bestimmung von Kochsalz und Harnstoff im Harn," *Annalen der Chemie und Pharm.* 85 (1853): 289–329.

21. Bischoff, *Der Harnstoff*, pp. 30–115, tables I and II, facing p. 160.

22. Ibid., pp. 7–8, 74–78, 148–151.

23. Ludwig Trost and Friedrich Leist, eds., *König Maximilian II von Bayern und Schelling: Briefwechsel* (Stuttgart: J. G. Cotta, 1890), p. 196; Max Pettenkofer to Liebig, 17 June 1851, Liebigiana, Staatsbibliothek, Munich.

24. Trost and Leist, *König Maximilian II*, p. 228; Laetitia Boehm, "Das akademische Bildungswesen in seiner organisatorischen Entwicklung (1800–1920)," in *Handbuch der Bayerischen Geschichte*, ed., Max Spindler (Munich: C. H. Beck, 1975), vol. 4, pt. 2, pp. 1012–1014, 1020–1021; Justus Liebig, *Chemische Briefe* (Heidelberg: C. F. Winter, 1844), p. iv; Peter Borscheid, *Naturwissenschaft, Staat und Industrie in Baden (1848–1914)* (Stuttgart: Ernst Klett, 1976), pp. 16–33.

25. Liebig to Max Pettenkofer, 17 November 1851, 18 April, 20 April, 21 May, 9 June, 17 June, 1852; Pettenkofer to Liebig, 10 November, 8 December 1851, 18 May, 30 June, 10 July 1852, Liebigiana, Staatsbibliothek, Munich; Blunt, *Liebig*, p. 194.

26. Th. Bischoff to Liebig, undated, 29 October, 15 November, 29 December 1852, 21 January, 10 February 1853, Liebigiana, Staatsbibliothek, Munich.

27. Bischoff, *Der Harnstoff*, esp. pp. 152–153; Fr. Th. Frerichs, "Das Maass des Stoffwechsels," *Archiv für Anatomie, Physiologie und Wissenschaftliche Medizin* (1848): 469–491.

28. See William Coleman, "Prussian Pedagogy: Purkyně at Breslau 1823–1839," chapter 1, this volume.

29. Documents concerning Siebold's appointment are contained in Akten des k. akad. Senats der Ludwig-Max.-Univ., Betreffend Physiologie, Archives of the University of Munich. See also E. Ehlers, "Carl Theodor Ernst von Siebold: eine biographische Skizze," *Zeitschrift für Wissenschaftliche Zoologie* 42 (1885): xvii.

30. Ehlers, "Siebold," pp. i–xxxi; Richard Hertwig, *Gedächtnissrede auf Carl Theodor V. Siebold* (Munich: Königliche Bayerische Akademie, 1886).

31. See Arleen Tuchman, "From the Lecture to the Laboratory: The Insti-

tutionalization of Scientific Medicine at the University of Heidelberg," chapter 2, this volume.

32. Bischoff to Liebig, 21 January, 4 March 1853, undated (no. 17), Liebigiana, Staatsbibliothek, Munich.

33. Bischoff to Liebig, 1 May 1853, ibid.

34. Bischoff to Liebig, 1 May 1853, undated (no. 12), undated (no. 13), 20 August, 4 October, 4 November, 2 December, 27 December 1853, ibid.

35. Bischoff to Liebig, 9 May, 15 May, 22 May, 10 June, 11 July, 22 July, 2 November, 23 December 1854, ibid.

36. Bischoff to Emil du Bois-Reymond, 16 October 1856, Darmstaedter Coll., Staatsbibliothek, Berlin; Ehlers, "Siebold," p. xviii.

37. Bischoff to du Bois-Reymond, 16 October 1856, ibid.; Frank, *Voit*, pp. 1, 5–7; Carl Voit, "Ueber die Entwicklung der Lehre von der Quelle der Muskelkraft und einiger Theile der Ernährung seit 25 Jahren," *Zeitschrift für Biologie* 6 (1870): 312.

38. "Gallenfistelhunde von Prof. Bischoff, Nr. I und Nr. II," Voitiana, no. 41, Staatsbibliothek, Munich; "Gallenblasen Fistel bei einer Katze: Nov. 1854," ibid.; Bischoff to Liebig, 11 July 1854, Liebigiana, ibid.

39. Karl Voit, "Beiträge zum Kreislauf des Stickstoffes im Thierischen Organismus," in *Physiologisch-Chemische Untersuchungen* (Augsburg: Rieger, 1857), pp. 3–5.

40. John E. Lesch, *Science and Medicine in France: The Emergence of Experimental Physiology, 1790–1855* (Cambridge, Mass.: Harvard University Press, 1984), pp. 211–214.

41. Voit, "Kreislauf des Stickstoffs," pp. 6–30.

42. Th. L. W. Bischoff and Carl Voit, *Die Gesetze der Ernährung des Fleischfressers durch neue Untersuchungen festgelegt* (Leipzig: Winter, 1860).

43. Ibid., pp. 1–27, 258–264.

44. Carl Voit, *Untersuchungen über den Einfluss des Kochsalzes des Kaffee's und der Muskelbewegungen auf den Stoffwechsel* (Munich: Cotta, 1860), pp. 26–27.

45. Carl Ludwig, *Lehrbuch der Physiologie des Menschen*, 2d ed. (Leipzig: Winter, 1861), 2: 692–711.

46. "Gallenfistelhund IV," Voitiana, no. 41, Staatsbibliothek, Munich; Rothschuh, "Bischoff," p. 161.

47. "Fehlblatt: Betreff Dr. Voit," 4 November 1860; Voit to Maximilian II, 23 February 1862, Akten des k. akad. Senats der Ludwig-Max.-Univ., Betreffend Physiologie, 292, Abtheilung III, Archives of the University of Munich.

48. Voit, *Einfluss des Kochsalzes*, pp. 29–147.

49. Ibid., p. 31.

50. Ibid., pp. 148–228.

51. Ibid., p. 6.

52. V. Regnault and J. Reiset, "Recherches chimiques sur la respiration des animaux des diverses classes," *Annales de chimie et de physique* 26 (1848): 299–519.

53. Max Pettenkofer, "Ueber die Respiration," *Annalen der Chemie und Pharmacie*, Suppl. Vol. II, pt. 1 (1862): 1–52.

54. Ibid., pp. 9, 12; Pettenkofer to Liebig, Munich, 12 October 1859, Liebigiana, Staatsbibliothek, Munich; Karl Kisshalt, *Max von Pettenkofer* (Stuttgart: Wissenschaftliche Verlagsgesellschaft, 1948), pp. 59–61; Otto Neustätter, *Max Pettenkofer* (Vienna: Springer, 1925), pp. 32–35.

55. Max Pettenkofer and Carl Voit, "Untersuchungen über die Respiration," *Annalen der Chemie und Pharmacie*, Suppl. Vol. II, pt. 1 (1862): 52–53.

56. Max Pettenkofer and Carl Voit, "Ueber die Producte der Respiration des Hundes bei Fleischnährung und über die Gleichnung der Einnahmen und Ausgaben des Körpers dabei," in ibid., Suppl. Vol. II, pt. 3 (1863): 365–366.

57. For Bischoff's role as defender, see Th. L. W. Bischoff, "Zur Frage nach den Harnstoffbestimmungen bei Untersuchungen über den Stoffwechsel," *Zeitschrift für rationelle Medizin* 14 (1862): 320–343.

58. Ehlers, *Siebold*, p. xviii.

59. Faculty Senate to Maximilian II, 9 April 1862, Akten des k. akad. Senats, Ludwig-Max.-Univ., Betreffend Physiologie, Archives of the University of Munich; Frank, *Voit*, p. 6.

60. The most comprehensive study formulated around this assertion is Robert E. Kohler, *From Medical Chemistry to Biochemistry: the Making of a Biomedical Discipline* (Cambridge: Cambridge University Press, 1982).

61. On the role of competition among German universities, see Joseph Ben-David, *The Scientist's Role in Society: A Comparative Study* (Englewood Cliffs, N.J.: Prentice-Hall, 1971), p. 123.

62. This view is expressed, for example, in Donald T. Campbell, "Ethnocentrism of Disciplines and the Fish-Scale Model of Omniscience," in *Interdisciplinary Relationships in the Social Sciences*, ed. M. Sherif and C. W. Sherif, (Chicago: Aldine, 1969), pp. 328–348.

63. F. L. Holmes, *Claude Bernard and Animal Chemistry: The Emergence of a Scientist* (Cambridge, Mass.: Harvard University Press, 1974), p. 449.

64. Voit to Maximilian II, 23 February 1862, Akten des k. akad. Senats der Ludwig-Max.-Univ., Betreffend Physiologie, 292, Abtheilung III, Archives of the University of Munich.

CHAPTER SIX

The Telltale Heart: Physiological Instruments, Graphic Methods, And Clinical Hopes 1854–1914

Robert G. Frank, Jr.

In late November 1865 an editor of *Lancet*, the leading and rather conservative London medical journal, wrote with uncharacteristic enthusiasm about a new instrument that might change medical practice.[1] It was a device that depended upon mechanical principles— hence "Physicians and Physicists" as the title of the editorial—and exemplified that extremely interesting trend in the "recent history of Medicine": the "remarkable ingenuity with which physical means of research have been brought to bear upon the hidden secrets of the body in health and disease." In previous decades the stethoscope of Laënnec had made manifest the hidden organs of the chest, the ophthalmoscope of Helmholtz had illuminated the eye, the laryngo-scope of Czermak had revealed the larynx, and in the hands of Wunderlich and his admirers the thermometer "is beginning to tell us its own story in the diagnosis and prognosis of disease." Now another "instrument of precision, of remarkable beauty and wide range of usefulness," had been devised:

> The sphygmograph of M. Marey is an exquisitely designed instru-ment, by the aid of which the pulse is armed with a pen, and at every beat writes its own diagram, and registers its own characters. In this diagram each part of every revolution, or "beat" of the heart is re-corded, so that the relation of the systole and diastole is inscribed in every curve, and the state of arterial tonicity on the one hand, and the impulsive power of the heart on the other, are automatically com-

pared. The finger is substituted by an instrument of precision, which replaces impressions by recorded facts self-analyzed.[2]

For some time, *Lancet* informed its readers, Drs. Francis Anstie and John Burdon-Sanderson had been pursuing a series of clinical and physiological observations using this instrument, and had recently given a presentation to the Medical Society of London on the sphygmographic differentiae between typhus and typhoid fever. The writer expatiated on the possible role of the sphygmograph in the diagnosis of other fevers and of conditions of the heart. He closed by echoing the hope of Burdon-Sanderson—"to whom, indeed, the idea of the investigation was due"—and Anstie that English physicians would take "to the immense field of fruitful observation which lies open to the investigation of observers who are willing to devote time and patience to the development of M. Marey's brilliant invention."[3]

The sphygmograph was not to remain unique. It was merely the first in a series of instruments, such as the capillary electrometer, the polygraph, the electrocardiograph, the phonocardiograph, and the sphygmomanometer, that were developed over the succeeding half-century and that aimed to make the salient features of the action and pathology of the human heart accessible to the physiologist and the physician.

The notion that the heart could be "armed with a pen" was a seductive one. For millennia the condition of the heart and blood vessels—and, by projection, the state of health of the entire body—had been judged by feeling the pulse.[4] Pulse lore was a key point in the diagnostic protocols not only of Western medicine but of a number of Eastern medical traditions as well. But the perception of the heart and blood vessels had always depended on the *cultivation of sense*, either the sense of touch as the finger was applied to an artery such as the radial or, by the 1820s and 1830s, the sense of hearing that discerned differences in the sounds of the heart valves as they were channeled through the conduit of the stethoscope. What Burdon-Sanderson, Anstie, and the *Lancet* foresaw were aids to diagnosis of circulatory disorders, or even febrile disease in general, that were *not* dependent upon the acuity of the cultivated sense of the physician. These new instruments would create visible and permanent records of great precision the factual contents of which, unlike the private knowledge of the pulse taker or the stethoscope user, would be so accessible to all that they would occasion no disagreement; such "facts" would indeed be "self-analyzed."

In this sense—the creation of a record—the *Lancet* was correct in seeing Wunderlich's thermometer as more of an analogue to the new sphygmograph than the microscope, stethoscope, ophthalmoscope, or laryngoscope. These last three especially had delighted the medical profession and even the public by showing to the eye that which was, at least technically speaking, *visible* but which, because of size or inaccessibility, was not *seeable*. These four instruments *sharpened* or *extended* a perception that already existed and presented their results in the same modality as that in which the information was generated.

But the thermometer took a human sense that was imprecise, variable, and fleeting and translated it into the movement of an instrument—in this case, the column of mercury. This movement could be measured, and the magnitudes so produced could be plotted to give a fever chart. Heat had been translated first into quantity, which could then be displayed as a visual pattern over time. The visual pattern, in turn, contained diagnostic and prognostic information. The thermometer, in ever so simple a way, made possible the rearrangement of sense experience into some new format. It was the forerunner of a host of laboratory instruments that created for the physiologist and the physician a pattern that was not a *picture* of reality but a *manufactured or constructed representation*.

Such representations were not natural modes of perception for the practicing physician of more than a century ago. They came to him out of the physiological laboratory. He learned to cope with them because, beginning in the 1850s, European countries and later America demanded an exposure to laboratory, or "practical," physiology as a sine qua non of clinical training and eventual licensure. But these statutory requirements alone would not have assured a competence in using physiological instruments, or in interpreting their records, much less a reorientation of the physician's perceptual modes. Many "theoretical" preclinical subjects could all too readily vanish from the mind of the busy professional. The graphic, or instrumental, mode of perception endured because modifications of laboratory instruments eventually proved, as *Lancet* had hoped, to be of varying degrees of usefulness in clinical medicine.

But the course of modification and adaptation, from the first physiological experiment and apparatus that reveals a phenomenon to the widespread adoption of an instrument in clinical practice, proved to be a much more convoluted process than the the simple "co-operation of a large number of careful and painstaking observers" that the *Lancet* naively thought necessary. To explore the historical and logical aspects of that transition, I would like to examine some selected episodes concerned with the graphic registration of the heart and arteries, some of the instruments that made this registration possible, and some of the laboratories and hospitals within which these ideas and instruments were developed, from the mid-1850s to the eve of the Great War. I have chosen the cardiovascular system because of its importance in the practice of medicine, because its action generates effects that are both perceivable (movement of heart and arteries) and imperceivable (electric field changes), and because its story has continuities of technique, locale, and personae that tie together a period of almost six decades.

In the course of my narrative I wish to highlight certain questions concerning the historical process of discovery, invention, modification, and exploration that binds physiology and clinical medicine.

- In what ways must a laboratory instrument designed to work with animals be modified to be appropriate for humans?

- Are there any categories of instrumental determinants that dictate whether a given laboratory procedure can be transformed successfully into clinical practice?

- How does the nature, quality, and ease of creation of the graphic record produced by an instrument relate to its acceptance by clinicians?

- What opportunities and pitfalls does the existence of a graphic record present to the physician who is attempting to understand disease?

- What categories of physiological phenomena lend themselves to successful transition from laboratory appearance to clinical datum?

- What types of scientific/medical personalities can carry out such translations from the laboratory to the clinic, and how do they function to bring it about?

- What kinds of institutional circumstances encourage, permit, or obstruct this process of moving techniques out of the physiological institute and into the clinical setting?

Such an approach, when applied to the graphic registration of the heart and arteries, provides me with several different points of comparison and contrast within the theater of European physiology: of venue—Paris, London, Leiden; of personality—Marey, Burdon-Sanderson, Waller, Einthoven, and Lewis; and of outcome—the relative failure of the sphygmograph versus the early inapplicability of the electrocardiogram, and its eventual clinical triumph. This essay makes no claim to being a full history of any of its component parts—sphygmography, electrocardiography, physiological instrumentation, or the use of clinical technology. Nor does it treat fully the lives of those physiologists and clinicians whose investigations I trace. Rather, my hope here is that by limiting my focus to coherent and related parts of each I can make some explorations of a topic that lies at the foundations of both modern physiology and modern medicine.

MAREY, BURDON-SANDERSON, AND THE SPHYGMOGRAPH

The sphygmograph, literally a "pulse writer," had its distant origins across the Rhine. Its forerunner was the kymograph, devised in 1846 by Carl Ludwig, then age thirty-one and in his first job as an anatomist-physiologist at Marburg and long before his move to Leipzig and rise to fame as a doyen of physiologists worldwide.[5] Ludwig's instrument consisted of a drum covered with smoked paper, which was rotated slowly and uniformly by a clock mechanism. Resting on the paper was a stylus, which could be attached to a float on a mercury manometer, which in turn could be connected via a flexible India rubber tube and metal cannula into an artery of an experimental animal. With each heartbeat the stylus would inscribe a small blip on a baseline that would slowly rise and fall as mean arterial pressure was raised or lowered following the changes in intrathoracic pressure caused by respiration.[6] Experiments measuring an animal's blood pressure by tapping directly into an artery or vein went back to Stephen Hales in the early eighteenth century; Ludwig's new twist was an instrument that recorded the changes in a permanent way, such that one could see how the pressure changed *dynamically* with time.

But human beings, unlike horses or dogs, can seldom be induced to have an artery cut open and a cannula inserted. Moreover, as a device for recording pulses—as opposed to the more slowly changing baseline blood pressure—Ludwig's kymograph was not always accurate. As Karl Vierordt, professor of physiology at Tübingen, pointed out, the pulse wave had to move a large mass of mercury in order to register a small excursion; this damping, plus the oscillatory movements possibly created, meant that Ludwig's kymograph could not estimate accurately even the frequency, much less the characteristics, of the pulse.[7] To obviate both difficulties and to produce a tracing of the human pulse without having to open a vessel, Vierordt therefore, in 1853–1855, redesigned Ludwig's kymograph. The moving drum was left unchanged, but the stylus was connected to the long arm of a lever the short arm of which rested, via a pad, on the radial artery. Every pulsation of the artery moved the lever, which inscribed its movement on the paper. By using a large drum that held a sheet of paper over 500 mm long, he could get eighty-five to ninety seconds of continuous record.[8] These graphic recordings could then be analyzed to look for different frequencies to be found in various diseases, or variations in frequency over the period of the recording in a case of a single disease. With gusto Vierordt set out to collect data on the pulses of the well and the sick.[9] His instrument, called a sphygmograph, was, he said, another example of the characteristic direction of modern medicine: the search for objective signs of diseases by the use of chemical, physical, and physiological techniques.[10]

As a pulse counter Vierordt's sphygmograph was useful and suggestive. But as a device to display visually the form of the individual pulse, its results were disappointing. The lever had to be weighted to keep it from overshooting, and thus the movement of the stylus was heavily damped. The instrument was large and relatively immobile. The pulse appeared in the record as a simple oscillation, with almost no features except frequency. Despite Vierordt's clever improvements, the first attempt to make the human heart and its pulse tell its own story foundered on the inherent inadequacies of the instrument; Vierordt's sphygmograph could not discriminate the obvious features of the individual pulse form as well as even the most rank amateur in clinical medicine.

Frenchmen are said to have a lighter touch than Germans, and so it was in this case. In February 1859 Étienne-Jules Marey, a Parisian physiologist who at age twenty-eight had just completed an inaugural thesis on the circulation of the blood, displayed a new version of the sphygmograph before the Société de Biologie. It was a system of levers with an exceedingly light writing arm attached to a small clockwork that moved a piece of smoked glass underneath the stylus during a period of about ten seconds. The instrument was so small and light that it could be strapped onto the arm of the subject. The key to the effectiveness of Marey's sphygmograph was that light tension was exerted by a spring arm only upon the artery itself, and thus the arm could in turn push a separate and freely moving stylus. The heavy damping that plagued Vierordt's instrument was largely eliminated. The redesigned device could write a short but clear record that seemed to contain some interesting characteristics of the normal pulse: a steep rise, a sharp peak, a slower decline sometimes punctuated with a notch, followed by a trough before the whole cycle began again.[11]

The author of this beguiling piece of machinery was born in 1830 in Beaune, Burgundy, and educated in the town at the Collège named after one of Beaune's most famous sons, the mathematician, engineer, and revolutionary Gaspard Monge.[12] Marey went on to study at the Paris Faculté de Médécine and to serve as an *interne* there at the Hôpital Cochin. But very early he turned to a career in physiology. He visited Germany and seems to have made the acquaintance of Ludwig, who was then at Vienna.[13] It was there that Marey became an enthusiast for what he was later to call "*la méthode graphique*," and which he used to great advantage in his thesis of 1859. His career thereafter flowed equably, albeit with a touch of that early poverty that often characterized continental scholars. Until 1868 his living quarters had to serve as his laboratory. In 1867 he was appointed assistant, and in 1869 professor, at that unique Paris institution, the Collège de France, succeeding Flourens in Cuvier's old chair of natural history of organisms. The position brought with it a stipend and a laboratory but no teaching responsibilities beyond an occasional course of public lectures.

It was in these early, struggling days that Marey explored the potentialities of the sphygmograph. He published his work in small increments as he went[14] and then integrated it in his first full-scale book, *Physiologie médical de la circulation du sang basée sur l'étude graphique des mouvements du coeur et du pouls artérial, avec application aux maladies de l'appareil circulatoire* (1863). It was a massive work of over 550 pages, with 235 figures, many of them kymograph tracings. But despite the prominence of words such as "medical" and "diseases" in the title, Marey's book was essentially a treatise on animal physiology. He gave several chapters on the sphygmograph and its characteristics, and tracings of patients with "senile pulse," fevers,

aortic and mitral insufficiency, but without any detailed clinical findings.[15] Marey's concerns were essentially hydrodynamic: he used
his sphygmograph to explicate how the contractile force of the heart
interacted with the tension of the arteries to produce a given pulse
wave. Sphygmographic tracings taken from humans were used
largely for comparison to experiments on animals—for example, the
horse—in which surgically implanted cannulas gave the investigator
much more direct access to the heart and arteries.

Finally, one should note that the *Physiologie médicale* was only the
opening fusillade in a lifelong campaign that Marey waged to establish *la méthode graphique* in physiology and medicine. He sketched
out the idea in his first series of lectures at the Collège de France in
1867–1868,[16] continued to develop it through the 1870s, and gathered together his scattered pieces on the subject in his highly influential monograph, *La méthode graphique dans les sciences expérimentales et
principalement en physiologie et en médecine* (1878). The object of this
method was twofold: first, to remedy "the defectiveness of our
senses for discovering truths, and secondly the inadequacies of language for expressing and transmitting the truths that we have acquired."[17] The graphic method, Marey argued, created a permanent
record, one that was not affected by the prejudices of the observer or
the rhetoric of the expositor. A graphic record could speak across
language barriers. Words changed their meanings with place and
custom; a graphic record did not. The instrument that created it
could retard or accelerate time. It could record more precisely those
phenomena that human sensation perceives with little discrimina-
tion, such as heat and cold. It could create a record of quantities that
we cannot sense at all, such as electricity, magnetism, and gravity.
Indeed, insofar as written language had its origins in pictographs,
civilization itself, he argued, owed its birth to *"l'expression graphique."*[18] Marey was clearly a salesman for more than simply a new
apparatus.

How was such an instrument, and the program implicit in it,
received in the world of English medicine, a world that prided itself
on its practicality, on its disdain for theorizing? When Marey's original description of the sphygmograph was reprinted in the *Gazette
médicale* in 1860, *Lancet* had summarized the article in a paragraph.
The London journal noted that the writing lever on the Marey instrument was lighter and the device easier to use than Vierordt's, but felt
it could "only indicate the frequency or the more or less regularity of

the pulse." It "may be doubted," *Lancet* concluded airily, "whether these instruments, though very ingenious, will ever prove actually useful in practice."[19] Why then, five years later, was this mouthpiece of English medicine trumpeting the instrument it had formerly dismissed? Because it had been taken up by a clinician, who happened also to be a physiologist and an Englishman—a perhaps not unimportant fact.

The clinician-physiologist was John Scott Burdon-Sanderson. Born in Northumberland in 1828 to a wealthy family of dissenters, the tall, rangy, and rather austere Burdon-Sanderson had received his M.D. from the University of Edinburgh in 1851. Immediately thereafter he spent some months in Paris studying botany, organic chemistry, embryology, and physiology—the latter with Claude Bernard—while also attending the Paris hospitals. He then settled in London in 1852. In a way typical of British medicine throughout most of the nineteenth century, Burdon-Sanderson had to cobble together a scientific career during this period of his life by combining some private practice, service as a medical officer of health (Paddington, 1856–1867), some consultantships at a few London hospitals (Brompton Hospital for Consumption, 1859–1863, 1865–1871; Middlesex Hospital, 1863–1870), part-time lecturing at a hospital medical school (St. Mary's, first on botany and then on medical jurisprudence, 1854–1862), and his own researches at home. His early scientific interests were mostly in botany and microscopic histology, and it was only in the early 1860s that he began investigations on physiological topics.[20]

In the autumn of 1864, most likely through his long-standing connections with the Parisian medical world, Burdon-Sanderson got his hands on a Marey sphygmograph and by November was using it to make records on his patients.[21] By early 1865 he brought another up-and-coming physician, Francis Edmund Anstie, then thirty-one years old, into the research.[22] Anstie, in turn, showed the instrument and its uses to Balthazar Foster, a young consultant physician and newly appointed professor of anatomy at Queen's Hospital, Birmingham.[23] All three worked intensely with the sphygmograph over the succeeding few years to clarify the possible uses the instrument might have within clinical medicine. Indeed, they worked so actively that something of a rivalry developed between the Londoners Burdon-Sanderson and Anstie on one side and Foster and his Midlands co-workers on the other. Medical journals also chose sides. *Lancet*, on whose editorial staff Anstie worked, sided with Burdon-Sanderson and his protégé. The upstart *British Medical Journal*, perhaps predict-ably given its connection with the British Medical Association and its championing of country physicians, sided with Foster.[24] For our pur-poses, however, we can treat the three, and their coworkers, as a single group and focus on questions of use and interpretation rather than on the question of who deserved priority for introducing the instrument into British practice.

From the very beginning it seemed likely to the English clinicians that the *shape* of the pulse record might help in the diagnosis and prognosis of acute fevers. In their presentation before the Medical Society of London in November 1865, for example, Anstie and Burdon-Sanderson reported that the sphygmograph might differenti-ate between, on the one side, typhus and typhoid fever and, on the other, "the ephemeral fevers which occasionally simulate them." The sphygmograph seemed to show that typhus and typhoid fever were characterized by a great reduction in arterial tonicity. As a result, when the pulse wave surged into an artery, it met little initial resistance. Thus the sphygmographic curve showed "a nearly verti-cal line of ascent, an acute summit, a sudden descent, and a very marked dicrotism, or double-beat." This continued all hours of the day, up to the time convalescence began, at which point the pulse curve returned to normal. On the contrary, if the pulse failed to return to normal, "dangerous sequellae may be feared." By way of contrast, in other febrile diseases although the pulse became more rapid, it did not change shape.[25]

Given that the presence of a weakened or unusually elastic por-tion of artery would change the shape of the pulse distally, the sphygmograph could also be used to detect and even to locate aneu-rysms. Early in 1866 Anstie reported a case each at King's College Hospital and St. Mary's Hospital, and Foster showed several cases at Queen's Hospital, Birmingham, in which the sphygmograph was used in this way. When an aneurysm was aortic, the right and left radial pulses would be approximately the same. However, when it was axillary or subclavian, the pulse tracings on the two sides would differ.[26] Anstie even went so far as to claim that he could locate the aneurysm from the pulse tracings alone.[27]

As was suggested by these diagnoses, the British emphasized that the sphygmograph could give the clinician a picture of the condi-tion of peripheral arteries. In old age, for example, the arterial walls lose some of their elasticity. Following the lead given by Marey, both

Anstie and Foster found that the resultant tracing in these cases tended to follow the pressure created by the contraction of the ventricle, thus showing a more extended summit and a sudden fall from the plateau. The sphygmograph gave a consistent and reproducible picture of this "senile" pulse.[28]

Even more important than the information that the sphygmograph yielded about arteries was the potential picture it gave of the condition of the heart. If the patient had, for example, aortic insufficiency, with the exit valve from the left ventricle closing incompletely, then blood would regurgitate back into the ventricle, the pulse would be felt as a jerking motion, and the stylus of the sphygmograph would trace an almost vertical line of ascent, with a great amplitude accentuated by a rapid fall in pressure after the pulse.[29] Conversely, if the opening from the heart into the arterial tree were narrowed—aortic stenosis—then the rise and fall of the pulse would be more gradual; the trace looked like a series of hillocks rather than a row of cliffs.[30] Left ventricular hypertrophy showed up, Burdon-Sanderson and Anstie found, as a pulse trace with a broad summit, usually with a pronounced dicrotism.[31] A different pattern seemed characteristic in mitral valvular disease.[32] An irregular and apparently distinctive pulse could be seen in gout.[33] A colleague of Foster's even took three tracings from a surgical patient during the amputation of his leg in order to assess the effect of shock upon the heart.[34]

By late 1866, within two years of the sphygmograph's introduction into Great Britain, it had gotten a favorable reception—at least from the establishment medical press. *Lancet* noted that the physiology of the circulation "has been revolutionized" by the "modern 'mechanical' school," of which Ludwig and Marey were "illustrious members." Progress had been won primarily "by the application of exact instruments" to the heart, circulation, and pulse.

> The fruits of these labors have yet to be gathered. There is reason to hope that a rich harvest of pathological discovery awaits those practical workers who are now applying the new physiological methods to morbid phenomena.

Anstie and Burdon-Sanderson were once again cited as leaders in this new effort.[35]

But Burdon-Sanderson was also a leader in pointing out the difficulties and uncertainties of the method.[36] Indeed, in retrospect it seems that the more he used the sphygmograph, the more he came to appreciate the complexity of the records it yielded. Most certainly the sphygmograph created exact, faithful, and permanent pictures of the phenomena of arterial movement that actuated it. Most certainly these records could capture "differences and peculiarities of the pulse so minute that the most delicate and practiced finger would fail to recognize them."[37] Most certainly these tracings showed, in the same individual but at differing times, an "amazing constancy of form"—but only "*under the same physiological conditions*" (Burdon-Sanderson's emphasis).[38] Change the person or change the conditions, and greatly differing tracings could result. The sphygmograph could be made useful "at the bedside or in the consulting-room" only if we understood the origins of these variations. It was a problem of deciphering:

> The difficulty lies in the fact that the record is written in a language which we are only beginning to understand. Without a proper knowledge of the physiological facts, of which they are the transcript, the oscillations of the lever are quite as meaningless as the vibrations of the telegraphic needle to one who is not furnished with a proper alphabet. If anyone imagines that he will discover in pulse-curves invariable characteristics of particular diseases, he is entirely mistaken; for he will occasionally find that very different tracings present themselves in morbid conditions which appear to be nearly the same, and similar tracings in states of the circulation which are entirely opposite.[39]

An interpretation of the sphygmographic trace, Burdon-Sanderson was saying, would always involve going back to first principles.

What were these first principles? Overall, one could conceive of rhe record as the temporal outcome of the interplay between the tension in the arteries and the force and timing of the beat of the heart. Even in health these could have an immense variation. True, the movement of the sphygmograph did reflect the movement of the artery to which it was attached. But that motion of the instrument depended upon at least four other variables: (1) the force and rate with which the heart ejected blood; (2) the resistance that this force met in the vascular tree as a whole; (3) the state of tonicity of the individual artery to which the sphygmograph was attached, which in turn might be related to its permanent (senile hardening) or transient (vasomotor contraction) condition; and (4) the pressure with which the lever is applied to the artery.[40] With relation to the heart especially, Burdon-Sanderson emphasized, the sphygmograph provided a very compound and indirect record.

Moreover the English investigators found that pulse tracings displayed many adventitious, and sometimes unpredictable, variations even in the state of health. Anstie, for example, found that his own sphygmogram taken in the morning differed from that recorded in the evening; and neither of them matched a tracing made, as he put it, "in a state of great depression from autumnal diarrhea."[41] A young man's pulse taken at midday differed from the trace obtained after a full dinner.[42] Alfred Henry Garrod, an older brother of Archibald Garrod who later became famous as a biochemist, found that the increase in frequency induced by normal exercise could, in turn, change the entire shape and appearance of the pulse wave excursions.[43]

Upon closer examination, febrile diseases also showed a great variety of traces. Some of the best research in this area was done by Frederick H. Mahomed, an Anglo-Indian who began sphygmographic researches in 1870 while a twenty-one-year-old student at Guy's Hospital. By the time he published his results in an extensive series of articles in 1872–1873, he had assembled pages of representative traces related to disease states.[44] Only a few of these, however, could be interpreted clinically with any degree of certainty or consistency. Indeed, even a friend acknowledged that it was "a common saying that no one but Mahomed could interpret all the teachings of the sphygmograph," and that perhaps the "study of its records led him to place too strong a reliance upon the faithfulness of a mechanical contrivance, without due allowance for its necessary imperfections."[45]

Through the 1870s and 1880s sphygmographic tracings continued to adorn articles in medical journals and to be used in medical textbooks.[46] However, they were often used not so much to indicate a visual pattern that invariably accompanied the disease state being discussed, and that could be read as such, but rather as a way of communicating in print what the clinician had felt and observed in *this particular case*. The renowned London clinician William Broadbent, for example, in his famous book on the pulse published in 1890, argued that learning to distinguish pulses with the fingers was more important—and more certain—than placing one's faith in an instrument. He too had shared Anstie's and Burdon-Sanderson's enthusiasm when they had taken up the sphygmograph in the 1860s and 1870s.

> It is not, therefore, from ignorance or want of familiarity with the sphygmograph that I have come to the conclusion that it is not specially useful in practice—that in any form known to me it is not a clinical instrument for everyday work. It is rarely necessary for diagnosis, and scarcely ever to be trusted in prognosis. The indications obtained from it are not, like those of the thermometer, independent of the observer.[47]

Too much hinged, he said, on the type of instrument, the state of the patient, and the skill and unconscious intentions of the sphygmographer. Yet despite these misgivings, Broadbent's book contained hundreds of sphygmographic tracings. Why? Their function was not to train the student to interpret sphygmograms but, rather, to provide a visual means of ensuring that the author and his reader were understanding and describing the same phenomena when they felt the pulse. Broadbent saw the graphic method mainly as a pedagogic tool, with which one could dispense after the apprentice had developed sufficient tacit knowledge.

Although sphygmography in the last decades of the nineteenth century did not fulfill the great expectations so enthusiastically announced in the 1860s, it did not disappear completely. As one can see in figure 6.1, which plots the number of articles and books published on the subject in Europe and America, interest grew rapidly in the 1860s, slowly in the 1870s, and declined in the 1880s. Interest was spread on both sides of the Atlantic, with the instrument being particularly well explored in the more intensely practical medical cultures of Great Britain and the United States.

In England, at least, sphygmography suffered because, by some coincidental twists of fate, it lost its most talented and active adherents. Burdon-Sanderson launched a career in academic physiology by becoming lecturer in that subject at Middlesex Hospital Medical School in 1866 and began to resign his more clinical posts and to cut back his private practice. In 1870 he was appointed professor of practical physiology and histology at University College, London, in the place of Michael Foster, who had left to take the newly created praelectorship in physiology at Cambridge.[48] At almost exactly the same time, British medical licensing bodies began to demand experience in laboratory physiology of candidates sitting examinations,[49] so Burdon-Sanderson's life rapidly filled with teaching and laboratory research. He continued to use the sphygmograph for physiological purposes and incorporated it into his laboratory manual for medical student teaching, but he did little to develop it as a clinical instrument.[50]

Other interests, and in some cases deaths, also depleted the store of workers. Anstie died at the age of forty in 1874. Garrod turned toward comparative anatomy after about 1872 and died of tuberculosis in 1878 at the age of thirty-three. Mahomed became interested in kidney disease; he also died young—aged thirty-five—in 1884. Foster's ambitions took him into politics as a Liberal, through which he became a Member of Parliament, was knighted, and eventually raised to the peerage.

In intellectual terms, the technique failed to gain further ground because there was little in the way of diagnosis that it could do that could not be done in other, more traditional, ways. Aneurysms, hypertrophy, stenosis, valvular incompetence—these aspects of the heart and great arteries could be explored using palpation, percussion, and auscultation. The sphygmograph could provide an interesting and permanent supplementary record, but it was clear by the 1880s that it could make no claims to any exclusive spheres of knowledge. Indeed, it lost one area of usefulness—as a device for measuring blood pressure—when noninvasive sphygmomanometers came into use in the 1890s. Nor did it provide new knowledge about the physiological function of the heart; much of what was known continued to be gleaned from experimental animals, using cannulas inserted surgically into arteries, and instruments that wrote more direct records of cardiac activity. In the 1890s sphygmography remained the purview of a small group of urban consultant physicians, often those who had had a particular enthusiasm for physiological research in their student days.

MAREY, BURDON-SANDERSON, AND THE ELECTRICAL ACTION OF THE HEART

If the sphygmograph proved by the 1880s to be something less than the revolutionary device it had been touted to be, at least it operated on a set of physical principles that any clinician could understand. Yet in the panoply of twentieth-century medical technology, the pulse-writer ended up being replaced by an instrument that recorded not something as obvious and palpable as the heart's beat but a physiological signal imperceivable to human sense: the electrical wave that causes that heartbeat. How did it come about that clinicians after World War I became so intensely concerned with a set of physiological events that were almost totally unknown fifty years before, when the sphygmograph seemed to promise so much? How were devices developed that were capable of recording these events? Once they were developed, how did clinicians come to accept them?

The history of this aspect of graphic recording of the heart is much more convoluted than that of the sphygmograph. In part, such complexity was dictated by biological phenomena. Whereas before 1860 the pulse had a fully defined and preexisting set of medical and physiological meanings, the nature and significance of electrical activity in the heart unfolded only very slowly. Coming to a clear picture of those events depended heavily upon the invention of improved instruments for electrical recording and upon better experimental techniques. Devices that might have potential clinical usefulness were at the same time the very laboratory instruments through which new experimental knowledge was gained. Yet often the accumulators of this knowledge, as well as those who developed the instruments, had their own unique configurations of education, preparation, setting, and agenda, which may or may not have included a commitment to clinical applications. Interestingly, the major figures who pioneered this new picture of the heart were once again Marey and Burdon-Sanderson.

Marey was a man always greatly interested in devices, and in 1875 he came across one that seemed to have great promise. It was an apparatus that used a new physical principle to measure electrical potential and its changes: the capillary electrometer. The concept behind the instrument was really quite simple and elegant and had been worked out in Kirchoff's laboratory in Heidelberg by a young Parisian physicist, Gabriel Lippmann.[51] Lippmann found that the surface tension of a liquid such as mercury, when covered with another electrolyte such as dilute sulfuric acid, was dependent in a complex way upon the *potential difference* across the phase boundary. Change the voltage by even a miniscule amount and one changed the surface tension, and hence the *shape* of the meniscus: it moved up and down. Converting this principle into an instrument was equally simple. One took a glass tube perhaps one-quarter inch across, pulled out one end into a capillary, filled it with mercury, inverted the capillary end into a bath of dilute sulfuric acid, and applied a potential across the mercury/sulfuric boundary. The tiny meniscus, no more than one-fiftieth of a millimeter across, could be viewed through a microscope and could be seen to move almost instantaneously with changes in electromotive force of as little as .0001 volt.[52] Lippmann published preliminary accounts of his experiments on electrocapillarity in 1874 and incorporated a full theoretical treatment into a *Thèse* he presented to the Paris Faculté des Sciences in April 1875 and printed in July.[53]

Marey was a member of that Faculté[54], and he saw immediately that the capillary electrometer had one very important feature that made it vastly superior to the standard galvanometer: it was both sensitive and *quick*. This was especially important in physiological studies of muscle activities, which had long foundered on inadequate investigative instruments.[55] The *jugend* work of Emil du Bois-Reymond in Berlin in the 1840s, based partially in turn upon the much less precise studies of Matteucci in the previous decade, had shown that if an investigator connected one electrode of a sensitive galvanometer to a cut part of a muscle and the other to an uninjured part, a "resting current" flowed. Moreover when the muscle was stimulated into contracting, this resting current was reduced—the so-called negative variation.[56] This change in electrical activity seemed to be an invariable concomitant of muscle contraction. But an experimental difficulty soon became apparent. The separate electrical variations, to which the galvanometer reacted, were very much faster than the response time of the instrument; hence it could give no indication of the time course of these electrical signals. A single electrical impulse was hopelessly distorted, and a rapid series of them was fused into a single excursion.

Marey, in the 1870s, knew this as well an any physiologist. He had worked on some problems of muscle physiology in the early 1870s, and especially on recording the electrical discharge of the torpedo. He was familiar with the properties of the standard galvanometer of the physicists.[57] As he argued cogently, the sensitivity of that instrument enabled it to indicate exactly the electrical state of resting muscle, but its inertia made it unable "to signal the quick variations of the currents" that were generated when a muscle was thrown into a tetanus.[58] Lippmann's new electrometer seemed to promise a way out of this dilemma. Marey joined forces with its inventor, and by April 1876 he could report that *"L'électromètre de*

Lippmann," with its *"mobilité remarquable,"* was able to distinguish individual muscle action potentials where the galvanometer could register only a fused signal.[59]

More important, the capillary electrometer could be applied to Marey's favorite organ, the heart,[60] because it had already been discovered that the heart too displayed a "negative variation" during activity. Two decades before, in 1855, at the modest Physiologisches Institut at the University of Würzburg, Albert Kölliker, friend and former Berlin colleague of du Bois-Reymond, and his colleague, Heinrich Müller, had demonstrated the suspected electrical activity of the vertebrate heart.[61] They placed the electrodes of a galvanometer on the apex and base of an excised frog ventricle, and the needle moved when the heart contracted. By laying the nerve of a frog nerve-muscle preparation (the so-called rheoscopic frog) onto the heart, they could sometimes see the limb twitching just before the systole of the ventricle, indicating perhaps that the electrical event preceded—and might indeed cause—the contraction of the heart.[62]

The experiments of Kölliker and Müller appeared at the time to be idiosyncratic, and were not followed up until 1874 in Utrecht. Franciscus Cornelis Donders[63] and his younger colleague and son-in-law, Theodor Wilhelm Engelmann,[64] a Ludwig student, were fitting out the lavish new Physiologisch Laboratorium there[65] and acquired the newest in electrical recording instruments—the differential rheotome. This exceedingly clever piece of apparatus had been designed and built by Julius Bernstein, working in Helmholtz's physiological laboratory in Heidelberg, to circumvent (at least partially) the sluggishness of sensitive galvanometers.[66] It allowed an investigator to stimulate an excitable tissue, such as a muscle, at a steady rate (for example, ten per second). Then, at some determined interval after each of the stimuli, the rheotome conducted to a galvanometer a brief "slice," as little as one millisecond (msec) long, of the current generated in the active, contracting muscle. The reading of the galvanometer, used in this case as a "ballistic" device bombarded at equal intervals by uniformly brief segments of currents, gave a steady reading that was proportional to the average magnitude of the "slices" of current. By changing the interval between stimulus and slice and recording the different magnitudes at different intervals, one could plot out a representation of the wave of excitation and thereby construct a picture of events less than 5 msec in duration, of which one could have no direct knowledge.[67] At Utrecht Engelmann applied the rheotome to an artificially stimulated frog heart, and from the values it produced he could plot out a wave form of the electrical activity at the surface of the organ. The curves were rather confused, but at least investigators could begin to get some sense of the *propagation* of electrical activity in the heart.[68]

Each instrumental approach to the heart had, however, its own defects. The galvanometer was sensitive but slow in reacting to electrical changes. The rheoscopic frog preparation was fast, but it had greatly variable sensitivity and gave information of only a presence-or-absence kind. The rheotome was the most sophisticated of the three, in that it provided magnitudes during relatively short time intervals, but it produced a picture that was constructed rather than real, of averaged events rather than individual ones, and of reactions evoked by stimulation rather than of natural ones.

Even in his first communication of April 1876 Marey could confirm that the capillary electrometer seemed to meet many of the objections raised against previous techniques and instruments. Attaching electrodes of the Lippmann electrometer to the auricle and apex of an excised frog heart, and viewing the mercury column through the microscope, he could see immediately that there was a potential difference between the two points. Moreover as the heart resumed its slow beating, Marey could watch the column move first one way to indicate a decrease in the voltage at the auricle and then in the opposite direction to indicate a voltage decrease in the ventricle. The two "jerks" in opposing directions had different characters; the first was quick and the second much slower—corresponding, he thought, to the contraction rates of the two chambers.[69]

But Marey was not content with merely observing. He and Lippmann were, he reported, already trying "to capture via photography the image of the movements of the column of mercury." They were seeking an electrical record the precision of which would parallel that of the mechanical record produced by the muscle contraction via the kymograph.[70] Within three months, by late July 1876, after "a great number" of experiments, they could report success in photographing the all-important *forme*, "the faithful expression" of the electrical variation."[71] Using a capillary with a mercury column no wider than $\frac{1}{20}$ mm, embedded in a metal plate, they could shine focused sunlight on one side of the screen four times each second and move a light-shielded photographic plate on the other, at the rate of about 1.25 mm/sec. As the column moved up and down in response to the changing potential in the contracting heart, it obstructed more or less of the light, thereby painting a rhythmically varying boundary between exposed and unexposed parts of the plate, "whose curves correspond to the changes of intensity of the electromotive force of the heart."[72] A tortoise and a frog were honored by having their hearts produce the first electrocardiograms. These techniques, Marey concluded, "open up a new domain to the graphic method."[73]

But it was a domain not without its problems. Some were technical. Marey's setup produced a moderately satisfactory record for the tortoise heart, but only because that organ had a contraction cycle some six to seven seconds long, and a recorded voltage change of a bit more than 20 millivolts. Even so, the record of an individual cardiac cycle was minuscule—8 mm long by 3 mm high. The auricle of a frog heart, beating once each second, with a quarter the amplitude, produced a record that resembled a fine saw blade. Because there was no magnification in the system, over fifty seconds of record was crammed onto 6.5 cm—about two and a half inches—of photographic plate.[74] Marey was indeed the first to produce a true record of the electrical activity of the vertebrate heart, but it was an exceedingly limited record of a very specialized set of circumstances.

Burdon-Sanderson was privy to these new developments from the very beginning—although by something of an accident. In the grand tradition of Victorian expositions, an exhibition of a "Loan Collection of Scientific Apparatus" had been arranged for May 1876 at the South Kensington Museum.[75] Among the special day-long conferences to be held in conjunction with this event were two on biology chaired by Burdon-Sanderson. Marey came over from Paris with his assistant, Charles A. François-Franck, to demonstrate his various instruments. He spoke at length (in French) about his newest modifications to the sphygmograph and about the mechanical cardiograph.[76] Then he, François-Franck, and Donders adjourned with many of the attendees to the Criterion Restaurant, Piccadilly Circus, for dinner and the first Annual General Meeting of the Physiological Society, not yet two months old.[77] It was during this exhibition that the London physiologist learned about the capillary electrometer.

That spring and summer of 1876 Burdon-Sanderson was in an unusually favorable circumstance to understand and appreciate Marey's innovation—favorable both with regard to his institutional resources and facilities, and with respect to the recent line of his research. In the early 1870s Burdon-Sanderson had had, as always, more projects and responsibilities than most men had careers.[78] In addition to his job as professor of practical physiology and teacher of histology at University College, he was appointed in late 1871 as professor-superintendent of the newly founded Brown Institution, where he and an assistant established an eight-room pathological laboratory as a research center for diseases of animals and humans. During the 1870s he wrote not only on his old topics of circulation and respiration but on a host of new ones, including the question of abiogenesis, and bacteria in their connection to pyaemia, inflammation, and infectious diseases of humans and animals. He was a stalwart of the Pathological and Clinical Societies of London, published a large and controversial textbook on laboratory physiology, and gave lectures on the state of the emerging discipline to the British Medical Association and to the British Association for the Advancement of Science. When the venerable William Sharpey retired in 1874, Burdon-Sanderson replaced him in a chair now dignified with an endowment of £7500, a name—the Jodrell Professorship of Physiology—and a grant from the donor of £500 to buy equipment.[79] Appropriately enough, it was at his house that a score of medical researchers had met in March 1876 to found The Physiological Society as a body for social and scientific exchange among physiologists, and as an action group to thwart the antivivisection legislation then threatening in Parliament.[80]

Inter alia, Burdon-Sanderson started applying the approach of an animal physiologist to a boyhood interest: botany. It had long been known that certain plants—for example, the Venus flytrap from the American South—had powers of movement analogous to those of muscle. Muscle, it was also known, had its intrinsic electrical activity that accompanied movement. Was the same concomitant also found in the contractile tissues of plants? To answer the question, Burdon-Sanderson had in 1873 obtained some flytraps, *Dionaea muscipula*, from Charles Darwin, who had long been carrying out experiments on insectivorous plants.[81] Burdon-Sanderson then recorded from them using a sensitive, but slow, Thomson astatic galvanometer. Within a few months he could show that potential differences—and hence currents—could be recorded from parts of the leaf and stalk and from cut surfaces. Moreover when a fly crept into a leaf during recording, the "leaf-current" first showed a "negative variation," and then the leaf snapped shut on the hapless fly. There was a delay of one-quarter to one-third second between the stimulus and the negative variation, and a refractory period of ten to twenty seconds before the leaf could be restimulated.[82] As Burdon-Sanderson emphasized in lectures before audiences both scientific and popular in 1873 and 1874, one of which occasioned a rare public appearance by Darwin himself, "these currents are subject, in all respects in which they have yet been investigated, to the same laws as those of muscle and nerve."[83]

Against the background of those kinds of recent investigations, it was natural that Burdon-Sanderson would want to learn how to use Marey's new toy. Before he had to return to Paris, François-Franck volunteered to help. Burdon-Sanderson's diary jottings in the next few months of 1876 reflect the transfer of technique:

    May 30: 10–3 Expt at Univ. Coll. with Dr. Frank
            6–7 Dr. F. to dinner
        31: Evening Dr. Frank—apparatus
    June 1: 2.30 At U.C. 4 Electromtrs
        2: 10–1 with Donders at S[outh] K[ensington]
        8: 6–7.30 Read Lippmann's Paper
        10: 2–5 Experiments on Dionaea First successful determination
            of time interval
    July 8: 12–3 Laboratory—Expt with Electrometer.[84]

Clearly the capillary electrometer was exactly the kind of instrument Burdon-Sanderson had sought, for in the succeeding months he used it not only at Kew Gardens on *Dionaea* but on muscle, nerve, and even heart:

    October 26: Afternoon—Lab Expts on the nerve variation of the
                Heart
            27: Aftn—Expts on H[eart] variation time measurement
            31: 1–4 Work at Laboratory—Expts as to Elect. Phenom. of
                Heart
    November 1: Afternoon—Expts on Heart & Muscles
            2:1–5 Laboratory—Continue Expt on Heart[85]

The experiments eventuated very quickly in two papers before the Royal Society, one on the electrical activity of the *Dionaea* leaf, which he finished in late November, and another, shorter one on the electromotive properties of muscles which he sent off two weeks later.[86] In both, Burdon-Sanderson used the Lippmann electrometer as a visual indicator of change in potential. In the first he and his collaborator gratefully acknowledged that they "became acquainted with this instrument through the kindness of Prof. Marey, who had already adopted it in physiological investigations relating to animal electricity."[87]

Given how quickly both Marey and Burdon-Sanderson pounced upon the new device and saw its applicability to the heart, it is genuinely curious that the Frenchman failed completely to follow up on the graphic aspects of his technique, and the Englishman did so only in a roundabout way. In 1877 Marey used the electrometer to inspect visually the electrical discharge of the torpedo, and in 1878 he published a brief note on ventricular systole studied with the Lippmann electrometer.[88] But beyond that, nothing. When, in 1881, he brought out a new edition of his already classic *La circulation du sang, à l'état physiologique et dans les maladies,* he inserted a section entitled "Electrical Variations that Accompany the Movements of the Heart"; but it contained only three brief paragraphs about electrical recording and the tortoise and frog electrocardiograms done five years previously.[89] Burdon-Sanderson, with his assistant at the Brown Institute, F. J. M. Page, worked steadily through the late 1870s on the excitatory process and its conduction in the frog's heart, but he did the investigations largely with the rheotome. He used the capillary electrometer in the circuit only as a way of making a preliminary visual observation on the nature of the deflection caused by artificial excitation—in other words, as a detector rather than as a recording instrument.[90]

To transform the capillary electrometer into a useful graphic instrument for actual recording, Burdon-Sanderson added to it an adequate optical and photographic system, one largely of his own design. He seems to have begun work on the apparatus about 1879 and did not bring it to the requisite perfection until mid-1881. His greatest problem was to amplify optically the minuscule movements of the mercury. He therefore arranged an apparatus that shone light from a powerful artificial source (an oxyhydrogen lamp with a condensing lens) across the top of the column, and then used another lens to focus the enlarged shadow on a blackened screen about twenty inches distant. This dividing line between light and dark fell upon a slit in the screen only a millimeter wide. Behind the screen ran an inclined railway with a small carriage to carry a photographic plate past the slit. A clock mechanism, with cords and pulleys, regulated the descent to move the plate at a uniform rate. His new apparatus therefore hitched the quickness and sensitivity of the capillary electrometer to a much more flexible means of creating records. Compared to Marey's rather makeshift photographic apparatus, the plate moved four times as fast, was twice as large, and registered excursions that had been optically amplified up to twentyfold.

To test his new system, Burdon-Sanderson used his old friend, the Venus flytrap. It had slow and powerful action currents and was relatively simple to use compared to animal tissues. His *Dionaea* responded beautifully when he stimulated their leaves with a camel-hair brush; they produced action currents that showed up as distinct diphasic spikes a second in duration and of sizable amplitude.[91]

By the late summer and fall of 1882 Burdon-Sanderson had improved the speed and sensitivity of the apparatus still further and added time markers and a signal for stimulation. He could now go back to the more fragile preparation: the heart. Burdon-Sanderson and Page made a series of recordings from the stimulated hearts of frogs and tortoises, duplicating some of the rheotome studies they had done almost five years before.[92] By varying the placement of the stimulating and recording electrodes, they could show—with direct visual rather than derived numerical proof—that contraction of the ventricle was accompanied by a negative electrical wave that radiated outward from the point of stimulus. It could last as long as two seconds and could be much shortened if the ventricle were stimulated directly rather than through the auricle; part of the time in the natural cycle was absorbed in the slow conduction of the stimulus through the auricle. The plates pictured clearly how the controversial diphasic action current of the heart occurred because the near electrode first became negative with respect to the more distant one, and then the more distant with respect to the near.

Perhaps more important in the long term were not Burdon-Sanderson's results but his records. The best of his plates, some 26 cm long and moving at almost 10 mm/sec., showed clearly the time marker at 20/sec., the dot at stimulation, and the sharply defined spikes some 6 or 7 mm high. Despite the acknowledged need for further refinements, which he promised, Burdon-Sanderson felt the case for his technique had been documented:

> The results of our experiments appear to us to establish the applicability of the Capillary Electrometer as an instrument of physiological investigation and the value of the photographic method as a means of recording electrical changes in living structures.[93]

The first thirty years of physiologists' "recording" the electrical activity of the heart, from 1854 to the mid-1880s, shows some interesting patterns underlying the leisurely, almost desultory pace characteristic of investigations into phenomena that have as yet no defined significance. One can see, for example, how it can take several generations of instrumentation before one instrument—in this case the capillary electrometer—overcomes enough of the inherent obstacles to begin to define the phenomena. One can see in the events of 1876 an instance of how instrumentally based techniques often need personal contact among investigators in order to be communicated effectively. Finally, one can see in the constant interplay between biological materials and instrumental capabilities an ever-present dialectic in the investigative enterprise; each must continually be fitted and refitted to the other; Venus flytraps and tortoise hearts had to be used as test subjects until the apparatus was sufficiently developed even to produce a record of a seemingly simple and lowly object, the frog heart. The path between phenomenon and graphic record, even at the zoological level, could be as convoluted in reality as it now seems straightforward in retrospect.

WALLER AND THE HUMAN ELECTROCARDIOGRAM

One very interested witness to these developments in the laboratory at University College was Burdon-Sanderson's youngest guest investigator, Augustus Désiré Waller. He came to physiology both by inheritance and by training. His father, Augustus Volney Waller, F.R.S., was a distinguished English anatomist/physiologist who spent most of his professional life in the stimulating medical ambience of Paris. There the younger Augustus was born in 1856, and there he was raised before being sent on to the Collège de Genève. It was the father whose name is preserved in the anatomical technique of "Wallerian degeneration," discovered in the year of the son's birth, and which is used to the present day as a way of tracing the course of neurons through the peripheral and central nervous system. When Augustus Désiré came to write a widely used *Introduction to Human Physiology* in the early 1890s, he dedicated it to his father's memory and emblazoned it with a list of discoveries: "Emigration of leucocytes, 1846; degeneration and regeneration of nerve, 1856; ciliospinal region, 1851; vaso-constrictor action of sympathetic, 1853." Augustus D. was intensely proud of his father's reputation; Hallibur-

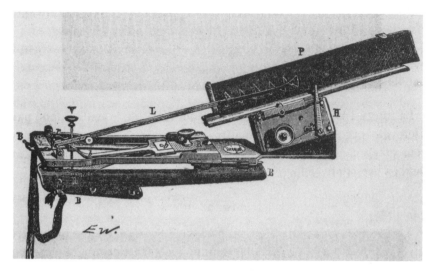

Marey's original illustation of his sphygmograph (1859)

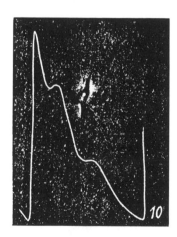

Sphygmographic tracing by Burdon-Sanderson and Anstie in a case of aortic regurgitation (1867)

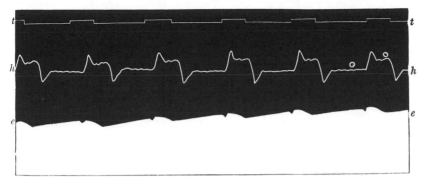

Waller's first published electrocardiogram of man (1887), showing tracings of the capillary electrometer (e), mechanical cardiograph (h) and time (t); actual size

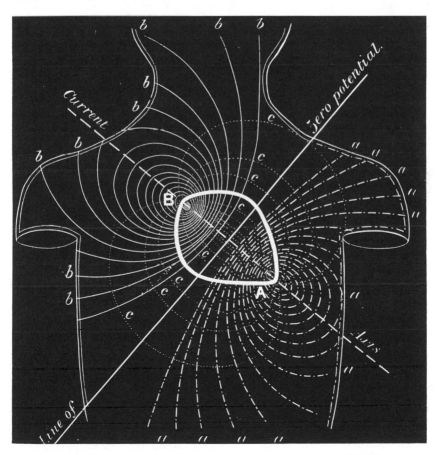

Waller's diagram of tilted electrical axes in the human heart (1887)

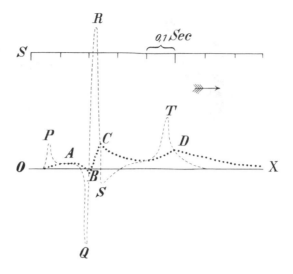

Einthoven's reconstruction of a true electrocardiogram PQRST from the distorted capillary electrometer tracing ABCD (1895)

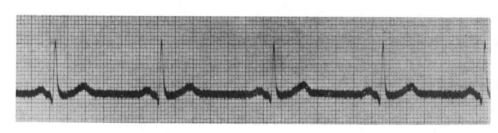

One of Einthoven's first published electrocardiograms using the string galvanometer (1903)

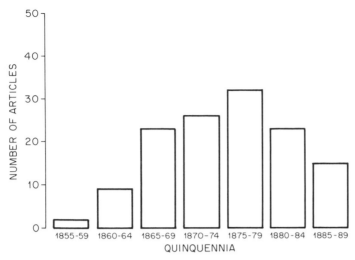

Numbers of journal articles under "Sphygmograph" in the Surgeon General-al's Catalogue

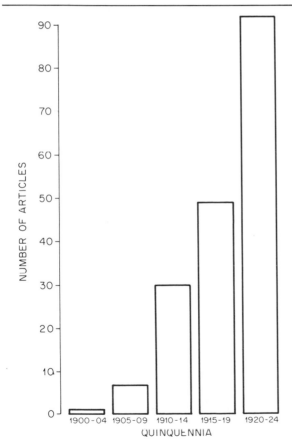

Numbers of journal articles under "Heart, Electrocardiography of the,"in the Surgeon General's Catalogue

ton recalled that in forty years of knowing Waller, he had seen him aroused to anger only when he thought his father's work was being misrepresented or depreciated.[94]

The elder Waller died in 1870, and mother and son returned to Aberdeen, where Augustus lived at home, read medicine at the university, and graduated M.B., C.M. in 1878. His father's friend William Sharpey had urged him into research, so he went immediately for about six months of laboratory training at Carl Ludwig's institute in Leipzig. As was usual with Ludwig's students, Waller learned by doing. In his *Arbeit* he used manometric techniques to investigate how pressure in the auricles of guinea pigs varied as a function of electrical stimulation of the spinal cord.[95] The experiments were typical of Ludwig's approach, and very likely—given both Ludwig's usual practices and the complexity of the German text—it was also the professor who wrote up the results.[96] But it was exactly this combination of solid training with self-effacing encouragement that brought so many of Ludwig's pupils into the discipline. Waller was no exception, and for many years he proudly counted himself as a pupil of the Leipzig master.

After some additional study at Edinburgh, Waller settled in London to practice in the autumn of 1879, and his ties with Sharpey and Ludwig naturally brought him into the orbit of Burdon-Sanderson at University College. Waller's first small piece of research there was done in 1879–1880 at the suggestion of the Jodrell professor, and showed Waller's talents to advantage. Using two Marey "tambours" to transmit both the heart's apex beat and the pulsation of a peripheral artery to a kymograph, he could measure the propagation rate of the arterial pulse wave and distinguish the time taken in propagation from the latency caused by the systolic pressure building up to equal the resisting aortic pressure.[97] It was an elegant piece of work, in which Waller took a confused question, analyzed it, and then mastered it with a set of experimental techniques that were simple, quantitative, and precise. As a clinical coda he discussed how his findings illuminated the nature of systolic murmurs and how the propagation rate of the pulse was affected by the recently discovered cardiac drug, amyl nitrate.[98]

With this kind of solid background, instrumental skill, clarity of thinking, and interest in human and clinical aspects of physiology, Waller was obviously a man worth encouraging. Burdon-Sanderson did exactly that. In 1880 he sponsored Waller for election to the

Physiological Society, at whose meetings in succeeding years Waller gave demonstrations on the electrical excitability of muscle and nerve.[99] In the same year Waller won a small research grant of £20 from the British Medical Association, most likely with Burdon-Sanderson's support, for "An Investigation on the Time and Relations of Muscular Contractions in the Human Body in Health and Disease."[100] Burdon-Sanderson also brought Waller into laboratory teaching at University College London. Waller responded by contriving many new exercises on the physiology of nerve and muscle. These were incorporated by Burdon-Sanderson into his book, *University College Course of Practical Exercises in Physiology* (1882), with credit on the title page and praise in the preface to Waller, "who devoted much time and thought to simplification of methods."[101]

This grooming of a physiologist came to a head in 1883 when Burdon-Sanderson stepped into the newly created Waynflete Professorship of Physiology at Oxford; his alter ego, Edward Schaefer, was promoted to the Jodrell professorship at U.C.L., and Waller got Schaefer's old position as lecturer in physiology at the London School of Medicine for Women. Waller stepped up to an even better situation a year later, when he received the lecturership at St. Mary's Hospital Medical School and a two-year concurrent appointment as one of the British Medical Association's first research scholars.[102]

It was his research project for that fellowship, on the process of fatigue and recovery in muscle, that led him back to his earlier interest in the heart, but with the new electrical-photographic methods that had been developed by Burdon-Sanderson at University College in the early 1880s. Waller apparently thought that during fatigue, the action current of a muscle might be altered.[103] The standard Thomson reflecting galvanometer gave him inconclusive results, so he redesigned it, by about the summer of 1885, into a galvanograph that could create permanent, kymograph-like records.[104] A small mirror was mounted on a coil suspended between the poles of a permanent magnet; a spot of light was shone on the mirror, and the beam reflected into a lightproof box, upon a slowly rotating drum covered with a bromide photographic paper. When a biological current was passed through the coil, the mirror moved minutely, with a deflection proportional to the strength of the current. It was a very slow instrument, but its new form of writing "stylus"—a beam of light—made it very sensitive. With this he could see in frogs' muscles a distinct decline of injury and action currents following fatigue.[105]

Given Waller's bent toward physiology of a more human type, it was natural that he should ask himself, "If this happens in cold-blooded animals, does it happen in warm-blooded ones as well?" He set out to make analogous recordings in frogs and mammals and to compare the three major classes of muscle: voluntary, involuntary, and cardiac.[106] It was this last combination, amphibian compared to mammalian cardiac muscle, that provided him with a surprising and tantalizing anomaly. As the excised mammalian heart died, *the electrical sign associated with contraction outlasted the contraction itself.*[107] In all other muscles electrical and mechanical activity had been indissolubly linked. Here was a biological circumstance that indicated not only the temporal but the causal primacy of electrical action.

By October 1885 Waller and his assistant in physiology at St. Mary's, E. Waymouth Reid, had started a series of kymographic and electrophysiological studies of the excised mammalian heart that continued into the summer of 1886. The aim of their dual approach, using both mechanical and electrical graphic recording, was to explore the relation between the two. They found, for example, that hearts of rabbits, cats, and dogs would give spontaneous beats for much longer after excision than had been thought—up to two hours in the case of a dog. Their kymograph records showed that in the dying heart, force and frequency declined regularly, often with a bigeminal beat (alternating strong and weak) appearing. Sometimes a beat would be dropped, with the following systole being of unusual force. Moreover the duration of systole would be lengthened, from a normal value of about 0.3 seconds to a maximum of 6 seconds. This, he found, was caused by cooling; cold had a preservative effect such that a cat's heart could even be frozen hard and recommence spontaneous beating after thawing. Lengthening of systole was accompanied by an increase in the delay before the heart responded to artificial excitation, the so-called latent period of stimulation.

By a double kymograph similar to the one they had used on the arterial pulse wave six years before, Waller and Reid could show clearly that contraction traveled as a mechanical wave from one part of the heart to another. But the wave of contraction in the mammalian ventricle was ten to one hundred times more rapid than that of the frog, a rapidity that decreased progressively after excision. Seemingly of more significance was a *reversed direction of propagation;* whereas the mechanical and electrical waves in the frog heart went from base to apex, the mechanical wave in a mammal's heart generally seemed to go from apex to base.[108]

Exactly the same kind of findings seemed to be confirmed by the very delicate and slow Thomson galvanometer—so slow, in fact, that each time they took a reading they had to wait half a minute for the needle to stop oscillating. When contractions were stimulated artificially, the electrical signs were often diphasic, indicating a propagated wave. Similarly, spontaneous beats were diphasic, but the galvanometer could show no uniform origin for the propagated wave; base to apex and apex to base occurred in equal numbers.[109]

These experiments were completed by late winter of 1886, so Waller and Reid took advantage of a meeting of the Physiological Society in Burdon-Sanderson's department at Oxford on 20 March to demonstrate some of their galvanometer findings. The spontaneously beating excised heart of a dog showed diphasic variations, which seemed to indicate "negativity at base (1st phase) followed by negativity at apex (2nd phase)." They also discussed some of their other results on excised mammalian hearts.[110]

Given the ambiguity of the galvanometer findings, Waller and Reid argued, an "examination by the electrometer of the electromotive changes, as revealed by the galvanometer," was "of obvious importance." The key feature of the Lippmann capillary electrometer was that it could "follow rapid changes of potential far more faithfully" than any other instrument. Its superiority could be fully used only by "recourse to the photographic method, by which a permanent record of the variations is made." Moreover Waller recognized that in the galvanometer "*magnitude* and *duration* of electromotive changes, such as occur with the action of the heart, are compounded and cannot be separated." (That is, one cannot distinguish y current flowing for x time from $\frac{1}{2} y$ current flowing for $2 x$ time). The electrometer could, "to some extent," estimate the two quantities separately. Waller had been schooled in just the apparatus needed: Burdon-Sanderson's version of the capillary electrometer, arranged to record photographically, although Waller modified it slightly, substituting focused sunlight for the oxyhydrogen lamp as a source of illumination. The recording electrodes were arranged as for the galvanometer, with one on the base and one on the apex of the excised beating heart.[111]

It was squarely in the middle of these new experiments with the capillary electrometer on excised mammalian hearts that Waller "discovered" the human electrocardiogram. The historical evidence is sparse indeed, consisting of two sentences in the published Proceedings of the Physiological Society for its meeting at Cambridge on Saturday, 15 May 1886:

> 1. Drs. WALLER and REID communicated further results of experiments on the mammalian heart with the capillary electrometer. Photographs were shown of the electrical variations of the cardiac contractions, both excited and spontaneous, also of the variations of the human heart.[112]

Clearly Waller had obtained capillary electrometer records of the electrical action of the human heart. If one is to credit retrospective evidence, it seems to have been one of those conjectural discoveries: "What if I try . . . ?" As he was thinking about how contraction ran from base to apex in the frog, and seemingly from apex to base in mammals, he thought of the human heart.

> Led on from thought to thought it occurred to me that it should be possible to get evidence of electrical action on man by connecting not the heart itself, which is obviously impossible, but parts of the surface of the body near the heart with a suitable instrument; having verified this supposition, the next step was to see whether or no the same evidence can be obtained by connecting the instrument with parts of the body at a distance from the heart, with the hands or feet.[113]

Indeed, it did work.

After his rather casual announcement to the Physiological Society, Waller did little to follow up on his discovery. When he published his second report on fatigue and recovery in July, work he had done on his B.M.A. research scholarship, he summarized in passing his and Reid's findings on excised hearts, noted that they had studied the electrical aspect by means both of the galvanometer and the capillary electrometer, and stated: "We have extended our observations from the excised to the heart *in situ*, and to that of man."[114] And in November, when Burdon-Sanderson communicated Waller and Reid's long paper to the Royal Society, it contained only a final paragraph dealing with the human electrocardiogram:

> A desire to obtain the variation of the absolutely normal and unexposed heart led us to the exploration of the human subject with the following result, viz., auricular followed by ventricular negativity anteceding respectively the auricular and ventricular events. We could

obtain no evidence of a diphasic ventricular variation, and we have yet to exclude the possibility of the observed variation being caused by alteration of contact by the heart's impulse.[115]

Waller repeated much the same wording in a brief précis of his and Reid's findings in a note he sent to Brown-Séquard to read before the Paris Académie des Sciences in the spring of 1887.[116] These few sentences, here and there, tucked into four disparate publications over an eleven-month period, hardly constituted a strong statement of an important discovery. Why should Waller, interested in the human aspects of physiology, be so desultory and obscure in announcing his findings?

Part of Waller's reticence becomes manifest in the structure and content of his first article that focused entirely on the phenomenon of graphic recording of the electrical activity of the human heart, "A Demonstration on Man of Electromotive Changes Accompanying the Heart's Beat," published about September 1887 in the *Journal of Physiology*. He started with the observed effects.

> If a pair of electrodes (Zinc covered by chamois leather and moistened with brine) are strapped to the front and back of the chest, and connected with a Lippmann's capillary electrometer, the mercury in the latter will be seen to move slightly but sharply at each beat of the heart. If the movements of the column of mercury are photographed on a traveling plate simultaneously with those of an ordinary cardiographic lever a record is obtained as under (figure 1) in which the upper line *h.h.* indicates the heart's movements and the lower line *e.e.* the level of the line in the capillary. Each beat of the heart is seen to be accompanied by an electrical variation.

Waller then went on to his main point: proving that this "electrical variation is physiological, and not due to a mechanical alteration of contact between the electrodes and the chest wall caused by the heart's impulse." If it were physiological, then the electrical signal ought to *precede* the heartbeat—a point he proved by meticulously comparing electrical and mechanical records to show that the variation appeared about 15 msec. before the mechanical effect of the beat. One could prove the same beyond doubt by plunging two hands, or one hand and one foot, into dishes of salt solution that were connected to the electrometer. The movement of the mercury, although less than when recording through the chest electrodes, could not have been created by the mechanical movement of the electrodes, and confirmed that this was a genuinely physiological phenomenon. In conclusion, Waller noted that there were "difficulties which arise in the interpretation of the character of the electrical variation of the human heart." One of these was the puzzling fact that among the seven possible leads (precordium, back, left hand, right hand, left foot, right foot, mouth), some combinations of two gave strong signals and some weak; some gave variation in one direction, and some in the opposite. "It is on account of these sources of doubt," Waller said, that he had "not thought it advisable at this stage to attempt a definite interpretation of the character of the variation."[117]

Yet by the early summer of 1886, Waller had arrived at a satisfactory interpretation of the human electrocardiogram, one that he pressed with great success, which won him much scientific fame in his own day and a place of respect in ours. How did this come about? Or, conversely, why did it take Waller two years to "discover" his discovery? The answer lies in an obstacle overcome and a picture "seen."

Sometime in the early summer of 1886, only a few months after Waller had discovered the phenomenon of the human electrocardiogram but before he had proved its physiological nature, he and Reid completed their electrometer studies of the excised mammalian heart.[118] Plates seemed to show more and more clearly that the spontaneous electrical signal was *monophasic,* and became *diphasic* only as the heart died. This was, as they put it, a fact "for which our previous experiments had not prepared us." Given that the capillary electrometer is an instrument of demonstrated rapidity, a monophasic variation "is proof of a practically single and simultaneous change taking place throughout the ventricle, and disproof, or at least failure of proof, of the passage of a wave of excitation in the contractile substance." Such simultaneity, in turn, "postulates the existence of nervous channels of conduction"—an interesting and significant new piece of evidence in the controversy raging during the 1870s and 1880s on whether the heartbeat was *myogenic* or *neurogenic.*[119] The mammalian heart seemed clearly different from the amphibian one. Yet the human electrocardiogram seemed, in turn, not to square with the properties of the mammalian heart. The amphibian heart seemed diphasic, the mammalian monophasic, and the human diphasic. Waller might well have wondered whether a retributive God had decided to annul vertebrate evolution. Little wonder that Waller, known to be a physiologist highly interested in the human and clinical side of his discipline—a set of programmatics based upon the belief that frogs and cats had something to say about man—hesitated and temporized.

The insight seems to have come about February or March 1888. The "master key," as Waller put it later that year, was the "curious and puzzling," the "unsymmetrical and irrational" ensemble of favorable and unfavorable leads.[120] Right and left hands in the basins gave a signal, as did right hand and left foot. But left hand and left foot gave none. Suddenly he saw why. The longitudinal axis of the human heart tilts to the left. If there were a dipole created between the base and the apex of the heart, then the current axis of this dipole would be similarly tilted, and there would be a line of zero potential perpendicular to the current axis. With the body acting as a volume conductor, only connections across the zero line would yield variations when the dipole was activated. Hence right arm and left leg gave a signal, whereas left arm and left leg gave none.[121]

But if a dipole existed, even ever so transiently, then a diphasic variation must also exist. So in March and April he went back and used the capillary electrometer to record from the cat heart *in situ.* First, he could show that certain distant leads, such as mouth, front paws, and back paws, were functionally equivalent to direct leads from the base or the apex. Moreover the potentials led off in this way showed symmetry with respect to the axis of the animal's heart. But more important, when recorded *in situ* the spontaneously beating heart of the cat showed a *diphasic* variation. In the majority of cases the apex became negative first, followed by the base. Monophasic variations came only as the result of injury, to which the mammalian heart was very prone; Waller could show in experimental detail how these injuries and artifacts could come about.[122]

Having cleared up the animal side, Waller could then interpret the human electrocardiogram, and its system of favorable and unfavorable leads, as evidence that "contraction of the ventricles is not simultaneous throughout the mass, but traverses it as a wave. . . . Inequalities of potential at different parts of the mass, are consequently established at the beginning and at the end of each systole."[123] To confirm his interpretation, he sought out medical cases of human *situs viscerum inversus,* a rare congenital circumstance in which the patient's heart tilted to the right. Exactly as he had expected, the pairs of favorable and unfavorable leads were reversed.[124]

Moreover the potential recorded on the plate of Waller's human electrocardiogram seemed to be diphasic and to represent the heart becoming negative first at the apex, then at the base. He could even infer that because the maximum of the first phase was reached in about 20 msec., the excitatory state traveled the 10 cm of the ventricle's length at about 5 m/sec. These, then, were the elements of Waller's discovery: (1) the recorded plate showed a true physiological variation of a diphasic nature, which (2) created a potential distribution that gave rise to favorable and unfavorable leads, which (3) indicated a propagated wave traversing the heart from apex to base.

If the foregoing reconstruction of Waller's thinking is correct, the human electrocardiogram emerged out of a tangled welter of hunches, notions, research lines and instrumental improvements applied to a range of animals in almost a bewildering variety of experimental circumstances. The thread connecting the bits and pieces was the belief that there exists a coherence in nature between the physiological phenomena of men and of animals. If instruments can be designed so as to yield, indirectly, graphic records of a kind that can be produced directly through experimental procedures on animals, then other points of congruence should validate this uniformity—this transitivity—of interpretation. In the case of the sphygmograph, the pulse was so clearly both a human and an animal phenomenon of precisely analogous nature that the question of nontransitivity was never raised. But electrical action of the animal heart was so new and still in the process of being defined that one had to use the instrument itself that revealed the human electrocardiogram—the capillary electrometer—to confirm this transitivity. For this reason the first electrocardiograms could not be, as we might like them to be, mere pictures. They had to be assigned meaning. To find that meaning they had to be linked up with the animal evidence, even if that meant, as in the case of Waller, having to discover it himself.

The story of the human electrocardiogram had developed very rapidly in the winter and spring of 1888, and Waller spent the next two years trumpeting his results. First came a half-page note of results sent off to the Paris Académie des Sciences in May.[125] The major piece of work was a paper to the Royal Society in June, once again communicated by Burdon-Sanderson, although it was not published in full for another eighteen months.[126] In October Waller made "the electromotive properties of the human heart" the subject of his introductory address to open the academic year at St. Mary's Hospital Medical School; the text was reprinted in full in the *British Medical Journal* and even in the *Times* of London.[127] He followed it up with a brief précis in *Nature* of the main points of his paper presented to the Royal Society, which was still in press.[128] In December he traveled to Paris, where he demonstrated the effect to Brown-Séquard, and where his memoir on the subject was awarded the Prix Montyon in physiology by the Académie des Sciences; Brown-Séquard chaired the committee that recommended the award, and Marey served on it.[129]

The year 1889 saw Waller's proselytizing activities unabated. He visited the reclusive but influential Edward Pflüger at Bonn, and with the skeptical physiologist coaxed a message out of the mercury of the capillary electrometer.[130] When the First International Congress of Physiologists gathered at Basel in September, Waller was there to demonstrate and explicate the human electrocardiogram.[131] Finally, in December he journeyed to Berlin, where his demonstrations were the centerpiece of an extraordinary session of the Berlin Physiologische Gesellschaft. In addition to a dog and a horse, the venerable du Bois-Reymond himself was an experimental subject on whom the favorable and unfavorable leads were demonstrated. The variations could even be magnified 1,250 times and projected upon a ground glass screen in a lecture room.[132] Such wide exposure, both of the phenomenon and of the man, led the Bologna Academy of Sciences to award Waller its Aldini medal in May 1892 and the Royal Society to elect him a fellow in the following month.[133] He was only thirty-five at the time.

Waller's papers of 1887 and 1888 are commonly cited as the beginnings of electrocardiography. They are indeed. But it is important to keep in mind that Waller took a fundamentally *physiological* approach to his subject. He was interested in *normal* function, whether of mammal or of man. His themes, as he developed them in lectures, demonstrations, and papers, were ones of *understanding* the variations. The graphic representations he produced and the instrument that created these images were of relatively secondary concern. Waller published—although often republished—only two human electrocardiograms in the era of initial discovery. Several of his articles contained no electrocardiograms at all; but every one had his favorite diagram of the potential distribution around the dipole of the heart.

As graphic records Waller's electrocardiograms were miserable. In their original form the plates show deflections of only a few millimeters on a time base of 2 cm/sec. Even using the best and most sensitive of several capillary electrometers in his laboratory, he could produce an image of only less than 3 mm deflections, on a time base of 5 cm/sec.[134] He never really improved the pictures; nor did he attempt to analyze them in detail. Nor did he ever seriously address the question of how much distortion his instrument introduced into these records. Nor is there any evidence that he saw potential diagnostic usefulness for the technique. In 1886, only a few months after recording the first puzzling human electrocardiograms, he noted that the Lippmann electrometer presented "great advantages when the difficulties which its employment first presents are overcome." One of these advantages was that it could be used as a photographic instrument. But this advantage was to be used only in the laboratory; "the technical difficulties are such as to prohibit its use as a clinical instrument."[135]

One can only speculate why Waller, once so anxious to pursue the clinical applications of physiological discoveries, should fail to press for a practical application of the electrocardiogram. Part of the answer was scientific. Electrical activity and conduction within the heart was such a new and ill-understood concept that no one had conceived of it as the basis of any disease state. But part of the answer was also institutional and organizational. Waller was of the second generation of English physiologists who had obtained for their discipline ever-broadening recognition. He had a new but firmly established post. He met a half-dozen times a year with colleagues in the Physiological Society. He journeyed to international congresses, not of medical men in general but of physiologists in particular. It was natural that in showing his wares he spoke to the concerns of what he now perceived to be his primary audience.

EINTHOVEN: ANALYSIS OF THE ELECTROCARDIOGRAM AND DEVELOPMENT OF THE STRING GALVANOMETER

Waller, as it turned out, did not follow the human electrocardiogram beyond the point to which he had brought it by the end of 1889. But when he demonstrated his discovery in the main lecture room of the Vesalianum at Basel on 12 September 1889, in front of the First International Congress of Physiologists, one member of the audience was mightily impressed with its possibilities. Willem Einthoven was then a twenty-nine-year-old professor of physiology at the Dutch University of Leiden. Reporting back to his colleagues in Holland, he called Waller's discovery "one of the most beautiful investigations communicated at the Congress." Einthoven recapitulated Waller's concept of the body divided into electrical poles by an inclined plane perpendicular to the axis of the heart, across which current flowed when first the apex, and then the base, became negative during the heartbeat—he detailed the presentation even down to Waller's red and blue diagram of the chest. But it was clearly the accompanying demonstration that really caught Einthoven's interest. Waller held one electrode in his left hand, the other in his mouth, and, after using his right hand to compensate for skin current, invited his colleagues to view in the microscope how the meniscus of the mercury moved up and down to the rhythm of his own pulse. Switching one electrode, Waller demonstrated the unfavorable lead of mouth/right hand. The congress, Einthoven concluded, valued Waller's work in no way less than the Académie des Sciences, which had awarded him the Prix Montyon the previous December; the assembled physiologists gave Waller a round of applause warmer than had been accorded any other communication.[136]

In many ways Einthoven was the perfect person to be inspired by this discovery.[137] Born in Dutch Java in 1860, he returned to Holland in 1870 after his father, a physician, died. Living at home to save money, Einthoven worked his way through medical school at Utrecht. There he took courses with Engelmann, who had worked on the electrical action of frog muscle and heart in the 1870s, and was ushered into physiology as a favorite student of Donders, who had done the same. Einthoven was no doubt familiar with this research, but by the 1880s, when he was a student, Engelmann had gone on to other subjects and Donders was concentrating on the physiology of vision. Hence Einthoven did the same.

Einthoven's thesis of 1885 on stereoscopy showed talent, but it was largely the strong recommendation of Donders that won Einthoven the chair of physiology at Leiden at the startlingly young age of twenty-five. With the position came a moderately large and well-equipped Physiologisch Laboratorium, a sturdy two-story brick building that situated Einthoven more within an academic than a medical context. The hospital was almost a mile away, and around the corner was the university Physics Laboratory, where future Nobelists H.

Kamerlingh Onnes and H. A. Lorentz had professorships in, respectively, experimental and theoretical physics.[138] Einthoven fit well into this environment. He had a quiet, scholarly temperament and a flair for languages—he read and spoke English, German, and French fluently. He liked instruments and experiments and in physiology valued them more than theory. He had a physicist's bent of mind and was not afraid of mathematics. He had the kind of patience that could focus on a single problem for months or years. Most of all, he was a young man who was looking for an important subject that would pay dividends on an investment of time, talent, and resources. At Basel in 1889 he found that subject.

Upon returning to his laboratory in Leiden, Einthoven seems to have begun immediately a five-part attack on the ambiguities surrounding the human electrocardiogram: (1) continued improvement of the mechanical, optical, and electrical characteristics of the capillary electrometer and its photographic apparatus; (2) an analysis of the distortions introduced into photographic records by the capillary electrometer, and development of techniques to correct these distortions and construct a true wave form; (3) experimental definition of the shape of the normal electrocardiogram and its different forms in normal individuals under physiological conditions of exercise, posture, and different systems of leads; (4) identification of distinctive and abnormal patterns in the electrocardiograms (ECGs) of patients known to be suffering from well-defined heart disease; (5) use of the capillary electrometer as a precision device to detect and register heart sounds. Although one can perceive some logical sequences in these five parts of his research program, and hence parts of one had to be carried forward before parts of others, they seem to have been carried out to a great degree concurrently rather than seriatim. Certainly each of the lines was well established—although pursued to different degrees of completion—by late 1892 or early 1893.[139]

Improvement of the instrument itself was an ongoing project, one compounded from theory and empirical trial.[140] Einthoven found, for example, that in pulling capillary tubes it was advantageous to make the transition from large bore to small bore as short as possible; this minimized the mechanical friction that slowed the movement of the mercury. Cleanliness was of the essence; the capillary had to be soaked for a day in strong nitric acid, rinsed with distilled water, and then dried in a special centrifuge. Even then the best tubes became unusable over the course of time.

To make the image as sharp as possible, he rearranged the optical system so that the shadow of the meniscus fell first on a slit only 0.2 to 0.3 mm wide, and then was further focused onto the plate by a cylindrical lens that reduced the line to a mere 0.075 mm wide. He then linked this arrangement to an improved projection system so as to magnify the movement of the meniscus eight hundred times and still retain clarity.

The photographic plates, some 30 cm long and 6 cm wide, were carried on a redesigned version of Burdon-Sanderson's "railway," by which the plate could be pulled at a constant speed with a velocity of up to 1 m/sec. Even at more moderate speeds of about 20 cm/sec., one could photograph clearly a tuning fork vibrating at 500 cycles/second. Finally, the apparatus was floated on a thin "lake" of mercury to avoid transmitting ambient vibrations to the system.[141] By the time it was fully developed, about 1895, Einthoven's capillary electrometer was an instrument whose definition was greatly in excess of the requirements for recording an electrocardiogram.

Einthoven's institute, modeled upon the generous facilities of German universities, served him well in this multiyear task of instrumental development. He had a trained mechanician at his beck and call; he had a regular budget to pay for the costs of apparatus and research; and he had friends among the physical scientists with whom he could discuss vexing problems. By the late 1890s his laboratory at Leiden had the most advanced instrumental setup in the world.

Such refinements left Einthoven only with the intrinsic shortcomings of the instrument itself. As far back as Lippmann, it had been recognized that although the meniscus *started* to move immediately upon the application of a potential difference, the mass and inertia of the mercury made it impossible for the meniscus to reach the final deflection within an arbitrarily short time period. Einthoven found experimentally, for example, that when an instantaneous voltage of about 5 millivolts was applied to one of his better instruments, it took the mercury about 60 msec. to reach half of its ultimate deflection; the full value was not reached until over 350 msec. had passed. In other words, the capillary electrometer would very badly distort any waveform whose variations were completed in less than a few hundred milliseconds. The human electrocardiogram—as opposed to that of a tortoise or a frog—fell exactly into that category.[142]

Through a combination of theoretical analysis and practical trial, however, Einthoven worked out an algorithm and a procedure that enabled him to calculate a true, derived waveform from the photographic record. For each capillary electrometer in his collection, with its own unique combination of bore, mechanical frictions, resistance, and so forth, he first determined experimentally a constant of distortion that characterized that instrument. He would then make a paper tracing of an electrocardiogram recorded with that electrometer and calculate the slope at a dozen or so points on the traced curve. Then Einthoven used the slope and the constant to calculate the true potential at each of the points. He then replotted the points and connected them into a corrected waveform. Einthoven arrived at the method about 1892 and continued to refine and defend it for almost a decade. It was laborious, but it served him well.[143]

Interestingly, an Englishman arrived at essentially the same conclusions independently, and published them first. After Burdon-Sanderson began his teaching at Oxford in 1883, there was a long hiatus in his own electrophysiological work as he organized the teaching there, solicited money to build a laboratory, and battled with the antivivisectionists. What progress he did make was by proxy. About 1886 he interested a gentleman-physicist living at Oxford, George J. Burch, into taking up the capillary electrometer as a theoretical and practical problem. Burch made hundreds of electrometer tubes over the next decade and arrived through an experimental approach at many of the same conclusions that the Dutch physiologist had reached with more aid from theory. He even worked out a geometrical method of correcting records that seems to have been faster than the numerical method used at Leiden.[144] Einthoven always recognized Burch's priority in publication, although once in 1895 their parallel paths caused a small contretemps when Burdon-Sanderson thought that Einthoven had not done so.[145]

With an improved instrument and the means of reducing the photographic record to a true waveform, Einthoven and his collaborators set out to do what Waller and others had not done: record enough electrocardiograms from a large sample of normal subjects to establish the true *form* of the ECG. By the autumn of 1894 he had taken almost 250 recordings. When a plate was made using a consistent set of leads (usually left hand/right hand), Einthoven found that the records showed a consistent set of four "points" (*Spitzen*), which he labeled A, B, C, and D. After applying the necessary mathematical corrections, the four apparent inflections could be resolved into five true ones, for which Einthoven proposed a different set of identifiers: an initial P wave, a rapid complex of Q, R, and S inflections, followed later by a more rounded T wave, the whole event taking place in about 0.5 seconds. It is a tribute to the care with which Einthoven worked that these same wave characteristics, with the same identifying letters, are recognized in electrocardiography to the present day.[146] Waller may have obtained the first records of the electrical activity of the human heart, but it was Einthoven's apparatus and analytic protocols that created the first true human electrocardiogram.

One can see here the intimate relationship between Einthoven's obsession with ever-improving instruments and procedures and the excellent results he obtained. In his first publication on the electrocardiogram, a lecture entitled "New Methods for Clinical Investigation" given in mid-1893 to a group of Dutch physicians, he did not identify the P and Q waves because his instruments were not yet able to record the slightly rounded hump that was their physical embodiment.[147] Within eighteen months, however, instrumental improvements gave better photographic methods, which in turn gave a truer picture. Moreover by 1895 Einthoven could begin to see the advantage of dealing with *corrected images* rather than the raw photographic records. Whereas every capillary electrometer produced electrocardiograms distorted in different ways by its own idiosyncratic constants, if the corrected records were reduced to a common standard of time and voltage, then *one corrected electrocardiogram could be compared to another*. As Einthoven emphasized strongly, "the variations of potential difference [are] absolutely independent of the instrument used."[148] For the first time one could get not merely a rough indication but a *precise picture* of electrical changes.

Once Einthoven had a set of corrected electrocardiograms for several subjects, he could measure each wave—P, Q, R, S, T—for length (duration) and height (voltage amplitude). These magnitudes could be tabulated so that for each of the five waves, an average amplitude and duration could be calculated. One could see graphically that the electrocardiogram for each subject was absolutely consistent; for each heartbeat each of the waves had the same duration and amplitude.

Most important of all, Einthoven could then attempt to correlate each of the waves with events in the cardiac cycle. As early as 1894 he tended to think that the first part of the ECG, the P and Q waves, represented the contraction of the auricles (atria) whereas the second part, the R, S, and T waves, represented the contraction of the ventricles.[149] In modern terms it was an explanation that was partially mistaken because the Q wave is considered to belong to ventricular rather than atrial contraction. Yet the very fact that Einthoven could assemble a large enough body of self-consistent corrected ECGs to attempt the correlation is remarkable.

About 1895–1897, as Einthoven and his coworkers became more adept at taking and analyzing electrocardiograms, they carried out a series of electrocardiograms on seventeen volunteers. The results served to refine the picture of *"das normale Elektrokardiogramm"* and to emphasize that the range of this normality, both in amplitude and in duration of the waves, was quite broad. Amplitudes differed the most. Among the seventeen subjects, the height of the P wave (atrial contraction) might range between 56 and 248 percent of its average value of 0.125 millivolts (mV). Durations tended to differ less from individual to individual. The quick and high R wave lasted between 20 and 30 msec., with an average of 24 msec. Moreover they could find an identifiable and consistent set of changes in the electrocardiogram of each subject when the heart rate was increased by exercise, when the position of the body was changed, and when different combinations of leads were used.[150]

In comparison to the attention Einthoven lavished upon establishing the features of the normal electrocardiogram, he spent relatively little time examining the ECGs of patients with heart disease. But it was indeed a concern. In March 1894, through the courtesy of his colleague at the University Hospital, Professor Rosenstein, Einthoven examined two patients who had been diagnosed for aortic insufficiency with different degrees of left ventricular hypertrophy. He found in each case that the R wave was much higher and longer than normal and that the T wave was almost flat in one case and inverted in the other.[151] In another case in June, Einthoven and his assistant found a wildly aberrant electrocardiogram with an inverted QRS complex that completely puzzled them at the time. Einthoven was able to come back to the same case thirty-one years later, record the same aberrant ECG with greatly improved instrumentation, and diagnose the cause as a block in the left bundle branch.[152] For the moment, however, Einthoven could do little more than make the plates, correct the records, and hope that a unified picture would emerge.

Einthoven saw that the capillary electrometer, with its rapid response and its ability to detect small signals, was an ideal indicator of heart sounds. His old teacher at Utrecht, Donders, had tried an indirect method of registering heart sounds back in 1866, but the intervening development of the telephone made the task easier for Einthoven. By mid-1893 he had a working setup. He took a commercial microphone and led it into his capillary electrometer. With the plate travelling at a moderate 20 cm/sec., he could get clearly etched records that were visually distinctive for the two heart sounds. He even arranged to write the mechanical record of the apex beat onto the same plate, so that the precise timing of the sounds could be compared to known benchmarks in the cardiac cycle.[153]

By the turn of the century Einthoven had taken the human electrocardiogram far beyond where Waller had left it. He had started with an ill-defined phenomenon and shown it to be quantitatively consistent. He had defined the *range of differences* that it displayed in normal human subjects and the short-term *variations* it showed in any individual man according to different physiological conditions. He had labored mightily to produce the best possible records and to develop techniques to correct those records so as to reveal their true forms. But he could not overcome the intrinsic limitations of the instrument. The capillary electrometer could never be standardized, and it would never produce records that could be "read" directly. Although the evidence is by no means clear, this seems to have been the impasse that drove Einthoven to consider other principles upon which a graphic device might be built.

One of these was the galvanometer. The French physicist-physiologist Arsène D'Arsonval had devised a new version of this old instrument in which a small frame carrying a mirror was suspended between the poles of a fixed magnet. When an electrical signal passed through the frame in the appropriate way it twisted, and a beam of light reflecting off the mirror would move. The instrument was very quick, responding within one-tenth of a millisecond. Moreover it operated on an appealing principle, because the amount of the deflection was proportional to the current passing through the coil; hence the movement of the beam of light, which could be recorded on a photographic plate, was a true representation of the magnitude of the event being measured. But, as Einthoven pointed out, the D'Arsonval galvanometer "cannot serve for physiological measurements" because it required very intense currents. A full ampere was required to get a deflection of 290 mm. The instrument had to be made more sensitive. It became clear from Einthoven's calculations that one needed to increase the strength of the magnetic field by replacing the permanent magnet with an electromagnet and to decrease the mass of the frame. The logical extension was to replace the frame with a single conducting filament and to observe its deflection through a microscope. The filament, as a consequence, had to be made as light and thin as possible.[154]

Einthoven's answer to all these constraints was an elegant new piece of apparatus, the *snaargalvanometer* (Dutch), or *galvanomètre à corde* (French), or *Saitengalvanometer* (German), or string galvanometer.[155] It is not clear when Einthoven began work on this new instrument, but about 1898 seems most likely; he brought it to a fair degree of technical perfection by the time of his first published account in November 1901. The "string" was a filament of drawn-out quartz only .0021 mm in diameter and 13 cm long, silvered at vacuum pressures to make it conductive. It was held in tension between the poles of an electromagnet that produced an intense magnetic field. The horizontal movement of the middle portion of the string was then optically magnified four hundred times and projected onto a photographic plate. Such an instrument was so sensitive that it would show a deflection of 5.6 mm in response to a minuscule 10^{-8} amperes of current, although the string did take almost a second to reach a full excursion. By increasing the tension on the filament, the speed of deflection could be greatly increased but with some loss of sensitivity. The instrument was, however, already so exquisitely delicate that Einthoven could afford to reduce the sensitivity to a microamp (10^{-6} amperes) in order to produce a similar deflection (5.6 mm) in three milliseconds.[156]

In its earliest form the string galvanometer had some noteworthy characteristics that both connected it to and contrasted with its predecessor.[157] The optical and photographic systems were identical to those used for the capillary electrometer, with the simple substitution of the shadow of the string for the shadow of the meniscus. But unlike the meniscus, the deflection of the string was, within the range of normal physiological recording, proportional to the current. Moreover the deflection for a given current was *adjustable* by changing the tension on the string, so that records adhering to a common scale—or to several standard scales, such as fast and slow—could be created automatically; by contrast, when one used the capillary electrometer, one had simply to accept what records the instrument produced and adjust them afterward. In sum, the string galvanometer promised to retain all the progress of the previous decade while dispensing with many of the difficulties that impeded widespread interest in the earlier instrument and in the human electrocardiograms that it produced.

Einthoven's initial brief announcement in 1901 of the physical characteristics of his instrument was followed by four years of steady work in two directions. His primary effort was to improve the quality and fidelity of the records produced by the string galvanometer; secondarily he sought to use it to record human electrocardiograms of both healthy and sick subjects.[158]

A waveform is most easily studied if it is projected onto a grid that gives amplitude and time at a glance. To produce this effect, Einthoven adapted a technique developed by Siegfried Garten, Ludwig's successor at Leipzig. Horizontal lines were obtained by mounting a glass millimeter scale in front of the slit so that the sharp shadows of the scale divisions fell on the photographic plate. To create vertical lines, a uniformly rotating disk of spokes interrupted the light falling on the slit. Every fifth spoke, and hence every fifth line of the millimeter scale, was made slightly thicker to mark off divisions of five millimeters. This arrangement meant that the speed of movement of the plate, the tension on the string, and the rotation of the timing spoke could each be separately adjusted so that a millimeter of photographic record had a value of 40 msec. horizontally and 0.1mV vertically. Records of uniform format could be produced directly rather than having to be derived post hoc. Because the image of the string was a line segment rather than an interface, the grid both above and below the signal could be seen easily and values of voltage and time read off directly. Both the instrument itself and the records it produced were of an elegance and precision more often found in the physical sciences than in physiology and medicine. Little wonder that Einthoven chose to publish the early and important descriptions of the string galvanometer and its properties in the prestigious *Annalen der Physik*.[159]

With this new instrument Einthoven could go on to the second phase of his program: to record immediately and directly the electrocardiograms that had taken so much effort to construct from capillary electrometer plates. In one case, the subject "Mr. v.d.W.," Einthoven could take a direct ECG with the string galvanometer and then compare it to the constructed ECG from a capillary electrometer plate taken from the same patient almost a decade before. The two had the same shape and magnitude. Einthoven may have been smiling at his own doggedness when he wrote wryly:

> It may give some satisfaction that the results formerly obtained by means of the capillary electrometer and more or less laborious calculation and plotting have been fully confirmed in a different and simple manner by means of the new instrument. For this affords us a twofold proof, first of the validity of the theory and of the practical usefulness of the formerly followed methods and secondly of the accuracy of the new instrument itself.[160]

By late 1904 and early 1905 Einthoven was ready to go to the third stage of exploration with his new instrument: application in the clinic. Because the instrument itself, large and immovable, was at the Physiologisch Laboratorium, and the patients were at the university hospital, 1.5 km distant, the two had to be connected by a section of telegraph wire. It was, as Einthoven entitled his lecture of November 1905 in which he described the results, a "Tele-Cardiogram."[161] The patient in the hospital sat in a chair, put his arms or left leg into the now standard containers of salt solution, and his electrocardiogram was produced in the physiological laboratory across town. The wires from the electrodes in the containers were arranged into three combinations: (1) right hand with left hand, (2) right hand with left foot, and (3) left hand with left foot. Although not yet named as "Leads I, II, and III"—or the "Einthoven Leads," as they have come to be known—these combinations were already established as the norm.

With such arrangements Einthoven and his collaborators could explore a host of clinical conditions. They saw the R wave greatly elevated in a case of mitral insufficiency. They could record the large and sometimes bifurcated P wave as the atrium pumped against a stenotic mitral valve. A case of *myodegeneratio cordis* showed the smaller R wave that would be expected of a smaller muscle mass. And they could see the electrical signs of various kinds of disturbances of cardiac rhythms, and even cases of heart block; there would be a clear P wave signaling atrial contraction but no QRS to show the ventricular contraction that should have followed. To a degree that had not been possible with the capillary electrometer, precise, self-scaling, undistorted, and rapid records could be produced.[162] One could even use the string galvanometer in conjunction with a microphone to record heart sounds with greater accuracy and fidelity than with the capillary electrometer.

One could even use the string galvanometer in conjunction with a microphone to record heart sounds with greater accuracy and fidelity than with the capillary electrometer. By 1907 Einthoven, with two of his assistants, had used this new "phonocardiographic" setup to discover a new—third—heart sound.[163]

The way was open for large-scale exploration of the relationship between the electrical action of the heart and the various maladies to which that organ was prone. The summary of Einthoven's early contributions came out in *Pflüger's Archiv* in mid-1908 under the title, "Weiteres über das Elektrokardiogramm" ("Further on the Electrocardiogram"), but by that time he was no longer working alone in the field he had pioneered.[164]

Einthoven had succeeded where others had failed—or, rather, where others had not even tried. What idiosyncrasies of apparatus, personality, and institutional circumstance entered into that ultimate success? In a sense the instrument was primary. Einthoven's string galvanometer produced records of such clarity, fidelity, and consistency that physiologists and clinicians could hardly ignore it. In the best sense of Marey's exhortations of three decades before, the Leiden instrument was the embodiment of the graphic method, producing records of uniform scale and reproducibility with little human intervention. It could do so because it possessed an *excess* of definition. For events lasting between 20 and 150 msec., such as occur in an ECG, it could offer resolution down to 3–5 msec. True, there was a cost for these properties. The original string galvanometer in Einthoven's Physiologisch Laboratorium weighed several tons, needed constant running water to cool the electromagnet, filled a room, and required highly trained technicians to run it. But it was built upon principles that could be scaled down to the dimensions of the office or clinic with only marginal loss of resolving power.

But in a further sense, the success of the string galvanometer was built upon the very limited usefulness of the capillary electrometer. That contraption of mercury and tubes was the stalking horse, the instrument that unveiled the phenomenon in the first place and provided Waller with the successful interpretation of its meaning. In Einthoven's hands the capillary electrometer revealed the universal P-QRS-T sequence, its consistency of form in one subject, and the range of differences from one individual to another. Most of all it defined the resolution that any subsequent instrument would have to achieve in order to be adequate. Einthoven's plotted ECGs of 1894, miserable though they were and bought at such great effort, at least established a reality that some successor instrument would have to define better and more easily.

The string galvanometer in turn would have been unthinkable without the resources of the Physiologisch Laboratorium at Leiden, or some institution like it. Certainly the development of that instrument would not have been possible in the context of British or French physiological laboratories, where individual inventiveness was expected to make up for inadequate and unpredictable financial support. No British laboratory could have afforded the long-term expenditure involved in building the string galvanometer. The London medical schools, as teaching units attached to hospitals, had little interest in or patience with such arcane efforts; nor would Oxford or Cambridge support such research with a fraction of the money the colleges spent each year on good port for the dining tables of the fellows. For years Waller subsidized his London laboratory out of his own pocket—a generosity that was ill-rewarded after the Great War, when the university proposed to close it entirely as an economy measure.

Perhaps the most extraordinary element in the mix was Einthoven himself. He was a man of regular, almost plodding habits, well suited to a quiet university town. He spent his eight, nine, or ten hours at the institute, six days each week, and his evenings reading French, German, or English. He would become so absorbed in a problem that he would occasionally forget about a lecture. Or worse, he would ring up an assistant a few minutes before the hour and ask him to give the lecture to the medical students; "I'm thinking," he would say. Part of Einthoven's absorption was with self-instruction. Finding that he needed to know more mathematics, for example, he worked his way through Lorentz's textbook on differential equations. Year in and year out he would write a few articles and perfect his instruments with little in the way of public ambitions or private distractions. Not for him the relentless hankering after novelties of Marey, or the committees and addresses of Burdon-Sanderson, or the avoidance of mathematics and physics of Waller. He developed a specialized instrument for a specialized purpose, and did it in such a way that it is hard to imagine that anyone else would have done the same—at least not before the advent of vacuum tube amplifiers and single-excursion cathode-ray tubes in the 1930s.

APPLICATION: LEWIS AND CLINICAL ELECTROCARDIOGRAPHY

After 1903, once Einthoven began publishing the first brief physiological studies using his string galvanometer, physiologists and clinicians started visiting Leiden to see Einthoven's setup. Several wanted to duplicate it, and in the case of his old friend, Augustus Waller, Einthoven agreed; he had one made for Waller's institute, the University of London's Laboratory of Physiology in South Kensington.[165] But Einthoven had no desire to turn the institute's workshop into a factory, so he arranged with a manufacturer of medical instruments, Edelmann and Sons of Munich, to build copies. For the first few Edelmann paid Einthoven the small ($25.00) royalty fee that had been agreed upon. But then after modifying the Einthoven design in several ways to make it smaller, Edelmann used the pretext of an earlier publication describing a primitive string galvanometer in telegraphy to stop paying the royalty.[166] These stripped-down Edelmann string galvanometers appeared on the German market about 1906. Einthoven felt ill-used and turned to the Cambridge Scientific Instrument Company in England, with whose chief partner, Horace Darwin (youngest son of Charles), he had been in contact since late 1903.[167] Darwin, a physicist-engineer of considerable talent himself, set a colleague to redesigning the Leiden behemoth to make it marketable. The first few Cambridge string galvanometers were delivered to physiological laboratories in 1905–1907, and the first complete cardiograph to Schaefer (later Sharpey-Schafer) in Edinburgh in early 1908. The instrument was improved rapidly over the next three years and very quickly surpassed the poor records produced by the Edelmann version;[168] by 1914 it had come almost to duplicate the fidelity of the Leiden original.

But the instrument, fascinating though it might be to physiologists, still needed to be proved as a clinical tool. Although there were groups in Berlin, Prague, and Vienna who were slightly quicker to apply the Edelmann instrument to cardiology, by 1914 it was reckoned by all that the emerging maestro of electrocardiography was Thomas Lewis, a clinician-physiologist at University College, London.

Lewis was a distinctively unusual man. Born in Cardiff in 1881, the son of a well-to-do collier, he was educated at home until age sixteen and allowed the run both of the nearby fields and of his father's library, well stocked with such Victorian standards of natural history and chemistry as Darwin, Huxley, Lyell, and Tyndall.[169] He learned to follow his own curiosity intensely. He did his basic medical sciences at University College, Cardiff, sweeping all honors, including a research apprenticeship in biochemistry that gave him the opportunity to publish his first paper at age nineteen.[170] In 1902 he went to London to do his clinical work at University College Hospital, directly across Gower Street from Burdon-Sanderson's old physiological laboratory, now directed by the new Jodrell professor, Ernest Starling. Lewis qualified as M.B., B.S., there in 1905, did his house officership in 1905–1906, his M.D. in 1907, and in 1907–1908 worked in Starling's laboratory. Although he collected other hospital appointments and practiced as a consultant in Wimpole Street for a few years after 1909, the center of his life was to remain University College.[171]

Lewis was a researcher to his core. He learned by investigating—whether it was a clinical problem or an almost purely scientific one. While still a medical student he worked in the Pathological Laboratory on the histology of the spleen and other hemolymph glands.[172] Then his interests turned to physiology. In January 1904, at age twenty-two, he was elected a member of the Physiological Society and became a regular attender of its London meetings.[173] His year as a house officer was not spent merely examining patients; he became strongly interested in the physiology of the pulse. He learned to use the sphygmograph and to interpret its peaks, plateaus, and notches. Most of all, he developed the approach of attempting to understand the graphic patterns he found in the clinic by experiments carried out on cats and dogs in the laboratory. By the autumn of 1906, when he started in practice, he had a clutch of a half-dozen first-rate articles reporting a host of new results in the fundamentals of sphygmography.[174] "His work on the pulse," his biographer wrote in 1945, "remains the standard on the subject and but little has been added to it since by others. In it can be seen the directness of approach, the clear-mindedness and the simplicity of crucial experiment to answer the points in question which became so abundantly manifest in his later work."[175] At University College, with the hospital on the west side of Gower and the Institute of Physiology on the east, Lewis truly worked both sides of the street.

Given his background and inclinations, the twenty-five-year-old Lewis was perfectly positioned to understand a set of new developments that, as he remarked later, were revolutionizing the study of the heart.[176] These centered upon the venous pulse. It had long been known that when the right auricle, and then the right ventricle, contract, they cause a small fluctuating increase in the pressure within the vena cava, which can be seen as a small movement, or pulse, in the jugular veins, especially the right. The venous pulse provided, therefore, a way to get access to the events of the right heart in a way not possible with the arterial pulse. It had been recorded graphically in humans by a colleague of Marey's back in the 1860s, but it was not until the 1890s that an English provincial physician, James MacKenzie, started exploring its clinical significance.[177] After the turn of the century Mackenzie moved to London and developed an instrument that could record both pulses at once: the polygraph. Marey-type tambours transmitted both the radial (arterial) and the jugular (venous) pulses to a mechanism whose two pens wrote the records on a long, continuous strip of paper. A clock mechanism added time markers every fifth of a second, and one could watch the two lines, venous above and arterial below, marching on for yard after yard of record.[178]

Lewis took to the technique with alacrity. It was just the kind of multiplicity of graphic evidence for which his studies in physiology had prepared him and yet which spoke to the characteristics of a single, unique individual. By a kind of dialogue between the two traces, one could puzzle out the contractile events of the two sets of chambers. But the polygraph proved to be more than just a new sphygmograph; it also provided the transition in Lewis's career between his focus on mechanical graphic records and on electrical ones.

The crucial year was 1908, when Lewis became associated with MacKenzie and started using his polygraph. A joint case showed unusual polygraph tracings in which the right auricle and left ventricle showed different rates. By analyzing the traces Lewis could show the way in which there were different kinds of relationship between auricular and ventricular action. Sometimes the auricle contracted twice for each ventricular systole, sometimes three times, and sometimes there was a complete dissociation between the two rates—a complete "heart block."[179]

As Lewis and a colleague at University College were writing up this work, they decided—by a process about which we have almost no evidence—to try to get some parallel electrical recordings of the same events.[180] On 12 November 1908 they took their patient over to Waller's laboratory in South Kensington and hooked him up to the Einthoven string galvanometer. It was an instrument that Waller had not used much—although, again, we do not know why. Waller and Lewis projected the radial pulse onto the same photographic plate and could see the way in which auricular P waves occurred independently of the ventricular systole that caused both the QRS complex and the radial pulse record. The electrocardiogram confirmed precisely, and with much greater clarity, the results of the polygraph.[181] It seems that this was the crucial turning point for Lewis, the juncture at which he realized that the electrocardiogram was a powerful tool for sorting out disturbances of rhythm in the human heart.[182] This enterprise, in turn, began to draw Lewis deeper into physiological questions about electrical conduction in the heart.

It had long been known from animal studies—including those of Engelmann and Burdon-Sanderson—that electrical excitation in the heart spread from the auricles to the ventricles, but the more precise knowledge of that process had come only very recently. In 1906 the anatomist at London Hospital School of Medicine, Arthur Keith, and a medical student, Martin Flack, had discovered in the mole a strange structure at the juncture of the superior vena cava and the right auricle. This clump of cells, the sino-auricular (now sino-atrial, or sinus) node could also be found in mammals and in man. This node correlated with several other sets of seemingly conductive tissue in the heart: the auriculo-ventricular node, described anatomically by Sunao Tarawa while working at Marburg in 1903–1906; the auriculo-ventricular bundle, discovered by Wilhelm His, Jr., at Leipzig in 1893; and the Purkinje system spreading out into the ventricular mass. The original definition of these structures was histological; through the microscope they could be seen to differ from surrounding populations of cells.[183] But beginning in the late 1890s experimental physiologists had used a series of lesion techniques—cutting and compressing—to define the conduction system more precisely.[184]

Lewis, at the end of 1908, was the one to see most clearly the interconnections between the conduction system in the heart, Einthoven's instrument, and the definition of cardiac arrhythmias as they were presented to the clinician. In early 1909 he bought an Edelmann string galvanometer, and in September he went over to Leiden for a visit, both to see Einthoven's setup and to talk shop.[185] When Lewis returned he began at once, with the massive energy few could equal, to use the string galvanometer to explore the relationship between cardiac conduction and arrhythmias.

One of his first successes was the explanation of the form of irregular pulse known before his work as *pulsus irregularis perpetuus,* in which the rhythm of ventricular beats is totally disordered and the size does not correspond to the intervals preceding them. The usual pulse curves could not explain the condition, but electrocardiograms could. They showed irregular and uncoordinated movement of the auricles at a high rate. This fibrillation would, at random intervals, produce a stimulus sufficiently coherent to excite the rest of the conduction system and cause the ventricles to contract. Auricular fibrillation correlated with the venous pulse record, which showed no auricular contractions, only the inflection associated with systole of the right ventricle.[186] Another condition, auricular flutter, in which the auricles contracted fully but at too rapid a rate for the ventricles to follow, was similarly elucidated by Lewis's combinations of pulse and electrocardiographic records.[187]

Another of Lewis's early successes was his explanation of the different forms of paroxysmal tachycardia. Using pulse records, electrocardiograms, and experimental studies on dogs producing the same effects, he could distinguish the set of symptoms into several types (which need not concern us) that could be identified using the clinical instruments.[188] He went through a similar type of analysis in explaining extrasystoles, defining the condition of nodal ventricular rhythms and explaining incomplete and complete heart block.[189] In each type of arrhythmia he used the full range of physiological tricks to gain access to the hidden clinical condition.

Lewis maintained a very conscious and successful program of fundamental research paralleling his clinical investigations. Indeed, the two were symbiotic. Much of his best work was done using the string galvanometer as a device to map out precisely the spread of excitation from the sino-auricular node, over the auricle, and through the rest of the conduction system. Because of the precision of the instrument, he could time portions of the traverse in intervals as small as 0.01 second. He could use electrodes attached to the string galvanometer as probes to localize electrical activities and prove what micrographs and lesion experiments could not prove: that the structure that seemed to be specialized for electrical generation and conduction did indeed function in that way.[190]

In his pursuit of these two paths, clinical applications and physiological research, Lewis was not alone in his use of the electrocardiograph. For each arrhythmia, or each idea concerning the heart's electrical system, one can construct a detailed story in which Lewis would be an important but not the only figure.[191] Yet the sum total of his work was much greater than that of any other person or group. Indeed, during the period of most intense activity, it equaled that of almost all other investigations *combined.* This occurred because Lewis was many things. He was not a surpassingly brilliant physiologist, but he was more physiologist than any other clinician. He was no intuitive and insightful diagnostician like MacKenzie, but he was more of a clinician than any other physiologist. His anatomical skills were only moderate but enough to let him see how the histological evidence related to function and dysfunction. He had no great love for understanding or tending complicated instruments, but the near-perfect one had already been put into his hands.

Most of all, Lewis was a doer and a writer. In an exploding field in which leisurely publication would leave one no original results to publish, he worked and wrote like a demon. In the six years between 1908 and 1913 he published sixty-five research articles. In 1911 he published his classic, *The Mechanism of the Heart Beat, with Special Reference to Its Clinical Pathology,* which he revised in 1920 and again in 1925. *Clinical Disorders of the Heart Beat,* published in 1912, went through seven editions by 1933. His primer of 1913, *Clinical Electrocardiography,* was published five more times by 1937. Both his journal articles and his books brought him fame. Clinicians came to University College in great numbers, especially from the United States and British Empire, to be inducted into this coterie that was leading scientific medicine.

One can see this dynamic at work in figure 6.2, which shows the growth of articles in electrocardiography. If one continued to plot the numbers, the graph would continue to mount because the more the electrocardiograph was used, the more it was found to be useful for. After the boom period initiated by the study of rhythmic disturbances, cardiologists began to see that it could yield important clues in diagnosing "heart attacks"—myocardial ischemia and infarction.[192] In addition to the classical three "Einthoven" leads, augmented and precordial leads were introduced to get a picture of the heart's activity "in the round." Today the cardiologist must make sense not of one or three simultaneous traces but of twelve, each providing a slightly differing characterization of the heart's electrical activity.

Such complexity Einthoven and Lewis might well have found to be too much. Lewis abandoned electrocardiography in the mid-1920s, perhaps for the very reason that its technical aspects were getting beyond his limited comprehension of physics and mathematics.[193] But together the two men began the process of increasing complexity—the one by creating the graphic device that recorded such elegant pictures, and the other by developing scientific and clinical principles for interpreting those records. When Einthoven received the Nobel Prize for Physiology or Medicine in 1924, he acknowledged that without Lewis's work such an honor might well not have come his way. Lewis, although no Nobelist, was equally indebted to Einthoven.[194]

CONCLUDING REFLECTIONS

What kinds of conclusions can one draw from these case studies of physiological instruments that produce graphic images, and their different courses of development into tools of the clinic?

First, on the instrumental side it seems clear that clinical medicine needs a piece of physiological apparatus with almost an *excess* of definition in the records that it produces. Enthusiastic as Vierordt was about his primitive sphygmograph, it did not attract the attention of clinicians because its dull, almost sinusoidal curves could capture nothing of the character of the pulse except its rhythm. Rather, it was the much more subtle instrument of Marey, with its ability to visualize what the finger felt, that aroused the interest of the more scientifically inclined physician. It was not Waller's technique of electrocardiography by capillary electrometer but Einthoven's vastly more accurate techniques of string galvanometry that made possible the real development of clinical electrocardiography.

There are some simple technical reasons for this desideratum of excess definition. Almost any instrumental technique has the quality of its graphic output degraded when it is transferred from the laboratory to a clinical application. The instrument must be made cheaper, hardier, easier to use, more forgiving of mistakes, and capable of coping with a less rigidly controlled set of circumstances of its subject. After all, human patients will not often put up with the treatment accorded the normal laboratory animal.

But perhaps more important, an excess of ready definition means that the graphic output does not have to be processed further. After all, Einthoven was capable of correcting a record from a capillary electrometer in such a way that its fidelity was indistinguishable from one made by the string galvanometer. But this was a laborious process, to be done for only one wave complex at a time. Not even Einthoven himself attempted to convince his colleagues that they should learn how to do this in order to diagnose their patients. Only when an instrument was capable of producing, on its own, a graphic record that was recognizably accurate and readily usable did it become capable of being carried into clinical applications.

Despite the contrast of a simple bit of clockwork and levers on one hand with a roomful of iron and lenses on the other, it seems that the level of complexity of the technology—high versus low—is not of itself a real and long-term determinant. One of the reasons that the sphygmograph was greeted with such enthusiasm at first was because it operated on obvious and easily understood principles. Yet the everyday accessibility of this "low technology" could not ultimately overcome some of the instrument's inherent limitations. The "high technology" of the string galvanometer, once developed and proved, could have its more complicated mechanical and electrical aspects simplified by the manufacturer and the complexities of its use moderated by the use of defined procedures. In his visit to America in 1924, Einthoven was amazed and quizzical to meet with a circumstance in which a technician, "who is not a physician can make a diagnosis of acute coronary thrombosis from the electrocardiogram, without seeing the patient."[195] One of the essences of the machine is that it can create automatically what once required art and experience.

The determinant seems to be rather the *exactness and clarity* of the relation between the *graphic evidence created* by the instrument and the *pathological process to be diagnosed*. The very fact that the sphygmograph told one about *both* the heart and the arteries meant that the number of possible combinations and variations rapidly became too great. There was too loose and too adventitious a relation between picture and pathology. The electrocardiogram told one a great deal less—in its early years, merely a set of results about the conduction and excitation systems of the heart. But the actions of that organ depend on those processes, and life in turn depends upon the resultant contractions. Such information is important to know. Moreover it seemed that when the electrocardiogram told the physician something, it told him precisely and directly. Small wonder that clinicians rapidly took notice. No other instrument provided so direct and seemingly certain access to life processes.

Before an instrument can have that usefulness, the phenomena it graphs must be defined. Thus if a laboratory instrument has some presumptive future incarnation in the clinic, it should have the capacity to illuminate the processes whose pathology it will expose. The capillary electrometer helped to define electrical processes in the heart during the 1870s and 1880s, but it never progressed beyond a specialty piece of physiological equipment. The string galvanometer, coming after the presumptive conduction paths had been defined anatomically, could confirm them physiologically in animal experiments—and thereby validate its use as an instrument on man.

If there are complex reciprocal relations between an instrument and its clinical use, so can one also see, especially in the case of electrical recording devices, an even more complex set of interactive relations between a laboratory instrument and the biological materials it is used to investigate. This occurs because the physiological phenomena can often be found in differing forms and to differing degrees in different organisms. The clinician has only one subject: man. The instrument has to be modified to bring it into physiological apposition with that invariant subject. One side of the equation remains fixed. But a laboratory investigator, such as Marey, Burdon-Sanderson, Waller, or Lewis, can explore bioelectrical activity in a venus flytrap, in a frog gastrocnemius muscle, or the heart of a frog, tortoise, dog, cat, or rabbit. Some organisms are harder to work with and some easier. The instrument that produces a good record in one experimental circumstance has to be modified or improved to produce an equally good one in another. The same instrument, whether rheotome, capillary electrometer, or string galvanometer, is tried first on one organism, then another. The same organ, whether frog heart or rabbit heart, is successively investigated with instruments built on different principles, or successive versions of the same instrument. Both sides of the equation are capable of variations, and a change on one side can often impose demands on the other. An important part of a laboratory investigator's genius is the ability to work within this subtle network of reciprocal dependencies between instrument and biological material.

Given the complexity of the instrument-subject relationship, whether in the laboratory or in the clinic, it is understandable that when information concerning instrumentation or technique is transmitted, this communication often takes place in person. In sphygmography the chain went from Marey to Burdon-Sanderson to Anstie to Foster. The capillary electrometer was passed along from Lippmann to Marey to Burdon-Sanderson to Waller. Waller's demonstration of the human electrocardiogram at Basel in 1889 was the event that started Einthoven on his life's work. His string galvanometer was in turn passed back to Waller, and from Waller to Lewis. Instrument-bound techniques, especially in their early stages of development, have such a large component of tacit knowledge that they are almost impossible to learn from printed descriptions.[196] It is only when the subject and the instrument have been standardized that the tacit knowledge communicated in person becomes less important. Or rather, a certain portion of it becomes reified in the instrument itself. The Cambridge string galvanometer was the embodiment, in iron and glass, of thirty years of electrocardiography. The task then becomes not merely producing the records or understanding them in physiological terms but teaching others, as Lewis taught a generation, to interpret pathological evidence from a new set of graphic images.

Any important physiological-clinical instrument requires the correlation of experimental and clinical evidence. Marey and Burdon-Sanderson did not have the temperaments or the interest to work out the relations between animal studies and human ones; perhaps each felt that such correlations would never be precise enough to satisfy the part of him that was the scientist. Lewis, however, is an exemplar of precisely the scientific personality that is needed for these kinds of correlations: well grounded in science, ambitious, indefatigable, committed to the clinical testing of physiological ideas and the physiological testing of clinical ideas. Such men are often neither great physiologists nor great clinicians. They lack the physiologist's committed search for biological principles and the clinician's genuine empathy with the individual patient. They look at a patient and see neither principles nor person but *disease*. They are intermediaries whose very failure to live comfortably in either world fits them admirably to mediate between the two. They can explore with gusto the power, dimensions, and limitations of an instrument. They have the patience to write the detailed papers, the manuals and the texts, and personally to train their fellow clinicians in a new way of looking and thinking.

Each of these instruments passed through a different set of locales and institutional environments in its development within the physiological laboratory, and transition into a role beyond it. Each history reflects some pertinent aspects of those environments. Although Marey was trained within the Paris medical world, he soon moved (at least mentally) outside of it. Independent institutions, such as the Collège de France, allowed Marey to make his physiology as little medical as he wished. In a sense Marey is most remembered for having exercised exactly that freedom; he is claimed by some to be the inventor of motion pictures, a technique he developed as yet another way to capture movement. Within his milieu he could continue to work with an instrument, as he did with the sphygmograph, or drop it entirely, as he did the capillary electrometer; there were few demands that could make themselves felt on him.

Burdon-Sanderson's environment was originally that of the hybrid clinician-scientist, *more Britannico*. But after the establishment of a true laboratory at University College, London, in 1870, a full-time career as a laboratory researcher opened up to him, and his contacts with patient care and clinical concerns became more attenuated. Waller followed the same pattern, but even more rapidly. By the time he made the first electrocardiogram in the spring of 1886, he was already a full-time physiologist; his marriage to a biscuit heiress a year later only accentuated his freedom from clinical concerns. Yet the London medical schools exacted tolls for such limited freedom. One was the seemingly tacit understanding that research would not get too "biological" and the other that it would not get too expensive. London physiologists, despite one endowed chair, seldom had enough resources at their disposal to develop complicated instruments.

Einthoven lived in perhaps the "purest" environment of all. The few Dutch universities, such as Utrecht and Leiden, supported physiology with generous facilities and budgets and with almost no constraints. One could, like Engelmann, become so biological as to write regularly on protozoans and silkworms, or, like Einthoven, so physical as to publish in the company of Einstein in *Annalen der Physik*. What clinical service that was demanded of him could be performed through intermediaries. It was perhaps the very purity of this environment—Germanic in institutional arrangements but without the driving competitiveness of the medical sciences in Germany— that allowed Einthoven the freedom and the resources to develop a massive and complex instrument. In addition Einthoven's cardiography consumed time with a prodigality unthinkable to a clinician, who measured his attention in hours and days, not months and years. What clinician would have spent ten years working on an instrument that did not prove useful, and another ten on one that did?

Lewis, too, had a setting congruent to his temperament. He was, after all, at University College *Hospital*, not at the college across the street. He had a sufficiently extensive laboratory training to have credit with and access to the physiologists; yet he remained essentially oriented to clinical problems. He self-consciously wanted to be a new type of investigator, the *clinical scientist*, and he found, certainly for his crucial period, the appropriate institutional niche in which to exercise his vision.

In the end, I might be tempted to say that these episodes most strongly emphasize that the process of creating an instrument, using it in the laboratory, and bringing it into the clinic is largely a problem of *translation*. First one creates an apparatus that produces as faithful a record as possible. That is, it translates physiological and pathological realities into a graphic display that is true to its source—a true "bildliche Darstellung," to use Vierordt's words. Next, that machine must be changed into a form that is applicable to the clinic; much must change, but the essential functions must be carried over intact.

But then comes the most difficult part: establishing a lexicon for the next translation, not of words into words or of movement into pictures but of graphic symbols into pathological meaning. This is what Burdon-Sanderson started to do in the late 1860s but put aside, both because he became a full-time physiologist and because he recognized that the translation was never going to be more than very loose and approximate. This is what Waller and Einthoven never did; but at least Einthoven bequeathed to his colleagues an instrument capable of supporting such a lexicon. And this is exactly what Lewis succeeded in doing between 1908 and the outbreak of World

War I. He also carried that process into the next stage: training a generation of practitioners to understand and to use that lexicon.

In many ways the process was a cumulative one. By 1900 the sphygmograph had a limited but secure place in clinical medicine and had trained several generations of physicians to be comfortable with graphic representations of clinically important physiological variations. They could feel such ease because the graphic records were of perceptible phenomena such as the pulse, which were known to them in other clinical terms. Thus when the Einthoven string galvanometer presented physicians with graphic records of nonperceptible phenomena, they were to some degree prepared to step up to the next level of required abstraction.

As Burdon-Sanderson said of the sphygmograph in the 1860s, the difficulty of such instruments lies in the fact that they wrote a record in a language that medicine was only beginning to understand. It strikes me as one of the most fascinating aspects of medicine in the subsequent century that it has learned to write and read a Babel of new graphic languages, languages both created and taught by physiological instruments.

NOTES

This research was supported in part by the National Institutes of Health, Research Grant LM 02956, and in part by the Academic Senate Research Fund, University of California, Los Angeles. A preliminary version of this essay was presented as the William Frederick Norwood Lecture at Loma Linda School of Medicine, Loma Linda, California, in February 1984.

1. "Physicians and physicists," *Lancet* ii: (25 November 1865), 599.

2. Ibid.

3. Ibid.

4. See, for example, Emmet Field Horine, "An Epitome of Ancient Pulse Lore," *Bulletin of the History of Medicine* 10 (1941): 209–249; D. Evan Bedford, "The Ancient Art of Feeling the Pulse," *British Heart Journal* 13 (1951): 423–437.

5. On Ludwig see Heinz Schröer, *Carl Ludwig: Begründer der messenden Experimentalphysiologie, 1816–1895* (Stuttgart: Wissenschaftliche Verlagsgesellschaft, 1967).

6. Ibid., pp. 104–114.

7. Karl Vierordt, *Die Lehre vom Arterienpuls in gesunden und kranken Zuständen. Gegründet auf eine neue Methode der bildlichen Darstellung des menschlichen Pulses* (Braunschweig: Friedrich Vieweg & Sohn, 1855), pp. 4–12.

8. Ibid., pp. 21–37.

9. Ibid., pp. 212–271.

10. Ibid., p. 1.

11. E. J. Marey, "Recherches sur le pouls, au moyen d'un nouvel appareil enregistreur, le sphygmographe," *Comptes rendus des séances de la Société de Biologie, Mémoires* 11 (1859): 281–309. For more on the sphygmograph and its use, see the series of papers by Christopher Lawrence, "Physiological Apparatus in the Wellcome Museum: 1. The Marey Sphygmograph," *Medical History* 22 (1978): 196–200; "2. The Dudgeon Sphygmograph and Its Descendents," ibid., 23 (1979): 96–101; "Alfred Henry Garrod and the Indirect Measurement of the Isometric Period of the Heart's Contraction," ibid., 24 (1980): 342–346.

12. The best introduction to Marey's work is H. A. Snellen, *E. J. Marey and Cardiology: Physiologist and Pioneer of Technology, 1830–1904* (Rotterdam: Kooyker Scientific Publications, 1980), which is largely a collection of reprints of selected Marey papers, but contains a good introduction and essays on particular topics of Marey's work. See also the obituaries that appeared after Marey's death: W. Einthoven, "In Memoriam: E. J. Marey," *Nederlandsch Tijdschrift voor Geneeskunde* i (21 May 1904): 1109–1113; "Etienne Jules Marey," *British Medical Journal* i (28 May 1904): 1289–1290; Otto Frank, "E. J. Marey," *Münchener medizinische Wochenschrift* 51 (8 November 1904): 2011–2013.

13. The anonymous obituary in the *British Medical Journal,* which quite likely was written by either Augustus D. Waller or Thomas Lauder Brunton, notes: "After visiting Germany and making the acquaintance of Ludwig in Leipzig, Marey returned to France. In 1860 he invented his well-known sphygmograph." The quotation is slightly wrong on two counts: Ludwig was still in Vienna around 1859–1860, and the instrument was announced in 1859, although the volume in which the publication appeared is dated 1860. However, so much other information in the obituary betrays personal knowledge of Marey that I am inclined to take the connection with Ludwig as fact, even if not precisely stated.

14. A highly useful bibliography of Marey's writings is in Snellen, *Marey,* pp. 235–259.

15. E. J. Marey, *Physiologie médicale de la circulation du sang basée sur l'étude graphique des mouvements du coeur et du pouls artérial, avec application aux maladies de l'appareil circulatoire* (Paris, 1863), pp. 369–370, 385–394, 410–422, 428–432, 442–452, 457–465, 511–517, 524–547.

16. E. J. Marey, *Du mouvement dans les fonctions de la vie. Leçons faites au Collège de France* (Paris: G. Baillière, 1868), contains discussions of the graphic method in general on pp. 81–202, with various topics of muscle movement treated graphically on pp. 222–460.

17. E. J. Marey, *La méthode graphique dans les sciences expérimentales et principalement en physiologie et en médecine* (Paris: G. Masson, 1878), p. i.

18. Ibid., pp. i–vi.

19. *Lancet* i (28 April 1860): 435.

20. Burdon-Sanderson very much deserves a modern, full-length biogra-

phy, although I fear such an effort would demand a scholar whose scientific and medical background matched Burdon-Sanderson's in breadth—quite a prerequisite! A good starting point is Lady [Ghetal] Burdon-Sanderson, *Sir John Burdon-Sanderson: A Memoir* (Oxford: Clarendon Press, 1911), although it contains little about his work in sphygmography. Overviews of his life are given in Arthur S. MacNalty, "Sir John Burdon Sanderson," *Proceedings of the Royal Society of Medicine* 47 (1954): 754–758, and Gerald L. Geison, "Burdon-Sanderson, John Scott," *Dictionary of Scientific Biography*, II: 598–599. Much biographical information not duplicated elsewhere, as well as judgments on Burdon-Sanderson's scientific work, is to be found in the obituaries and appreciations that appeared immediately after his death: London *Times*, 25 November 1905, p. 8 and 29 November 1905, p. 9; *British Medical Journal* ii (2 December 1905): 1471, 1481–1492; *Lancet* ii (2 December 1905): 1652–1655; *Nature* 73 (7 December 1905):127–129, and 73 (14 December 1905):150; *Proceedings of the Royal Society of London, Series B* 79 (1907):iii–xviii; *Practitioner* 80 (1908):849–856; *Dictionary of National Biography*, Supplement 1901–1911, pp. 267–269.

21. "The Sphygmograph in English Medical Practice," *Lancet* i (26 May 1866):579.

22. Ibid. On Anstie see the obituaries in *Lancet* ii (19 September 1874): 422, 433–434; and *British Medical Journal* ii (19 September 1874):380, 392; also G. H. Brown, *Lives of the Fellows of the Royal College of Physicians of London, 1826–1925* (London: Published by the College, 1955), p. 144.

23. Balthazar W. Foster, "On the Use of the Sphygmograph in the Investigation of Disease," *British Medical Journal* i (17 and 31 March 1866):275–278, 330–333; thanks to Anstie on p. 275. On Foster see Brown, *Lives*, p. 214.

24. See, for example: *Lancet* i (26 May 1866):579; ibid., i (9 June 1866):634; ibid., i (16 June 1866):671; *British Medical Journal* ii (14 July 1866):(review of Foster's monograph; no pagination).

25. "Physicians and physicists," *Lancet* ii (25 November 1865):599.

26. *Lancet* i (20 January 1866):65–66; ibid., i (17 February 1866):176; Foster, "Use of the Sphygmograph," pp. 331–332; *British Medical Journal* i (13 April 1867):433; ibid., ii (26 October 1867):375.

27. *Lancet* i (17 February 1866):176.

28. Foster, "Use of the Sphygmograph," pp. 277, 330–331.

29. Ibid., p. 332. Burdon-Sanderson and Anstie summarized their results in J. Burdon-Sanderson and Francis E. Anstie, "On the Application of Physical Methods to the Exploration of the Movements of the Heart and Pulse in Disease," [three parts], *Lancet* ii (10 November 1866):517–519; ii (22 December 1866):688–691; i (9 February 1867):170–172. Also J. Burdon-Sanderson, "Characters of the Arterial Pulse, in Their Relation to the Mode and Duration of the Contraction of the Heart in Health and Disease" [three parts], *British Medical Journal* ii (13, 20, and 27 July 1867):19–22, 39–40, 57–58. Burdon-Sanderson used the material from the foregoing six articles in his monograph, *Handbook of the Sphygmograph* (London: Hardwicke, 1867); reviewed in *British Medical Journal* i (4 January 1868):11. On aortic insuffi-

ciency, see Burdon-Sanderson and Anstie, "Application of Physical Methods," p. 689; Burdon-Sanderson, "Characters of the Arterial Pulse," pp. 40, 57.

30. Foster, "Use of the Sphygmograph," p. 332.

31. Ibid., p. 330; Burdon-Sanderson and Anstie, "Application of Physical Methods," p. 690; Burdon-Sanderson, "Characters of the Arterial Pulse," pp. 21, 57.

32. Foster, "Use of the Sphygmograph," p. 332; Burdon-Sanderson and Anstie, "Application of Physical Methods," p. 689; Burdon-Sanderson, "Characters of the Arterial Pulse," pp. 21, 57.

33. Burdon-Sanderson, "Character of the Arterial Pulse," p. 57.

34. Furneaux Jordan, "Shock after Surgical Operations and Injuries," *British Medical Journal* i (23 February 1867):191–192.

35. "The Pulse in Health and Disease," *Lancet* ii (3 November 1866):501.

36. Especially in "Application of Physical Methods," pp. 517–518, and "Characters of the Arterial Pulse," pp. 19–21.

37. Ibid., p. 517.

38. Ibid.

39. Ibid., pp. 517–518.

40. Ibid., pp. 517–519; pp. 19–21.

41. Burdon-Sanderson and Anstie, "Application of Physical Methods," p. 171.

42. Ibid.

43. A. H. Garrod, "On Sphygmography, Part II," *Journal of Anatomy and Physiology* 7 (November 1872):98–105, esp. pp. 100–102.

44. F. A. Mahomed, "The Physiological and Clinical Use of the Sphygmograph" [twelve parts], *Medical Times and Gazette,* 1872 and 1873, passim. On Mahomed see Brown, *Lives,* p. 276; *Lancet* ii (29 November 1884):973–974; *Dictionary of National Biography,* 35:333.

45. *Lancet* ii (29 November 1884):973.

46. See, as a random example, Charles Murchison, "Pyrexia," *British Medical Journal* i (3 February 1872):118.

47. W. H. Broadbent, *The Pulse* (Philadelphia: Lea Brothers, 1890), p. 32.

48. Ghetel Burdon-Sanderson, *Sir John Burdon-Sanderson,* pp. 91–98.

49. See the excellent discussion of this issue in Gerald L. Geison, *Michael Foster and the Cambridge School of Physiology: The Scientific Enterprise in Late Victorian Society* (Princeton: Princeton University Press, 1978), pp. 150–160, 329–330.

50. J. Burdon-Sanderson et al., *Handbook for the Physiological Laboratory,* 2 vols. (London: J. & A. Churchill, 1873). On the furor it caused, see Richard D. French, *Antivivisection and Medical Science in Victorian Society* (Princeton: Princeton University Press, 1975), pp. 47–50, 98–99.

51. Lippmann (1845–1921) later became professor of experimental physics at the Sorbonne, and in 1908 was awarded the Nobel Prize in physics for a method that used interference phenomena to produce color photographs. See I. B. Hopley, "Lippmann, Gabriel Jonas," *Dictionary of Scientific Biography,* VIII: 387–388.

52. Gabriel Lippmann, "Beziehungen zwischen den capillaren und electrischen Erscheinungen," *Annalen der Physik und Chemie* 149 (1873):546–561; translated in *Philosophical Magazine* 47, 4th ser. (April 1874):281–291.

53. Gabriel Lippmann, *Thèses présentées a la Faculté des Sciences de Paris . . . 1ʳᵉ Thèse.—Relations entre les phénomènes électriques et capillaires* (Paris: Gauthier-Villars, 1875).

54. The Bakken Library in Minneapolis has a copy of Lippmann's *Thèses* inscribed by him to Marey.

55. For a stimulating recent discussion of some of the problems of instrumentation in nineteenth-century electrophysiology, see Timothy Lenoir, "Models and Instruments in the Development of Electrophysiology, 1845–1912," *Historical Studies in the Physical and Biological Sciences* 17 (1986):1–54.

56. For an overview, see K. E. Rothschuh, "Emil Heinrich DuBois-Reymond," *Dictionary of Scientific Biography*, IV: 200–205; idem, "Emil du Bois-Reymond (1818–1896): Bibliographie," *Acta Historica Leopoldina* 9 (1975):113–136, contains a full listing of writings by and about du Bois-Reymond; a recent collection, Gunter Mann, ed., *Naturwissen und Erkenntnis im 19. Jahrhundert: Emil Du Bois-Reymond* (Hildesheim: Gerstenberg, 1981), treats him in a larger context.

57. See especially E. J. Marey, "Du temps qui s'écoule entre l'excitation du nerf électrique de la torpille et la décharge de son appareil," *Comptes rendus hebdomadaires des séances de l'Académie des Sciences, Paris* 73 (9 October 1871):918–921; idem, "Détermination de la durée de la décharge électrique chez la torpille," ibid., 73 (16 October 1871):958–961; idem, "Mémoire sur la Torpille," *Journal de l'anatomie et de physiologie* 8 (1872):468–499.

58. E. J. Marey, "Des variations électriques des muscles et du coeur en particulier, étudiées au moyen de l'électromètre de M. Lippmann," *Comptes rendus hebdomadaires des séances de l'Académie des Sciences, Paris* 82 (24 April 1876):975–977.

59. Ibid.

60. In the months immediately after Lippmann presented and printed his thesis, Marey was working specifically on the contraction cycle and refractory period of the heart. See E. J. Marey, "Des mouvements que produit le coeur lorsqu'il est soumis à des excitations artificielles," *Comptes rendus hebdomadaires des séances de l'Académie des Sciences, Paris* 82 (14 February 1876):408–411; idem, "Le coeur épouve, à chaque phase de sa révolution, des changements de température qui modifient son excitabilité," ibid., 82 (28 February 1876):499–501.

61. Kölliker (1817–1905) and Müller (1820–1864) were both fundamentally histologists, although they worked frequently on the nervous system; see their work in this period in Royal Society of London, *Catalogue of Scientific Papers* (London: Eyre & Spottiswoode, 1867–1872), III: 720–724, IV: 518–520.

62. Since the experiments were prompted by some earlier ones of du Bois-Reymond, Kölliker sent the first paper to du Bois-Reymond to read in Berlin: A. Kölliker and H. Müller, "Ueber das electromotorische Verhalten des Froschherzens," *Monatsberichte der Königlichen Preussischen Akademie der*

Wissenschaften zu Berlin, 1856, pp. 145–148; it also appeared as "12. Nachweis der negativen Schwankung des Muskelstromes am natürlich sich kontrahierenden Herzen," pp. 528–533 in "Zweiter Bericht über die im Jahr 1854–1855 in der physiologischen Anstalt der Universität Würzburg angestellten Versuche," *Verhandlungen der physikalisch-medizinischen Gesellschaft in Würzburg* 6 (1856):435–533.

63. For an overview of the work of Donders (1818–1889), see Rodolphine J. Ch. V. ter Laage, "Franciscus Cornelis Donders," *Dictionary of Scientific Biography*, IV: 162–164.

64. See K. E. Rothschuh, "Theodor Wilhelm Engelmann," *Dictionary of Scientific Biography*, IV: 371–373. Some of his papers on the heart from a later period, 1893–1903, as well as a complete bibliography, are to be found in Frits L. Meijler, ed., *Th. W. Engelmann, Professor of Physiology, Utrecht (1889– 1897)* (Amsterdam: Rodopi, 1984).

65. See the description by Donders, "Het Physiologisch Laboratorium der Utrechtsche Hoogeschool," in *Onderzoekingen, gedaan in het Physiologisch Laboratorium der Utrechtsche Hoogeschool* 1, 3rd ser. (1872):i–xii.

66. On Bernstein, see Armin von Tschermak, "Julius Bernsteins Lebensarbeit. Zugleich ein Beitrag zur Geschichte der neueren Biophysik," *Pflüger's Archiv für die gesamte Physiologie des Menschen und der Thiere* 174 (1919):1–89.

67. Ibid., pp. 9–20, on his invention and early use of the differential rheotome. For a full treatment of the rheotome in its historical context, see H. E. Hoff and L. A. Geddes, "The Rheotome and Its Prehistory: A Study in the Historical Interrelation of Electrophysiology and Electromechanics," *Bulletin of the History of Medicine* 31 (1957):212–234, 327–347.

68. Theodor W. Engelmann, "Ueber das electrische Verhalten des thätigen Herzens," *Pflüger's Archiv für die gesamte Physiologie des Menschen und der Thiere* 17 (1878):68–99.

69. Marey, "Variations électriques des muscles et du coeur," p. 977.

70. Ibid.

71. E. J. Marey, "Inscription photographique des indications de l'électromètre de Lippmann," *Comptes rendus hebdomadaires des séances de l'Académie des Sciences, Paris* 83 (24 July 1876):278–280.

72. Ibid., p. 280.

73. Ibid.

74. Ibid.

75. On the exhibition see the series of stories in the *Times* of London in the spring of 1876: 12 April; 1, 4, 5, 11, 12, 13, 15, 16, 17, 18, 19, 20, 24, 27, 31 May; 1, 3, 5, 6, 8, 12, 14, 26 June. Burdon-Sanderson's activities in connection with the biological part of the exhibition are mirrored in his diary for 1876, entries for 7, 8, 10, 18, 20, 21, 22, 25, 29 April; 2, 5, 10, 11, 12, 13, 15, 25, 26 May: University College, London, Archives MS. Add. 179/32.

76. The sessions on biology were held on 26 and 29 May; Marey spoke on 26 May: see the *Times*, 31 May 1876, p. 6, and "Biological Conference at South Kensington," *British Medical Journal* i (17 June 1876):767–768.

77. Burdon-Sanderson also had invited Marey and François-Franck to dinner the previous night, 25 May: Diary for 1876, entries for 25 and 26 May,

MS. Add. 179/32; Edward Sharpey-Schafer, *History of the Physiological Society during Its First Fifty Years, 1876–1926* (London: Cambridge University Press, 1927), p. 15.

78. Ghetel Burdon-Sanderson, *Burdon-Sanderson*, pp. 78–98.

79. Burdon-Sanderson was conferring with Sharpey and Jodrell about the endowment in the autumn of 1873. See the entries in his diary for that year on 4, 10, 19, 20, 21, 29 November; 4 December: MS Add. 179/29.

80. Sharpey-Schafer, *Physiological Society*, pp. 5–8.

81. Burdon-Sanderson's relations with both Charles Darwin and his son Francis at the inception of the work on *Dionaea* can be seen in entries in his diary for 1873: 24 March; 25 June; 4, 5, 28 July; 13 August; 12 September ("Work at Electrical phenomena of Dionaea—Telegraphed Results to Darwin"), 13, 16, 29 September; 1, 3, 4, 6, 7, 8, 9, 10, 11, 13, 14, 18, 21, 30 October; 19, 20 November: MS. Add. 179/29. Burdon-Sanderson's first report on this work was to the meeting of the British Association for the Advancement of Science, at Bradford, 17–24 September 1873: J. Burdon-Sanderson, "On the Electrical Phenomena which Accompany the Contractions of the Leaf of *Dionaea muscipula*," *Nature* 8 (2 October 1873):479.

82. J. Burdon-Sanderson, "Note on the Electrical Phenomena which Accompany Irritation of the Leaf of *Dionaea muscipula*," *Proceedings of the Royal Society of London* 21 (20 November 1873):495–496 [received 13 October 1873]; J. Burdon-Sanderson, "Venus's Fly-Trap (*Dionaea muscipula*)," *Nature* 10 (11 and 18 June 1874): 105–107, 127–128 [lecture at the Royal Institution, 5 June 1874].

83. Darwin attended Burdon-Sanderson's lecture at the Royal Institution. The quote is from *Nature* 8 (2 October 1873):479.

84. Burdon-Sanderson, Diary for 1876, MS Add. 179/32.

85. Ibid.

86. J. Burdon-Sanderson, "On the Mechanical Effects and the Electrical Disturbance Consequent on Excitation of the Leaf of *Dionaea muscipula*," *Proceedings of the Royal Society of London* 25 (14 December 1876):411–434 [received 23 November 1876]; idem, "Note on the Electromotive Properties of Muscle," ibid., pp. 435–439 [received 6 December 1876].

87. Burdon-Sanderson, "Mechanical Effects and Electrical Disturbances," p. 418.

88. E. J. Marey, "Sur la décharge de la Torpille, étudiée au moyen de l'électromètre de Lippmann," *Comptes rendus hebdomadaires des séances de l' Académie des Sciences, Paris* 84 (19 February 1877):354–356; Snellen, *E. J. Marey and Cardiology*, p. 247, has a citation of the following article: E. J. Marey, "La systole ventriculaire étudiée avec l'électromètre de Lippmann," ibid., 88 (1878):278. The reference seems to be erroneous, as I can find no such paper by Marey in the *Comptes rendus*, but it may have been published in a medical journal.

89. E. J. Marey, *La circulation du sang, a l'état physiologique et dans les maladies* (Paris: G. Masson, 1881), pp. 25–27.

90. J. Burdon-Sanderson and F. J. M. Page, "Experimental Results Relating to the Rhythmical and Excitatory Motions of the Ventricle of the Heart of

the Frog, and of the Electrical Phenomena which Accompany Them," *Proceedings of the Royal Society of London* 27 (23 May 1878):410–414 [received 6 May 1878]; idem, "Notice of Further Experimental Researches on the Time-Relations of the Excitatory Process in the Ventricle of the Heart of the Frog," *Proceedings of the Royal Society of London* 30 (13 May 1880): 373–383 [received 31 March 1880]; J. Burdon-Sanderson, "On a New Rheotome," ibid., pp. 383–387 [received 6 May 1880]; J. Burdon-Sanderson and F. J. M. Page, "On the Time-Relations of the Excitatory Process in the Ventricle of the Heart of the Frog," *Journal of Physiology* 2 (1880):384–435; use of the capillary electrometer on pp. 393–394.

91. J. Burdon-Sanderson, "On the Electromotive Properties of the Leaf of Dionaea in the Excited and Unexcited States," abstract in *Proceedings of the Royal Society of London* 33 (15 December 1881):148–151 [received 27 October 1881]; full text in *Philosophical Transactions* 173 (1883):1–55; Burdon-Sanderson displayed his apparatus and photographic records in a lecture at the Royal Institution, 9 June 1882: see "The Excitability of Plants," *Nature* 26 (14 September 1882):483–486.

92. J. Burdon-Sanderson and F. J. M. Page, "On the Electrical Phenomena of the Excitatory Process in the Heart of the Frog and of the Tortoise, as Investigated Photographically," *Journal of Physiology* 4 (1883–1884):327–338.

93. Ibid., p. 338.

94. Biographical information about Waller is contained in obituaries in *British Medical Journal* i (18 March 1922):458–459; *Lancet* i (18 March 1922):555; [W. D. Halliburton], "Augustus Désiré Waller, 1856–1922," *Proceedings of the Royal Society of London, Series B* 93 (1922):xxvii–xxx. There is no good bibliography for Waller's writings; references must be chased down in a variety of sources. He has attracted almost no scholarly attention; see only Zachary Cope, "Augustus Désiré Waller (1856–1922)," *Medical History* 17 (1973):380–385; Edwin Besterman and Richard Creese, "Waller—Pioneer of Electrocardiography," *British Heart Journal* 42 (1979):61–64; George E. Burch and Nicholas P. DePasquale, *A History of Electrocardiography* (Chicago: Year Book Medical Publishers, 1964), pp. 27–29, 77–78.

95. A. Waller, "Die Spannung in den Vorhöfen des Herzens während der Reizung des Halsmarkes," *Archiv für Anatomie und Physiologie. Physiologische Abtheilung* ([c. December] 1878):525–534.

96. See Warren P. Lombard, "The Life and Work of Carl Ludwig," *Science* 44 (1916): 363–375, esp. p. 369.

97. Augustus Waller, "Note of Observations on the Rate of Propagation of the Arterial Pulse-Wave," *Journal of Physiology* 3 (1880):37–47.

98. Ibid., pp. 41–42, 44–45.

99. Elected 14 October 1880: Sharpey-Schafer, *Physiological Society*, p. 53.

100. "Report of the Scientific Grants Committee," *British Medical Journal* ii (6 August 1881):240–241.

101. J. Burdon-Sanderson, *University College Course of Practical Exercises in Physiology* (London: H. K. Lewis, 1882), p. i; Waller designed the experiments on muscle and nerve contained in pp. 1–31.

102. *British Medical Journal* ii (8 September 1883):487; ibid., ii (13 September 1884):525; "Scientific Investigations," ibid., ii (25 July 1885):160.

103. Augustus Waller, "Report on Experiments and Observations Relating to the Process of Fatigue and Recovery" [first report], *British Medical Journal* ii (25 July 1885):135–148; his experiments were obviously considered important, as they were given an editorial summary on pp. 156–157.

104. Details of the photo-galvanograph are ibid., pp. 135–136.

105. See the full set of records ibid., pp. 137–146.

106. Augustus Waller, "Report on Experiments and Observations Relating to the Process of Fatigue and Recovery" [second report], *British Medical Journal* ii (17 July 1886):101–103.

107. Ibid., pp. 102–103.

108. Augustus Waller and E. Waymouth Reid, "On the Action of the Excised Mammalian Heart," communicated by Burdon-Sanderson to the Royal Society on 18 November 1886, abstract in *Proceedings of the Royal Society of London* 41 (16 December 1886):461–462, published in *Philosophical Transactions, Series B* 178 (1888):215–256; kymographic studies on pp. 216–231.

109. Ibid., pp. 232–235.

110. Proceedings of the Physiological Society, Oxford, 20 March 1886, in *Journal of Physiology* 7 (1886):x.

111. Waller and Reid, "Action of Excised Mammalian Heart," p. 235; the capillary electrometer experiments themselves occur on pp. 235–241.

112. Proceedings of the Physiological Society, Cambridge, 15 May 1886, in *Journal of Physiology* 7 (1886):xiii.

113. Augustus D. Waller, "The Electromotive Properties of the Human Heart," *British Medical Journal* ii (6 October 1888):751–754; quote on p. 751.

114. Waller, "Fatigue and Recovery" [second report, 1886], p. 103.

115. Waller and Reid, "Action of Excised Mammalian Heart," p. 243.

116. Augustus D. Waller and E. Waymouth Reid, "Étude de la contraction du coeur excisé chez les animaux mammifères," *Comptes rendus hebdomadaires des séances de l'Académie des Sciences, Paris* 104 (31 May 1887):1547–1549, esp. p. 1549.

117. Augustus D. Waller, "A Demonstration on Man of Electromotive Changes Accompanying the Heart's Beat," *Journal of Physiology* 8 (1887):229–234.

118. Waller and Reid, "Action of Excised Mammalian Heart," pp. 235–241.

119. Ibid., pp. 237–239.

120. Waller, "Electromotive Properties," pp. 751–752.

121. Ibid., p. 752.

122. Augustus D. Waller, "On the Electromotive Changes Connected with the Beat of the Mammalian Heart, and of the Human Heart in Particular," received and read at the Royal Society by Burdon-Sanderson, 21 June 1888; abstract in *Proceedings of the Royal Society of London* 44 (1888):331, and full text in *Philosophical Transactions, Series B* 180 (1890):169–194; direct recording from mammalian hearts on pp. 170–184.

123. Ibid., p. 185.

124. Ibid., pp. 187–188.

125. Augustus D. Waller, "Détermination de l'action électromotrice du coeur de l'homme," *Comptes rendus hebdomadaires des séances de l'Académie des Sciences, Paris* 106 (28 May 1888):1509.

126. Waller, "Electromotive Changes."

127. Waller, "Electromotive Properties": London *Times*, 2 October 1888, p. 13.

128. Augustus D. Waller, "On the Electromotive Variations which Accompany the Beat of the Human Heart," *Nature* 38 (25 October 1888):619–621.

129. Augustus D. Waller, "Détermination de l'action électromotrice du coeur de l'homme," *Archives de physiologie normale et pathologique* [5th Series] 2 (1890):146–155; this is the full text of the communication which Brown-Séquard had presented to the Académie des Sciences in May 1888. The report recommending award of the prize is in *Comptes rendus hebdomadaires des séances de l'Académie des Sciences, Paris* 107 (1888):1090–1091.

130. A. D. Waller, "Prof. E. F. W. Pflüger," *Nature* 83 (12 May 1910):314–315.

131. J. Gad, "Der erste internationale Physiologencongress in Basel. 10. bis 12. September 1889," *Centralblatt für Physiologie* 3 (12 October 1889):305–324; summary of Waller's demonstration, given 11 September 1889, on p. 317.

132. Verhandlungen der Berliner physiologischen Gesellschaft (Ausserordentliche) Sitzung am 27. December 1889, *Archiv für Anatomie und Physiologie. Physiologische Abtheilung* (1890):186–190; a recounting of the event was given in "The Electrical Phenomena of the Human Heart," *British Medical Journal* i (11 January 1890):91–92, and in *Nature* 41 (23 January 1890):288.

133. *British Medical Journal* i (21 May 1892):1098; elected Fellow of the Royal Society on 2 June 1892, admitted 16 June 1892: *Proceedings of the Royal Society of London* 52 (1893):1, 70.

134. Waller, "Demonstration on Man," pp. 229–230; Waller, "Electromotive Changes," pp. 189–190.

135. Waller, "Fatigue and Recovery," [second report], p. 101.

136. Willem Einthoven, "Het eerste Internationale Physiologen-congres te Bazel," *Nederlandsch Tijdschrift voor Geneeskunde* ii (5 and 12 October 1889):457–462, 496–503; the account of Waller's presentation is on p. 497.

137. The only full-length study of Einthoven is A. de Waart, *Het levenswerk van Willem Einthoven, 1860–1927* (Haarlem: Erven F. Bohn, 1957). H. A. Snellen, *Selected Papers on Electrocardiography of Willem Einthoven, with a Bibliography, Biographical Notes and Comments* (The Hague: Leiden University Press, 1977) reprints twelve of Einthoven's most important papers on the subject in their original languages of French, German, and English; the bibliography on pp. 25–42 is the most complete one available.

138. De Waart, *Einthoven*, pp. 1–30.

139. The earliest complete overview of Einthoven's research on the human electrocardiogram occurs in a lecture he gave at Dordrecht to the Dutch Association for the Advancement of Medicine (Nederlandsch Maatschappij ter bevordering der Geneeskunst) on 4 July 1893, "Nieuwe methoden voor clinisch onderzoek," *Nederlandsch Tijdschrift voor Geneeskunde* ii (19 August 1893):263–286.

140. Willem Einthoven, "Eine Vorrichtung zum Registrieren der Ausschläge des Lippmann'schen Capillar-Elektrometers," *Pflüger's Archiv für die gesamte Physiologie des Menschen und der Thiere* 79 (18 January 1900):26–38, which describes the apparatus "welche seit mehreren Jahren im hiesigen physiologischen Institute angewendet worden ist."

141. Willem Einthoven, "Een isolatie-inrichting tegen trillingen der omgeving," *Verslagen der Zittingen van de Wis- en Natuurkundige Afdeeling der Koninklijke Akademie van Wetenschappen te Amsterdam* 4 (25 May 1895):38–41; communicated by Kamerlingh Onnes.

142. Einthoven, "Nieuwe methoden," pp. 264–269.

143. Willem Einthoven, "Het meten von snel wisselende potentiaalverschillen met behulp von Lippmann's capillair-electrometer," *Maandblad voor Natuurwetenschappen* 18 (1893):109–120; published in German as "Lippmann's Capillar-Electrometer zur Messung schnell wechselnder Potentialunterschiede," *Pflüger's Archiv für die gesamte Physiologie des Menschen und der Thiere* 56 (26 May 1894):528–541. Einthoven, "Over den invloed, dien de geleidingsweerstand uitoefent op de bewegingssnelheid von den meniscus in Lippmann's capillair-electrometer," *Maandblad voor Natuurwetenschappen* 19 (26 January 1895):61–69; published in German as "Ueber den Einfluss des Leitungswiderstandes auf die Geschwindigkeit der Quecksilberbewegung in Lippmann's Capillarelectrometer," *Pflüger's Archiv für die gesamte Physiologie des Menschen und der Thiere* 60 (20 February 1895):91–100. Einthoven, "On the Theory of Lippmann's Capillary Electrometer," *Koninklijke Akademie van Wetenschappen te Amsterdam, Proceedings of the Section of Sciences* 2 (30 September 1899):108–120; published in German as "Beitrag zur Theorie des Capillar-Elektrometers," *Pflüger's Archiv für die gesamte Physiologie des Menschen und der Thiere*, 79 (18 January 1900):1–25.

144. See, for example, George J. Burch, "On a Method of Determining the Value of Rapid Variations of a Difference of Potential by Means of the Capillary Electrometer," *Proceedings of the Royal Society of London* 48 (22 May 1890):89–93; "On the Time-Relations of the Excursions of the Capillary Electrometer, with a Description of the Method of Using It for the Investigation of Electrical Changes of Short Duration," ibid., 50 (19 November 1891):172–174; and "On the Calibration of the Capillary Electrometer," ibid., 59 (21 November 1895):18–24. Burch also wrote the best introduction to the instrument in English: *The Capillary Electrometer in Theory and Practice, Part I.* [no further parts published] (London: George Tucker, [1896]); the text was reprinted from a series of articles published in *The Electrician* in 1896.

145. Willem Einthoven, "Vertheidigung gegen J. Burdon Sanderson," *Centralblatt für Physiologie* 9 (29 June 1895):277–278.

146. Willem Einthoven, "Ueber die Form des menschlichen Electrocardiogramms," *Pflüger's Archiv für die gesamte Physiologie des Menschen und der Thiere* 60 (8 March 1895):101–123.

147. Einthoven, "Nieuwe methoden," pp. 272–274.

148. Einthoven, "Ueber die Form des menschlichen Electrocardiogramms," p. 107.

149. Ibid., pp. 108–110.

150. Willem Einthoven and K. de Lint, "Ueber das normale menschliche Elektrokardiogramm und über die capillar-elektrometrische Untersuchung einiger Herzkranken," *Pflüger's Archiv für die gesamte Physiologie des Menschen und der Thiere* 80 (4 May 1900):139–160.

151. Ibid., pp. 156–160; the date is to be found in the Dutch version by Willem Einthoven, M. A. J. Geluk, and H. W. Blöte, "Onderzoek van eenige lijders aan hartziekten met den capillair-electrometer," *Nederlandsch Tijdschrift voor Geneeskunde* i (2 June 1900):1031–1035.

152. Willem Einthoven, "The String Galvanometer and the Measurement of the Action Currents of the Heart," in *Nobel Lectures, Including Presentation Speeches and Laureates' Biographies: Physiology or Medicine, 1922–1941* (Amsterdam/London/New York: Elsevier, 1965) pp. 94–111; on pp. 304–305.

153. Willem Einthoven and M. A. J. Geluk, "Die Registrierung der Herztöne," *Pflüger's Archiv für die gesamte Physiologie des Menschen und der Thiere* 57 (9 August 1894):617–639; an earlier discussion making many of the same points is in Einthoven, "Nieuwe methoden," pp. 274–284.

154. Willem Einthoven, "Un nouveau galvanomètre," *Archives Néerlandaises des sciences exactes et naturelles* 6 Série II (1901):625–633, especially pp. 625–629.

155. In the following account I treat the technical development of the string galvanometer for electrocardiographic purposes largely in the context of Einthoven's own lines of physiological research. For an approach that emphasizes its characteristics as an instrument of physics, see John Burnett, "The Origins of the Electrocardiograph as a Clinical Instrument," in *The Emergence of Modern Cardiology*, ed. W. F. Bynum, C. Lawrence, and V. Nutton [*Medical History*, Supplement No. 5] (London: Wellcome Institute for the History of Medicine, 1985), pp. 53–76.

156. Einthoven, "Un nouveau galvanomètre," pp. 630–633.

157. Burnett emphasizes that Einthoven's string galvanometer, as a physical instrument, used so many recently invented components and processes that it would have been "unthinkable" twenty years before: Burnett, "Origins of the Electrocardiograph," pp. 53–54.

158. Willem Einthoven, "The String Galvanometer and the Human Electrocardiogram," *Koninklijke Akademie van Wetenschappen te Amsterdam, Proceedings of the Section of Sciences* 6 (21 June 1903):107–115; published in German, with additional remarks on the capillary electrometer, in "Die galvanometrische Registrerung des menschlichen Elektrokardiogramms, zugleich eine Beurtheilung der Anwendung des Capillar-Elektrometers in der Physiologie," *Pflüger's Archiv für die gesamte Physiologie des Menschen und der Thiere* 99 (3 November 1903):472–480.

159. Willem Einthoven, "Ein neues Galvanometer," *Annalen der Physik* 12 (24 November 1903):1059–1071; "Ueber eine neue Methode zur Dämpfung oszillierender Galvanometerausschläge," ibid., 16 (25 January 1905):20–31; "Weitere Mitteilungen über das Saitengalvanometer. Analyse der saitengalvanometrischen Kurven. Masse und Spannung des Quarzfadens und Widerstand gegen die Fadenbewegung," ibid., 21 (20 and 27 November 1906):483–514, 665–700.

160. Einthoven, "String Galvanometer and Electrocardiogram," p. 114.

161. Willem Einthoven, "Het tele-cardiogram," *Nederlandsch Tijdschrift voor Geneeskunde* ii (1 December 1906):1516–1547; a short abstract was the first publication, ibid., i (6 January 1906):48–50.

162. Willem Einthoven, "Le télécardiogramme," *Archives internationale de physiologie* 4 (September 1906):132–164.

163. Willem Einthoven, A. Flohil, and P. J. T. A. Battaerd, "Het registreeren van menschelijke hartstonen met den snaargalvanometer," *Nederlandsch Tijdschrift voor Geneeskunde* ii (22 September 1906):818–826; in German as "Die Registrierung der menschlichen Herztöne mittels des Saitengalvanometers," *Pflüger's Archiv für die gesamte Physiologie des Menschen und der Thiere* 117 (18 April 1907):45–60.

164. Willem Einthoven and B. Vaandrager, "Weiteres über das Elektrokardiogramm," *Pflüger's Archiv für die gesamte Physiologie des Menschen und der Thiere* 122 (13 May 1908):517–584.

165. This is the one he used in A. D. Waller, "The Electrocardiogram of Man and of the Dog as Shown by Einthoven's String Galvanometer," *Lancet* i (22 May 1909):1448–1450.

166. Burch, *History of Electrocardiography*, pp. 114–115.

167. Burnett, "Origins of the Electrocardiograph," pp. 61–65.

168. Burch, *History of Electrocardiography*, pp. 114–115. Most of the electrocardiograms in Thomas Lewis, *The Mechanism of the Heart Beat* (London: Shaw & Sons, 1911), were done with the Edelmann instrument; in that year he switched to one on lease from Cambridge Scientific Instrument Company.

169. A. N. Drury and R. T. Grant, "Thomas Lewis, 1881–1945," *Obituary Notices of Fellows of the Royal Society* 5 (1945):179–202, is the best single source on Lewis's life; it contains a complete bibliography of his writings. There is no full-length biography, and little scholarship on Lewis, although Joel Howell, in the articles cited later, has much to say *en passant* about Lewis that is insightful and illuminating. See also Howard Burchell, "Sir Thomas Lewis: His Impact on American Cardiology," *British Heart Journal* 46 (1981):1–4; H. A. Snellen, "Thomas Lewis (1881–1945) and Cardiology in Europe," ibid., pp. 121–125; A. Hollman, "Thomas Lewis—The Early Years," ibid., pp. 233–244; A. Hollman, "Thomas Lewis: Physiologist, Cardiologist, and Clinical Scientist," *Clinical Cardiology* 8 (1985):555–559.

170. Swale Vincent and Thomas Lewis, "The Proteins of Unstriped Muscle," Proceedings of the Physiological Society, 26 January 1901, *Journal of Physiology* 26 (28 February 1901):xix–xxi; Swale Vincent and Thomas Lewis, "Observations upon the Chemistry and Heat Rigor Curves of Vertebrate

Muscle, Involuntary and Voluntary," *Journal of Physiology* 26 (14 June 1901):445–464.

171. Drury and Grant, "Lewis," pp. 180–181.

172. Thomas Lewis, "The Structure and Functions of the Haemolymph Glands and Spleen," *Internationale Monatsschrift für Anatomie und Physiologie* 20 (1902):1–56; Thomas Lewis, "Further Observations on the Functions of the Spleen and Other Haemolymph Glands," *Journal of Anatomy, London* 38 (January 1904):144–152; Thomas Lewis, "Observations upon the Distribution and Structure of Haemolymph Glands in Mammalia and Aves, Including a Preliminary Note on Thymus," ibid., 38 (April 1904):312–324.

173. Sharpey-Schafer, *Physiological Society*, p. 129.

174. Thomas Lewis, "The Influence of the Venae Comites on the Pulse Tracing, with Special Reference to Valsalva's Experiment, and Dicrotism; a Note on Anacrotism," *Journal of Physiology* 34 (29 October 1906):391–413; Thomas Lewis, "The Factors Influencing the Prominence of the Dicrotic Wave," ibid., pp. 414–429; Thomas Lewis, "The Interpretation of the Primary and First Secondary Wave in Sphygmograph Tracings," *Journal of Anatomy, London* 41 (January 1907):137–140; Thomas Lewis, "The Pulse in Aortic Disease; The Relation of Pulse Curves to Blood Pressure," *Lancet* ii (15 September 1906):714–717; Thomas Lewis, "Note on the Estimation of Blood Pressure," *British Medical Journal* ii (27 October 1906):1091; Thomas Lewis, "The Pulsus Bisferiens," ibid., i (20 April 1907):918–920.

175. Drury and Grant, "Thomas Lewis," p. 180.

176. Thomas Lewis, "The Normal Venous Pulse," *British Medical Journal* ii (30 October 1908):1482–1486.

177. On MacKenzie see Alexander Mair, *Sir James MacKenzie, 1853–1925: General Practitioner* (Edinburgh: Churchill Livingstone, 1973).

178. J. MacKenzie, "The Ink Polygraph," *British Medical Journal* i (13 June 1908):1411.

179. Thomas Lewis and A. Salusbury MacNalty, "A Note on the Simultaneous Occurrence of Sinus and Ventricular Rhythm in Man," *Journal of Physiology* 37 (15 December 1908):445–458.

180. One possible contact between Lewis and Waller would have been Starling, with whom Lewis was in daily contact, who was more of Waller's generation and who had used the capillary electrometer to record from mammalian hearts in the 1890s.

181. Ibid., "Addendum," pp. 457–458, where one record is reproduced and where Lewis writes: "It is with pleasure that I express my gratitude to Professor A. D. Waller, in whose laboratory the curve was taken, and to Mr. Symes for the trouble he has taken in rendering me conversant with the management of the apparatus." In a typographical error—which is perfectly understandable—the plate is labeled as having been "obtained with a strong [sic] galvanometer at a later date (Nov. 12, 1908)."

182. The incident may also have caused Waller's interest in the clinical use of the ECG to quicken. A few months later, during Easter vacation 1909, Waller visited Leiden and reviewed "the extensive collection of human electro-cardiograms gathered together by Professor Einthoven during the

last ten years." Although he praised the way that Einthoven's ECGs brought out "various forms of atypical heart beat" and "throw light not otherwise obtainable upon obscure clinical manifestations of disorderly cardiac action," he did not imagine that the string galvanometer was "likely to find any very extensive use in the hospital as affording means of physical diagnosis more searching than those in daily use." Waller, "The Electrocardiogram of Man," pp. 1448–1449. Waller did, however, return to the study of the electrical action of the heart, a subject he had largely ignored since the early 1890s.

183. Lewis, *Mechanism of the Heart Beat*, pp. 1–8; Burch, *History of Electrocardiography*, pp. 134–137. Useful information and comments are also to be found in Thomas N. James, "The Development of Ideas Concerning the Conduction System of the Heart," *Ulster Medical Journal* 51 (1982):81–97.

184. Lewis, "The Occurrence of Heart-Block in Man and Its Causation," *British Medical Journal* ii (19 December 1908):1798–1802.

185. H. A. Snellen, *Two Pioneers of Electrocardiography: The Correspondence between Einthoven and Lewis from 1908–1926* (Rotterdam: Donker Academic Publications, 1983), pp. 28–32.

186. Thomas Lewis, "Auricular Fibrillation: A Common Clinical Condition," *British Medical Journal* ii (27 November 1909):1528; Thomas Lewis, "Auricular Fibrillation and Its Relationship to Clinical Irregularity of the Heart," *Heart* 1 (30 March 1910):306–372; Thomas Lewis and E. Garvin Mack, "Complete Heart-Block and Auricular Fibrillation," *Quarterly Journal of Medicine* 3 (April 1910):273–284; Thomas Lewis, "Bigeminy of the Ventricle and Auricular Fibrillation," *Quarterly Journal of Medicine* 3 (July 1910):337–342. Aspects of Lewis's work on arrhythmias are mentioned in Dennis M. Krikler, "The Development of the Understanding of Arrhythmias during the Last 100 Years," in *Emergence of Modern Cardiology*, pp. 77–81.

187. Thomas Lewis, "Observations upon Disorders of the Heart's Action," *Heart* 3 (1 June 1912):279–300.

188. Thomas Lewis, "Paroxysmal Tachycardia," *Heart* 1 (1 July 1909):43–72; idem, "The Experimental Production of Paroxysmal Tachycardia and the Effects of Ligation of the Coronary Arteries," ibid., 1 (1 November 1909):98–137; idem, "Paroxysmal Tachycardia, the Result of Ectopic Impulse Formation," ibid. 1 (1 January 1910):262–282; idem, "Paroxysmal Tachycardia, Accompanied by the Ventricular Form of Venous Pulse," ibid. 2 (November 1910):127–142.

189. For a recent detailed study of experimental and clinical research on heart block, and Lewis's place within it, see Arthur Hollman, "The History of Bundle Branch Block," in *Emergence of Modern Cardiology*, pp. 82–102.

190. Thomas Lewis, "On the Electro-Cardiographic Curves Yielded by Ectopic Beats Arising in the Walls of the Auricles and Ventricles," *British Medical Journal* i (26 March 1910):750; idem, "Galvanometric Curves Yielded by Cardiac Beats Generated in Various of the Auricular Musculature. The Pace-Maker of the Heart," *Heart* 2 (30 July 1910):23–40; Thomas Lewis, B. S. Oppenheimer, and Adele Oppenheimer, "The Site of Origin of the Mammalian Heart-Beat; The Pace-Maker in the Dog," ibid., 2 (November

1910):147–169; also see the studies in 1914, 1915, and 1916, by Lewis with various coworkers, of the excitatory process in the mammalian heart.

191. See Burch, *History of Electrocardiography*, pp. 137–162.

192. This transition in the use of the instrument is admirably analyzed in Joel D. Howell, "Early Perceptions of the Electrocardiogram: From Arrhythmia to Infarction," *Bulletin of the History of Medicine* 58 (1984):83–98. For Lewis and his activities in the post-1914 period, see also Howell, " 'Soldier's Heart': The Redefinition of Heart Disease and Speciality Formation in Early Twentieth-century Great Britain," in *Emergence of Modern Cardiology*, pp. 34–52. The broader context of physiological concepts in the definition of heart disease as a special object of study is elegantly and provocatively explicated in Christopher Lawrence, "Moderns and Ancients: The 'New Cardiology' in Britain 1880–1930," ibid., pp. 1–33.

193. Drury and Grant, "Thomas Lewis," pp. 185.

194. Burch, *History of Electrocardiography*, p. 134.

195. Ibid., pp. 63–64.

196. I make some similar points in Robert G. Frank, Jr., "The Columbian Exchange: American Physiologists and Neuroscience Techniques," *Federation Proceedings* 45 (1986):2665–2672.

CHAPTER SEVEN

Epilogue

William Coleman and Frederic L. Holmes

The chapters in this volume derive from the ongoing scholarly work of their authors. In keeping with their individual points of view, the authors place different emphases on the role of scientific ideas, research programs, pedagogical objectives, and the interests of the state or other institutions in the shaping of investigative enterprises or institutional structures.

Nonetheless certain recurring themes disclose an underlying unity in these essays. In each of the episodes involving the origins of an institution, we find congruence between the scientific or medical vision of one or more founders and the interests of the professional, social, or political agencies whose support was essential to the success of the venture. Purkyně's pedagogical model; Pariset's belief in the importance of experimental physiology; Henle's program for a scientific medicine; Ludwig's conception of an integrative physiology; Liebig, Bischoff, and Voit's metabolic research program—each provided a driving force, shaping from within the activities carried on in an institute or an academy. In some instances an outside vision matched the inside closely enough so that the institution was designed from the start to implement a mutually desired program. This pattern was manifested particularly in the case of the institutes of physiology at Heidelberg and Leipzig. In other cases, such as in Munich, the institutional goals were not defined so clearly at the outset and only gradually came to be accommodated to the dominant activity within. Personal career, social, and political interests were at stake in the establishment of each of these institutions; but at the heart of what took place within each of them was a creative investigative enterprise.

Each of the German institutes considered in this volume carried out both educational and research functions. These were not coincidental but symbiotic enterprises. It has been argued, particularly by Rudolf Stichweh and Kathryn Olesko, that the combination of education and the pursuit of knowledge is essential to the survival of scientific disciplines.[1] The histories of the institutes described here illustrate the close connection between teaching and research. They also suggest, however, that the nature and extent of this relationship varied greatly with particular circumstances. In Purkyně's Breslau Institute pedagogy and investigation were interwoven so closely as to constitute two faces of the same activity. In Munich, conversely, a specialized research program in quantitative metabolism developed under the direction of scientists who taught a standard array of courses in anatomy and physiology. For these men teaching was not integrated with research in the way it had been for Purkyně, but was closer to being a service function.

This volume rests on the proposition that the complex interplay between the various factors that figure in the stories told here can be examined to special advantage in localized settings. We must keep in mind, however, that the events described cannot be understood from local perspectives alone. The research programs, the pedagogical approaches, the distinctive schools that emerged within local institutions were only nodal points within a network of interactions linking them with similar activities in other localities. None of the research or teaching programs described in our essays originated and grew to maturity entirely within a single institution. Some of them began in one place and flourished in another: Henle brought his program to Heidelberg and Ludwig brought his to Leipzig. Theodor Bischoff and Justus Liebig moved their metabolic investigations from Giessen to Munich. Successful research programs also spread from one institution to another when those who had participated in the work of one institute moved from assistantships to independent positions in other institutes. The investigative forefront in the quest for methods to depict the heart beat moved from setting to setting, from country to country, as various local situations proved favorable to certain phases of this long development but unsuited for subsequent stages.

Scientists work within two kinds of environment, both immediate to them, but in different dimensions. One is their local institutional surroundings; the other is the geographically dispersed social networks that comprise their disciplines or research areas.[2] Research programs are shaped by demands emanating from both contexts. Locally, success depends upon gaining the support of authorities in an organizational hierarchy that may include a rector, a minister of education, or a head of state. Within the context of the dispersed network a research program advances only if it is recognized as successful by colleagues in the same research area at other institutional centers. The kinds of research programs that are initiated are not determined by local opportunities and limits alone. Although shaped in part by these factors, research programs must in the first place be structured in keeping with the state of a discipline, or a portion of one, and the vision that their proponents entertain of the frontiers of opportunity that lie within those areas. A successful research program is one that can accommodate both sets of requirements.

This interplay between local factors and the broader state of a scientific field is clearly visible in the situations described in this volume. Purkyně's efforts to establish a physiological institute independent of anatomy prevailed in part because he was able to persuade the Prussian Ministry of Culture that this foundation was appropriate for the University of Breslau, but also because physiology at that time was emerging in several centers in France and Germany as a distinct and promising field for experimental investigation. Purkyně's focus on the microscopical examination of animal tissues put him in the forefront of an area of investigation that was just then becoming important in other places as well. The histologically oriented research program that Henle brought to Heidelberg fit that university's plans to revitalize its medical school but was fruitful in large part because it came in the wake of the great stimulus to such studies that Theodor Schwann's cell theory had imparted a few years earlier. Liebig and Bischoff's metabolic research program was productive because Liebig was in a position to provide support for it both in Giessen and in Munich, and also because he had previously had the insight to see how recent advances in organic chemistry could be brought to bear on certain central problems in physiology. The three component investigative approaches that Ludwig integrated into his Leipzig Institute— experimental physiology, physiological chemistry, and microscopical anatomy—may have fit his personal vision and research experiences as well as the objectives the Saxon minister of culture entertained for the University of Leipzig. They also comprised a viable institutional framework because each component represented a field of activity that was generally flourishing in that period and that intersected with the others at many common points.

NOTES

1. Rudolf Stichweh, *Zur Entstehung des modernen Systems wissenschaftlicher Disziplinen: Physik in Deutschland 1740–1980* (Frankfurt: Suhrkamp, 1984); Kathryn M. Olesko, "Review of Rudolf Stichweh, *Zur Entstehung des modernen Systems wissenschaftlicher Disziplinin,*" Isis 76 (1985): 607–608.

2. See Diana Crane, *Invisible Colleges: Diffusion of Knowledge in Scientific Communities* (Chicago: University of Chicago Press, 1972).

CHAPTER EIGHT

Commentary: On Institutes, Investigations, and Scientific Training

Kathryn M. Olesko

One thing an institution should be is a setting for a dialogic encounter in which limiting norms necessary for life in common are put to tests that may strengthen or transform them. . . . The difficulty is to create the material and intellectual conditions in which such an exchange is actually possible.[1]

During the nineteenth century the investigative techniques of the natural sciences matured within the context of increasingly sophisticated teaching, research, and clinical institutions that had been created in response to local disciplinary requirements on the one hand, and larger social, economic, and political needs on the other. The essays in the present volume explore the ways in which the investigative techniques of one science—physiology—were generated, taught, used, and canonized in institutions of various types in France, England, the Netherlands, and the German states of Baden, Bavaria, Saxony, and Prussia. Coleman and Tuchman explain when, why, and to whom exploratory investigative techniques were taught in physiology at two universities: Breslau in authoritarian and highly centralized Prussia and Heidelberg in constitutional and liberal Baden. Holmes and Lenoir examine some of the conditions under which quantitative and other investigative techniques of physiology were institutionalized in the teaching and research laboratories of the universities of Munich and Leipzig, equally contrasting in their political contexts. In fine detail, Lesch relates how in practice the accuracy and precision of investigative techniques were judged and evaluated in a closed institutional context, the Paris Academy of Medicine. Finally, Frank demonstrates how investigative instruments and their graphical results were interpreted in physiology and then translated and canonized for clinical use. A correlation might be drawn between the elaborateness of investigative endeavors and the complexity of the institutional structures that housed them. Several of the essays in this volume suggest, however, that such a conclusion would grossly and prematurely undervalue the equal importance and sometimes pivotal role of simpler settings, especially instructional and clinical institutes, in shaping the techniques, such as microscopy, used in physiological investigations. Despite the difference in function of the several institutes discussed in this volume, in each one the standards of physiological investigation were nonetheless articulated and refined, thus confirming the breadth of the investigative enterprise.

Of special historiographical significance is the examination, undertaken by four authors in this volume, of the investigative techniques employed for teaching and research in German university institutes. These essays manifest the changes that have occurred in this genre of scholarship since 1971 when monographs by Joseph Ben-David and R. Steven Turner appeared, providing powerful categories of analysis that could be used to examine historically the institute phenomenon within German universities.[2] Their work made older studies—such as Billroth's on medical education, Lorey's on mathematical instruction, and especially the vignettes on science institutes in celebratory and Whiggish university histories—seem outmoded in their narrative and hagiographical approaches, for they introduced ostensibly more sophisticated sociological categories of analysis such as competition, the research imperative, and productivity in order to retell the past.[3] Supported by German archival sources (the examination of which has become for some an obsession), fine-grained local studies devoted to one natural science in a single institutional context have begun to supplement and refine considerably global surveys of the natural sciences in the entire university system.[4] Although more remains to be done, it is clear that the institute phenomenon as a whole will not be understood in any other way than through local studies—and the syntheses based upon them— that explore the interactions between local disciplinary conditions, state goals and ideologies, and the research efforts of the larger scientific community. In recent times studies of university institutes have been enhanced greatly by the maturation of the socioinstitutional history of German education, as well as by the analysis of Germany's *Sonderweg* to establishing the "liberal" professions through state control of certification and advancement.[5] As is the case with most of German history, these histories of institutes project forward to later developments. Even though the institute phenomenon spanned a century and a half, from slow beginnings in cabinets, collections, and the certification of the learned professions at the end of the eighteenth century to its maturation first in large-scale university institutes and later in such research organizations as the Physikalisch-Technische Reichsanstalt, the Kaiser Wilhelm Gesellschaft, and the Notgemeinschaft der Deutschen Wissenschaft in the late nineteenth and early twentieth centuries, until recently historians of science have shown a preference for the period after 1860 when most of the larger institutes appeared.[6]

Archival sources and a more detailed historical context turned out to be mixed blessings. They vividly embellished the complex history of institutes and of the sciences practiced in them. But the more one used these "original" sources and the closer one came to the past of an institute, the more complicated matters became. Archival material, it has been found, cannot be taken as the last word. Strip mining quotations from original documents is not always enlightening. Proving itself not to be the end of a long causal chain or a specially designated privileged source of information, archival material in fact demanded the same kinds of skepticism and critical analysis applied to other sources more commonly used. Ironically, the most direct documents from the past proved at times also to be the most refractory. Often laden with rhetorical statements of intention framed to gain immediate support and favorable evaluations, they could not always be taken literally as programmatic prescriptions or even factual descriptions.

Nevertheless, with archives mined, categories of analysis honed, educational contexts explained, and professional and social changes mapped out, we have come closer to understanding historically both institutes and the investigative practices in them. As the essays in this volume show, this has not been accomplished without challenging or even abandoning some of the principles contained in studies that started it all. Neohumanism has predictably come under attack.

In an era that has challenged severely the legitimacy of doing intellectual history,[7] neohumanism seems to be a particularly appropriate victim in reassessing our understanding of the institute phenomenon. What had formerly been the foundation of our understanding of the modern research university now seems too diffuse and intangible to account for the fine structure of the smaller research institute within it. This situation resulted in part from examining more closely the growth of the natural sciences in the university, and in part from recognizing that standard background sources, such as Fritz Ringer's *The Decline of the German Mandarins*, did not consider university scientists or the medical faculty.[8] The essays on physiological institutes in this volume demonstrate that when dealing with the natural sciences, especially those in the medical faculty, it is essential to depart in some way from the historiographical tradition that uses the philosophical faculty, its humanistic institutes, and its ideologies as paradigmatic models for the analysis of all disciplines and institutes of the German university.

Historians of science have carried over to the study of university institutes their historiographical preference for discontinuities, ruptures, and change, all residues of the prior dominance of intellectual history. In institutional history, that preference has translated into the examination of origins, beginnings, and "firsts." Four essays in this volume deal with origins. Although no historiographical templates have been forged by them, the authors do approach their subject matter similarly, through a sectorial analysis. They look at several factors, such as personal visions, research programs, teaching styles, student clienteles, educational ideologies, material and economic constraints, ministerial policies, and state interests. They analyze the origin of an institute in terms of how well these factors fit together. Naturally, variations in the relative contributions of each factor, as well as in how they combined with one another, occurred from institute to institute. Yet despite local differences, we find that university institutes emerged in environments that were devoid of neither tradition nor modernity.

The circumscription of neohumanism and the more sensitive treatment of origins are potent contributions to a revisionist historiography of university institutes in Germany before 1870. They also raise several related issues that suggest avenues for future research. Two are especially important. First, studies of other scientific institutes, especially those in the medical faculty, undoubtedly will reveal new factors that gave rise to the institute phenomenon. They will also show additional limitations on the contributions of neohumanism to the evolution of university institutes, and such limitations deserve to be examined. In order to qualify our perspective, however, it seems necessary to ask if scientific institutes were singular in their challenge to neohumanism, or if the humanities and their institutes, principally seminars, also challenged the very ethos they were supposed to exemplify, and if so, in what way. This seems to be required if institutional historians are to explain how, if at all, the humanistic seminar and the scientific laboratory were related to each other.

Second, as several of the contributors to this volume have hinted, we need to go beyond origins to a study of the *operation* of institutes. A structural analysis that weighs the contributions of multiple factors is eminently suited for a study of origins, but that approach seems too mechanical if one wishes to capture the dynamics of an institute and to convey its *Alltagsgeschichte*. The everyday reality of an institute's operation requires a revised perspective: from considering the activity of research as the principal category of historical analysis to viewing research and teaching as equally important complementary institutional functions that promoted and sustained investigation. Several contributors to this volume have argued for the importance of the teaching function of university institutes. Still, we need to know the fine structure of how teaching and learning took place, especially in the exercise session and in the laboratory. Only in this way will we learn how students were trained to undertake investigations. The essays by Frank and Lesch offer suggestions here, for they demonstrate that scientific institutions are settings for dialogues that challenge and evaluate the intellectual and instrumental norms of science, especially the experimental and other skills that constitute techniques of investigation. What kind of dialogue, it might be asked, occurred during teaching? What skills were taught in laboratory or other exercises, and how were they related to the techniques of original investigation in research? How, precisely, was scientific training related to scientific practice, to the labor of science?

I

Existing literature projects a conventional image of the nineteenth-century university seminar. Drawn principally from Prussian examples, it links the seminar to the ideology of neohumanism, which found its strongest expression in the Prussian educational system. It pictures the seminar as an elite institute composed of exceptional students dedicated to two ideals: the ideal of *Bildung*, or cultivation; and the ideal of *Wissenschaft*, or the pursuit of knowledge through original research. Seminar statutes accordingly described the seminar as an arena in which *Wissenschaft* "could be preserved, propagated, and expanded." In principle, these two ideals were linked to each other, for in the seminar one achieved *Bildung* through *Wissenschaft;* building character took place through self-instruction of the most difficult type.

Hence, the activity that occurred in the seminar was in principle dependent not only upon the successful pursuit of research but also upon the personal qualities and traits of the students who participated in it. Consequently, during the early years of the seminar system, before 1815 or so, the student's personality seems to have been very important. On those rare occasions when early seminar statutes mentioned prerequisites for entry, for example, they did so in terms of personal qualities. Students were expected to possess an *innere Beruf*, an inner calling, that motivated them to attend the seminar in the first place. This inner calling was associated less with professional interests than with the seriousness and diligence with which a student took up a field of study. Through participation in the activity of the seminar, one's inner calling was drawn out and cultivated in a way that enabled the fullest expression of personal potential.

Lacking or feigning an inner calling was believed to lead eventually to failure in seminar exercises. In this way the pedagogical premises and objectives of neohumanism were institutionalized in the university seminar. From the perspective of this conventional image of the seminar, then, it appears likely that a neohumanist ethos did contribute substantially to the origin and operation of the seminar system, especially in the promotion of original research.[9] Lacking a comprehensive and comparative history of the seminar system, we still do not know to what extent seminars actually upheld this ideal. Evidence suggests that at least some did. Gesner's, and then Heyne's, eighteenth-century philological seminar at Göttingen and Wolf's at Halle remain, for better or for worse, the principal models of the seminar system as a whole. They seem to exemplify most clearly the institutionalization of the tenets of neohumanism. They were the first to incorporate into instruction the techniques used in original research and to base training for the *Lehrerberuf*, the profession of secondary school teaching, upon disciplinary knowledge rather than pedagogical theory as had been done earlier. The rapidity with which they were imitated (by 1812 twelve German universities had philological seminars of which Boeckh's at Berlin became the new ideal model) suggests that their operating principles were readily accepted and easily integrated elsewhere. The combination of *Bildung, Wissenschaft,* and *innere Beruf* that they promoted paralleled practices in the older seminars of the theological faculty, where it was assumed that a *wissenschaftlich* or scholarly consciousness, achieved through the critical application of a research methodology, was the way to gain accurate knowledge of Christianity's original truths. Just as preachers had been trained less through writing homilies than through conducting original theological research, so teachers were trained in principle through the pursuit of original investigations.[10]

For many seminars, however, the ideals of *Bildung, Wissenschaft,* and *innere Beruf* were impractical or irrevelant or appeared infrequently. Seminars were not always formed principally to engage students in original research. Many seminars, including several in the natural sciences, had evolved from exercise sessions and student societies. Sessions and societies stemmed from increased faculty sensitivity to student laxness and to what was considered to be, before the 1830s or so, the inadequate preparation received by students at secondary schools. Members of the medical faculty also complained about ill-prepared students, a sign that they wanted to teach at a higher level or in a different way.[11] The issue of student laxness was especially pronounced in Prussia, where Humboldt's original proposal to coordinate secondary school and university instruction could not always be implemented because of a shortage of properly trained secondary-school teachers, and where the introduction of the Abitur or Gymnasium-leaving examination in 1812 (made mandatory in 1834) helped to transfer part of the burden of preparation for university studies to the Gymnasium.[12] Existing alongside lecture courses but at the institutional fringes of universities, sessions and societies were unofficial classes (often offered as variations on or supplements to private lecture courses) created by professors to enhance university teaching and to assist student learning. They were conducted in a manner similar to what today are called recitation sections or problem sessions, and were not at first identifiable as colloquia or seminars.

Exercise sessions held by the mathematicians Wrede and later Jacobi at Königsberg during the 1820s, for example, functioned as review and problem sessions where material that had been introduced in class as well as homework problems were discussed. Similar sessions were held in mathematics under Dirichlet at Berlin and in physics at Halle. The most famous of these exercise sessions was offered by Ranke in history at Berlin after 1827. His private exercises were instrumental in creating what he later called his "historical family," the members of which collectively considered themselves to be a part of "Ranke's school." Professional matters were also handled in societies and sessions. At Bonn in the 1840s the philosopher Brandis offered, in his home, private exercises in logic, giving special consideration to how logic was taught in the Gymnasium so that he might train better Gymnasium teachers. *Gymnasiallehrer* and teaching candidates who wished to improve their scholarly training were invited to attend sessions and seminars at other universities. When Ranke moved to Bonn, he and the historian Sybel proposed transforming their historical society, established in 1844, into a seminar for training *Gymnasiallehrer*.[13] Like Purkyně's pedagogical innovations at Breslau, these sessions and societies were not a manifestation of neohumanism but were the consequence of a desire to change didactic practices, although not necessarily along the lines prescribed by Pestalozzi. Unlike Purkyně, the directors of sessions and societies did not necessarily aspire to instruct in the process of discovery. When societies and sessions were institutionalized and officially recognized as seminars, research was frequently introduced; but it always supplemented and rarely replaced the original educational function of instruction in more elementary matters. In this way the influence of neohumanism upon the promotion of student research was preceded or preempted by pedagogical and even professional exigencies.

The impact of sessions, societies, and the seminars that some of them eventually became goes beyond the behavioral corrective for student laxness that these faculty-initiated institutes offered. In transforming the nature of instruction at universities, sessions, societies and seminars engaged, and sometimes enticed, students into an intellectual dialogue with professors who were quite ready to monitor more closely the activity of their clientele so that more sophisticated teaching and more serious learning could take place. Through this opportunity for "closer and more fruitful scholarly contact . . . than occurs in lectures,"[14] these pedagogical goals were attained by tactics more imaginative than the periodic testing that merely would have required learning by rote. Constructing meaningful exercises in the humanities and workable problems in the sciences were tedious tasks not undertaken by all professors. When these exercises were framed carefully, however, they could assist the systematic learning of disciplinary knowledge. Moreover, when students used them to master fundamentals, such exercises could also train them to do research and lead sometimes to original investigations.

What happened in sessions and societies by design occurred in seminars by trial and error. Most seminars were created to promote *Wissenschaft* through the transmission of the techniques of original investigation and the application of these by students to novel, unsolved problems. But preparing students to do research was a considerable pedagogical task. Expecting eighteen- or nineteen-year-olds to possess as a matter of course knowledge of background literature and the requisite skills to manage intellectual curiosity in a disciplined way was unrealistic. Their secondary-school education certainly did not prepare them for the task, although the situation improved somewhat in Prussia when year classes, a standard curriculum taken by all students in the same grade, finally in the 1830s superseded the subject class system that allowed students with exceptional talent to move ahead in certain subjects and those with limited abilities to drop a subject altogether. The creation of year classes was one of several pedagogical changes that made it possible, in principle, to draw more than the talented into higher studies and, it was hoped, into research. Even after the 1830s, however, an unevenly prepared student clientele could be expected because regional variations in teaching persisted (even in the local adaptations of ministerial recommendations) and because no standard course of study had been introduced into the university, where the principle of *Lernfreiheit*, the freedom to choose what one studied, reigned.

Seminar directors gradually accepted the task that lay before them and attempted to bridge the gap between the school and the university, as well as to develop the pedagogical foundation for higher educational goals. Often with reluctance and some complaint, they developed programs of learning and eventually even recommended curricula and standardized exercises, thereby violating in effect the principle of *Lernfreiheit*. They set up entrance requirements that lent credence to the notion of *Vorkenntnisse*, or prerequisites. Oral and written entrance examinations, evidence of possessing preparatory knowledge in auxiliary fields, and mastery of *Gymnasium*-level textbooks were often required.[15] Each of these defined the sense in which the student was "qualified" to participate in the seminar. Even so, once they gathered their students together, they found that not all of them could be treated in the same way. They therefore created introductory and advanced divisions in their institutes; lower divisions often became proseminars. Sometimes the separate divisions of seminars were defined by topic rather than by level of accomplishment. In Greifswald's history seminar, for example, there were three divisions. Two of them, ancient history and medieval history, defined historical periods. The third, geography, provided an auxiliary subject for students of history. Together they constituted a curriculum (all students had to register eventually for all sections) and potential areas of specialization. Seminars in theology had divisions for the Old and New Testaments, or for philological and historical methods; in physics, for mathematics and physics; in the natural sciences, for all sciences represented by the directors.[16] Some seminars were bound to a series of lecture courses that then became a local syllabus for the field.

Seminar exercises engaged students in learning more than lecture courses did. Lecture courses had the potential to convey the principal ideas of a field, to outline its boundaries, and to convey impressionistically its problem structure. Seminar exercises did that and more. They trained students in the methods and tools of a field; they inculcated skills and techniques; and they instilled the habits of mind essential for the practice of scholarship or a profession. Furthermore, through seminar exercises dialogue was promoted in two ways. Evaluated by seminar directors, exercises brought teacher and student together; reviewed by peers, exercises created a sense of community among students. All of these activities were premised upon the assurance that certain foundations had been established. Only then could the student engage in the dialogue of the seminar, where he was expected "to ask questions about what still remains in darkness."[17]

Hence, the introduction into the classroom of scholarly and critical techniques did not necessarily entail the activity of student research because an intermediate step, the reorganization of knowledge and skills into teachable sequences and learnable forms, was required. Seminar instruction thereby contributed to curriculum development or the pedagogical consolidation of disciplinary knowledge,[18] as well as to the notion that the practice of scholarship consisted of separable skills that could be learned and that, when implemented properly, could lead to an original investigation. For students that meant accepting requirements: regular attendance, recommended or mandatory courses, exercises, homework, and active participation in general. Discipline building was premised in part upon disciplined learning. In this way the seminar was not a neutral institute but one with a particular ideology of teaching and learning.

Not everyone accepted its ideology. At Bonn the establishment of a history seminar was delayed until 1861 in part because the Prussian minister of finance, von Patow, viewed seminars as infringements upon *Lernfreiheit* that, he felt, differentiated the school and the university.[19] In principle, a seminar seemed appropriate for studying another subject, philosophy, for in it creative, critical, and disputatious thinking could challenge the status quo and sharpen the powers of philosophical argumentation. But representatives of philosophy at Bonn saw matters otherwise. "Philosophy appears to be left less frequently to seminar exercises and less suited for them than other disciplines [*Fächer*]," they argued. They upheld the "widely held view that philosophy cannot be learned by textual reading, textual criticism, and factual explanation," and they believed that "philosophical ability [*Begabung*] must be inborn."[20] In rejecting the seminar format, Bonn philosophers also rejected the notion that individuals could be trained to perform an intellectual task. For them the perpetuation and pursuit of philosophical knowledge was dependent upon the appearance of those with talent rather than upon the transmission of knowledge and skills in a systematic way. Eventually, however, they did establish a seminar, not wanting to pass up its social advantage in promoting dialogue in learning.

Where Bonn philosophers saw disadvantages others saw advantages to using seminar instruction to transform a field of knowledge socially and intellectually. When a seminar for experimental psychology was established at Berlin in 1893, it was not designed to promote original research because its directors felt that "in the case of such a young field of research with so few proven methods, so many sources of error, [and] so many difficulties in the exact construction and presentation of arguments, the main purpose [of the seminar] cannot be that of permitting students to prepare the greatest number of dissertations." Accordingly, exercises for this seminar were fundamental and foundational. Its practical exercises handled basic methods of psychological experimentation, while in its theoretical exercises, its directors explained, "questions from all areas of special and general psychology as well as intersecting issues [*Grenzfragen*] from epistemology, ethics, pedagogy, and jurisprudence (matters concerning volition) are thoroughly discussed, mostly with reference to investigations recently made known." "The principal emphasis," they continued, "is placed on rigorous accuracy in the interpretation of observations, in the cultivation of ideas, and in the certification of arguments."[21] Lacking a well-defined field of knowledge, Berlin experimental psychologists intended to use seminar exercises, which fell short of original research, to assist them in achieving conceptual consolidation and methodological certainty.

In practice, then, seminars in many respects belied the ideal image of them that has persisted to the present. Original research was only a part—probably a relatively small but highly rewarding part—of a seminar's activity. Out of necessity, seminar instruction contributed to "the tightening, in some cases, of curricular requirements"[22] that gradually came to characterize German university education in the nineteenth century. Despite their professed allegiance to the advancement of *Wissenschaft*, many seminars broke up learning not only by field but also by subfield, and introduced important graduated patterns of learning that made obvious the hierarchical (or at least topical) arrangement of knowledge and skills in each of them. The pedagogical emphasis in instruction thereby shifted from *Bildung* to *Ausbildung*, from cultivation to training in a manner contrary to neohumanism.

This result was not unanticipated by those active in the early years of the seminar system. The eighteenth-century Göttingen philologist Georg Christoph Lichtenberg implicity pointed to the limitations of neohumanism in building character, and to the realities of the new kind of university instruction, when he concluded that "a teacher at schools and universities cannot educate individuals; he educates only types [of individuals]."[23] Recent scholarship on the German university system has reaffirmed Lichtenberg's observation. Referring to the curricular changes of the university, Charles E. McClelland has claimed that "university graduates, too, were trained technicians of a sort" and that this result "collided with the traditional assertion of German neohumanist pedagogical theorists that classical and university *Bildung* shaped an independent, flexible mind capable of creative thought."[24] That German university education, especially the seminar system, had been viewed otherwise, doubtless stemmed from the obvious historical significance of the birth of the modern research university. Yet research was not its only new function. Pedagogically, the nineteenth-century university was a world apart from its eighteenth-century predecessor. The birth of the modern research university was also the birth of the modern teaching university with its prescribed or recommended courses of study, its exercises and homework assignments, and its expanded opportunities for dialogue between professors and students.

All of this led rather quickly to the disappearance of the notion of *innere Beruf*. It was an ideal notion, and probably one not often encountered in practice. Not unexpectedly, few students ever heard, much less responded to, an inner voice. Many had to be drawn or lured to seminars by the privileges and awards they provided. Free meals and better living quarters were two incentives offered initially, but they were replaced later by special library privileges and financial premiums for exceptional performance. By the late 1820s, precisely when the research imperative was institutionalized, a different notion of *Beruf* became relevant to seminar instruction. Even in seminars known for the research productivity of their students, many members nonetheless prepared for the *Lehrerberuf*. Wolf's philological seminar at Halle and Neumann's physics seminar at Königsberg, to name two of the best known, turned out primarily secondary-school teachers.[25] The training of teachers through scholarly instruction was directly and most strongly promoted by the Prussian state, which was interested especially in producing teachers of the natural sciences and mathematics. Significantly, as the seminar system expanded the Prussian state teaching examination became more sophisticated. Yet as seminar instruction was adapted to the needs of students, the relationship between knowledge and professional training changed. At first the way to the *Lehrerberuf* was in principle through *Wissenschaft*. By the end of the century, however, seminars offered to provide "a methodical introduction to fruitful and independent work," but to do so "under proper consideration of the needs of *Gymnasien* and other secondary schools."[26] So, for example, in Kiel's history seminar, established in 1882, "free lectures . . . for the purpose of giving direction to practical training [*Ausbildung*] for future historical instruction" supplemented the seminar's regular exercises.[27]

University histories abound with lists of the many professions taken up by seminar graduates, confirming the observation that seminar instruction was meaningful to students who did not have scholarly aspirations. The state's promotion of certain professions as a means of increasing its power through the training of individuals for politically and socially sensitive occupations also contributed to the relevance of seminar instruction. Technology and industrialization supplied the context within which Berlin's seminar for English philology, for example, could justify its existence. "The study of English should, without losing its foundation in the Middle Ages, be directed more at the needs of the present," its directors believed. They viewed their institute as strategic because "especially from England one can learn much about social concerns, for there the state preceded ours in its development, having been for some time transformed from an agricultural state to one of mass production."[28] For a country whose leaders practiced social imperialism and worked ceaselessly to keep democracy at bay, there was indeed something to be learned about "social concerns" from the English experience. Similarly, Berlin's seminar for oriental languages, founded in 1887 at a time when Germany's colonial movement was closely aligned with its social imperialism, functioned as more than an institute for learning languages. Its directors claimed that while "official interests were decisive in the founding of the seminar," there was also the imperative to consider "the collective interest of the German nation in foreign lands, especially Asia and Africa." The seminar therefore catered not only to individuals entering Germany's foreign service, but also to "other categories of students . . . who seek in the seminar specific preparation for a definite profession in service of our fatherland."[29] Hence knowledge in these seminars served not only *wissenschaftlich* and *beruflich* objectives but *staatlich* ones as well.

The notion of *Beruf*, once internalized in students' inclinations and predispositions preceding their seminar experience, was now externalized, embodied in the seminar exercises that constituted training for the professional activities that would be undertaken after leaving the seminar. Whereas previously the *wissenschaftlich* activity of the seminar related in vague ways to the cultivation of personality, now, with *Ausbildung* incorporated, seminar learning related in more direct ways to professional activities or functions. The transformation in the notion of *Beruf* evolved from the pedagogical consequences of trying to prepare students for research. For secondary school teaching, the concern of seminars in the philosophical faculty, that meant a shift from viewing knowledge as the epistemological foundation of the professional identity of the *Gymnasiallehrer* to viewing knowledge as something that was transmitted in Gymnasium instruction.

There is an irony in the importance of *Ausbildung* in seminar instruction to a professoriate that earlier had been critical of *Brotstudien* (courses taken to prepare for a profession), for they had created in effect its nineteenth-century functional equivalent. In the end they had to admit that their seminars were successful in part because students accepted their programs of learning as relevent to their intended *Berufe*. In seminars the tension between *Bildung* and *Ausbildung*, between an instructional philosophy that claimed to be able to form character from within and one that attempted to mold qualifications from without, was also a tension between *Wissenschaft* and *Beruf*, between the promotion of knowledge for its own sake and the formation of a professional, especially a learned one. For these reasons the promotion of research, no matter what its motivating source, was an ideal incompletely realized in seminar instruction. Institutionalizing research was in other ways an important factor in transforming university teaching and learning.[30]

II

Because humanistic seminars were among the first university institutes, it is often assumed that seminars in the natural sciences were modeled upon them, and even that both kinds of seminars were in some sense the institutional predecessors of laboratory-based scientific institutes. Structural similarities among seminars, especially the outward functional similarity in promoting research, and the fact that directors of scientific seminars either attended or were familiar with humanistic seminars, are two points most often cited in this regard.[31] Although a final assessment of this issue must await detailed studies of the origins of more seminars and institutes than now exist, it seems unlikely that any strong causal connection between seminars and institutes will surface. That several seminars in the natural sciences

and mathematics shared with humanistic seminars a common pedagogical origin in sessions and societies; that laboratories existed alongside scientific seminars without always being fully incorporated into
them; and that the seminar and the laboratory-based scientific institute were very different administrative units are some of the reasons
why an evolutionary model for scientific institutes might not work.
Finally, any assessment of the origin of university institutes for the
natural sciences will have to consider the indebtedness of scientists to
the very important institutional precedents set by clinical institutes,
cabinets, collections, and especially university observatories. An
early and strategic institute, the university observatory housed intellectual, pedagogical, and professional activities and had financial and
administrative ties to the state, all of which exemplified to some natural scientists—particularly physicists—precisely what a university institute could be and do.[32]

When we turn from the origins of scientific institutes to their operation, however, we find that the model of the humanistic seminar can
be used advantageously as a source for the kinds of questions that will
help gain access to the everyday reality of an institute's activities.
Some parameters of the daily operation of several institutes have been
outlined already in the literature. Administrative, financial, and architectural details are the best known, as are the essential features of
research programs practiced in their laboratories and the gross details
of courses taught in their classrooms.[33] Less well known are the students who were the lifeblood of an institute's daily activity, although
recent studies of student clienteles show promise of leading to more
detailed analyses.[34] Yet the most time-consuming function of institutes—instruction—is the one we know least, even though teaching
was the *raison d'être* of most (if not all) German university institutes.
One way to explore the teaching that took place in them would be
through a comparison with seminar instruction. Because both humanistic seminars and scientific institutes tried to encourage student research, both probably shared similar teaching problems, as well as
their solutions. While there was some curricular tightening in humanities seminars, prescribed courses of study became far more common,
and necessary, in medicine and the sciences. Although research skills
were taught in humanities seminars, the investigative techniques of
the sciences—especially experimental and mathematical ones—were
undoubtedly more thoroughly represented in student exercises because they could be broken down into simple tasks more easily. And

while many students in the humanities found their seminar experience relevant to their later careers, science and medical students came to depend upon their instruction as essential for career preparation.

We know little about the origin and implementation of science curricula and the codification of knowledge upon which they depended. We know less about the composition and purpose of student exercises and how they constituted training for research. Exploring both of these will require revising received views about the role of education in the history of the sciences. We know from our own personal experience both that teaching is not a static institutional activity and that its efficacy cannot be taken for granted. Yet too often as historians we treat it as though it were a derivative enterprise, changing only in response to external factors, such as the influx of new knowledge from research, the advent of new ideologies, or the influence of social, economic, and political forces. Sociologists of science also have tended to view scientific training as a function issuing unproblematically from the intellectual structure of a field. Ludwik Fleck, for example, acknowledged that the professional judgments exercised in the construction of scientific knowledge were themselves products of scientific education, but he did not address how scientists acquired the "professional habits" needed to become what Fleck himself called a "trained person."[35] Likewise, Joseph Ben-David considered "systematic training and the division of labor" to be "important factors of scientific growth." Because in his view research was the primary function of educational institutes such as seminars and laboratories, he believed that knowledge had to be assembled in a form suitable for instruction before training programs could be inaugurated. With the appearance of organized scientific knowledge, he argued, "science . . . could be used as an educational discipline."[36]

Much suggests that matters concerning scientific instruction are more complex than either Fleck or Ben-David recognized. In their description of scientific practice as something that is in part tacitly learned, Kuhn, Polyani, and Ravetz have isolated one side of that complexity. Their conclusions, however, must be regarded as tentative until more detailed examinations of scientific education demonstrate what can be learned by systematic training and what must be acquired in other ways.[37] In addition, the relationship between the conceptual content of a field of knowledge and its pedagogical representation needs to be examined. To the extent that the evolution of seminar instruction can serve as a historiographical model for instruction in other university institutes, it seems more likely that in the early years of scientific institutes, organized scientific knowledge was not at first completely available but was shaped in the course of dealing with pedagogical problems and student needs. As the essays in this volume demonstrate, changes in instruction were not always automatic responses to new ideas in a field. Independently of the appearance of new knowledge, even textbooks can promote new perspectives, and training exercises can have an impact upon professional qualifications (and hence upon the social structure of a discipline) as well as upon the execution of scientific investigations.

In order to expand upon the arguments in this volume and to view teaching as a creative enterprise in its own right, some historiographical imagination will be needed. The educational historian Konrad Jarausch has recently identified the content of instruction and the nature of classroom experiences as "research lacunae."[38] Historians of science have an opportunity to take the lead in this area, constructing a history quite different from the kind to which they are accustomed. The history of classroom experiences and of laboratory exercises will not examine radical change alone but will delineate the steadiness of repetitive daily operations and the intellectual, pedagogical, and professional reasons for them. In scientific pedagogy, tradition and stability cannot be taken for granted; the forces of inertia require explanation as much as do the forces of change. If we want to visit the classroom and to portray it in as intimate detail as possible, we should probably not look at it only through the eyes of teachers interested in the research productivity of their students; we should also view it through the eyes of students who entered the classroom with enthusiasm, curiosity, and in need of intellectual discipline, practice, and training in fundamentals. Where and how did students begin their intellectual journeys?

Often as German natural scientists argued for the relevance of the scientific disciplines to a neohumanist educational ideology and to the cultivation of *Bildung*, they failed for the most part to establish their case. Their own educational programs had other sources, as contributors to this volume have pointed out, including the pedagogical desire to engage students in the process of discovery and the professional tasks of training teachers, scientists, and physicians. Whether by design or by trial and error, natural scientists found themselves involved in the construction of curricula designed in part to achieve these ends. As was the case for humanists, they found their goals difficult to achieve. The needs of students—their level of accomplishment, their untrained abilities, and their career plans—shaped solutions to pedagogical problems in the sciences just as they had done in the humanities. At Göttingen, for example, because the student clientele for lecture courses in mathematics and physics changed every year, these courses rarely went beyond an introductory level. That university's mathematico-physical seminar was therefore established in 1850 not only as a place for instruction in fundamentals, but also as a center where students could find a "connected, systematic course of instruction."[39] Similarly, lacking a cadre of well-prepared students, the mathematico-physical seminar at Königsberg survived only because its directors were able to suspend, in some cases, fulfillment of their lofty goal of original student research and to construct a curriculum based on instruction in geometry and mechanics, which served as entry-level courses, and in physics, on exercises emphasizing precision measurement.[40]

Medical students figure prominently among the factors shaping physiological instruction at the institutes discussed in this volume. To accommodate them, Purkyně divided physiological instruction at Breslau into two levels. He placed medical students who intended to practice with beginning students in physiology, basing their instruction on "the art of physiological experimentation and observation of various types." This "art" must have consisted of fundamental exercises because he separated both medical and beginning students from a more advanced group requiring a higher level of physiological instruction, including exposure to original investigations.[41] According to Tuchman, Henle's educational innovations drew a greater number of medical students to Heidelberg, thus producing exactly the result the state wanted. It is worth noting that Henle, like Purkyně, introduced his innovation first in the form of exercises in microscopy in 1846, waiting four years to introduce physiological experimentation.

The fate of Carl Lehmann's 1849 proposal for an institute for physiological chemistry at Leipzig, outlined in detail by Lenoir, can be interpreted partly in terms of the pedagogical needs of medical students. While Leipzig's faculty apparently agreed with Lehmann's proposal to use advanced laboratory instruction as a means of introducing research results, the scientific method, and especially the analysis of causes to medical students, they did not agree with him on how it should be accomplished. Despite Lehmann's criticism of the dry-as-dust technical expertise often conveyed through laboratory instruction, the faculty apparently recognized more clearly than Lehmann did that an institute of the type described by him would work only if more elementary instruction were available. For that reason they approved an institute for chemistry first, before Ludwig arrived to direct Leipzig's new physiological institute.

Although the nature of physiological instruction was not explored by Holmes, it seems reasonable to assume that similar pedagogical adjustments for medical students occurred at Munich, where Siebold's familiarity with Purkyně's routine at Breslau probably guided his conception of medical instruction.[42] Later pedagogical innovations at Munich no doubt occurred when the working cooperation between chemists and physiologists fostered by Liebig, Bischoff, and Voit led to simultaneous instruction in both fields. Even if laboratory instruction for medical students at these institutes had remained at the level of elementary exercises in research techniques (as it probably did in most cases), its impact was nonethless profound. Frank has surmised that laboratory instruction with instruments in medical education was one factor that created greater interest in, and that made possible the more thorough analysis of, the patterned graphical data that these instruments produced. Episodes similar to the one discussed by Frank might be rare, but overall it cannot be denied that physiological instruction, especially in the laboratory, led to fundamental changes in medical theory and practice.

The needs and abilities of medical students were persistently troublesome factors to consider in the construction of science courses and exercises not only in physiology but in other sciences as well. In physics, accommodating medical students was one reason for the emergence of a two-track system of introductory instruction: a simpler experimental physics for all those who were taking physics as a *Nebenfach*, and the more difficult theoretical physics for those who intended to become physicists or physics teachers.[43] Despite Justus Liebig's success at Giessen in accommodating students with various interests, the problem of chemical instruction was not solved so easily elsewhere. The Tübingen chemist Lothar Meyer was still complaining about the problems involved in teaching an introductory chemistry course to a diverse audience of medical students and others in the 1870s. Although he blamed the student privilege of *Lernfreiheit* (which, he felt, obligated a professor to teach a necessarily diverse audience), he did not acknowledge that other solutions, such as that achieved in physics, infringed upon that freedom.[44] Medical students in some cases found seminar instruction useful and enrolled in the Bonn and Königsberg seminars for the natural sciences, the only Prussian seminars that covered the biological sciences. In part to accommodate their needs, the directors of both seminars requested funds for microscopes. In 1838–1839 the Königsberg natural sciences seminar offered anatomico-morphological exercises that used a Plössl microscope; some students were able to conduct their own investigations on the basis of these exercises.[45]

What the precise requirements of medical students were, and how they impinged upon the pedagogical construction of knowledge in these and other "basic" sciences, remain significant gaps in our understanding of the constitution of scientific instruction and its relation to the structure of disciplinary knowledge, as well as to medical training and practice. That student needs appear to have figured so heavily in the construction of courses suggests that the structure and content of scientific knowledge in the classroom did not derive exclusively from above, from the distillation and reorganization of the results of research, but also took into account what existed below, the pedagogical needs of students. Teaching science was by no means straightforward or easy. What Holmes has pointed out in the case of Bischoff at Munich holds as well for natural scientists at other institutes: teaching was a pressured and time-consuming but nonetheless essential task.

Textbooks provide the easiest and most accessible entry into one side of the dialogue that took place in classrooms. Even though textbooks with codified and systematically presented knowledge had been more common in the sciences than in the humanities for some time, we know little about the evolution of the modern science textbook, especially its exercises. From 1800 to 1850 the press of new pedagogical needs—including the desire of several university scientists to replace talent with training as a way to bring students into the practice of science—seems to have led to revised formats for science textbooks and to the incorporation into them of skill-oriented considerations, such as chapters or sections dealing with scientific instruments. To consider them as documents conveying a pedagogical reality, however, will mean abandoning the view expressed by both Kuhn and Fleck that textbooks, like other tools of teaching, were shaped exclusively by research.[46] Other factors, such as student needs, clearly came into play in their construction. In addition, textbooks were in some cases self-consciously designed as instruments of discipline building, as Emil du Bois-Reymond argued in 1852 to Carl Ludwig, then writing his own textbook in physiology. To bolster Ludwig's spirits, du Bois-Reymond reminded Ludwig that "there are epochs in the sciences when it is just as worthwhile to write a textbook as it is to do the most significant work of one's own. I see such an epoch now in physiology. It is due to the fact that our school sees things in a completely new light." In a statement that momentarily separated the contents of textbooks from the results of research, and that pointed to the independently powerful role of scientific pedagogy, du Bois-Reymond explained that "even if there were no new material not yet contained in old textbooks, a whole new science results simply by compiling the old knowledge according to our way of thinking." Three years later, Ludwig's textbook in his hands, du Bois-Reymond proceeded to reorganize his lecture courses, using Ludwig's book as their foundation.[47] To his institute in Leipzig a decade later Ludwig brought the structure for physiology that he had already worked out in his teaching.

Often compiled from actual lecture notes, textbooks thus seem to display most directly what was transmitted to students. But as John Harley Warner has pointed out, they are a "treacherous source," marked by an exaggerated internal consistency that tends to belie actual teaching practices. As a corrective to relying on them, Warner advocates consulting lecture notes taken by students.[48] In these notes, I would add, one can hear the whispers of the other side of the dialogue that took place in the classroom. Student lecture notes are an abundant source in German archives, but they seem to be little read and less frequently cited. Their strength as a historical document lies principally in the comparative perspective they offer. When compared to published textbooks based on lectures, they provide information on a teacher's actual classroom style. In other ways, they are the voices of students. When compared to notes from the same course taken by other students, they reveal individual student habits and interests through the relative differences in the density of detail and in marginal notes. Their advantage as a historical source extends beyond the corrective they offer for textbooks. As we know from our own experience, even when a teacher instructs from a textbook, the density of detail in lectures exceeds that in a corresponding textbook section. This difference is especially important in science education, where problems and issues outlined in textbooks are often derived and explained in greater detail in class using mathematical and other techniques appropriate to them. Hence lecture notes not only convey knowledge; they also show how the skills constituting techniques of investigation were employed.

Fleck believed that the "technical skills required for any scientific investigation" could not be "formulated in terms of logic."[49] Nevertheless, just as there was a pedagogical imperative to represent knowledge in a form appropriate for the classroom, there was a similar imperative to break up the investigative techniques of science into rudimentary skills that could be learned in student exercises. It seems that both Purkyně and Henle would have had to construct such skill-based exercises for their students if they were serious about bringing the average student into the process of discovery. At a later time Ludwig and the Munich group could have drawn upon new investigative techniques for their exercises, but they still had to assign and build upon the elementary exercises first developed in physiology by Purkyně, Henle, and others. In all cases uncovering those exercises and the skills they taught is a formidable historical task. Often one can reconstruct from archival or other documents the instruments that were purchased for instruction, but one is still left with the problem of determining how they were used in the classroom. Sometimes the task is eased considerably by the existence of exercise handbooks, such as Justus Liebig's *Anleitung zur Analyse organischer Körper* or Friedrich Kohlrausch's *Leitfaden der praktischen Physik*.[50] Like textbooks, however, these handbooks are rationalized presentations of ideal classroom practices, and hence as sources they can function only as first approximations, not exhaustive representations.

The most reliable source for uncovering the skills and techniques taught may come from the students themselves. They often reveal in their first published papers the techniques of investigation taught in the classroom. I have found that first papers tend to be less polished and less formal than those written after years of experience. In them students were more apt to apologize in print for their shortcomings when they were well aware (almost too aware) of the standards to be met. They were also more inclined to be verbose, explaining their every step as a teacher would do in a lecture, and to vent their frustrations when things did not work out as planned. Embodying residues of educational experiences, first papers reveal in direct ways the investigative techniques that earlier had been learned. For some students, especially those whose employment did not allow direct contact with a disciplinary community, educational experiences resonated in papers sporadically published until late in their careers. For that reason it is often necessary to read all papers published by students who attended an institute in order to capture the fullness of their educational experiences. In these and in other ways, student papers are windows on the activity of the exercise session, the seminar, or the teaching laboratory of an institute. Naturally, because these students have published, they represent an elite among the clientele of an institute. How other students—including those who became practicing physicians and those who did not publish—learned and assimilated investigative techniques can be accessed only in indirect ways through other traditional sources, such as letters, diaries, and the like, if they exist (and often they do not).[51]

These student sources supplement but do not replace more traditional ones that outline the activity of an institute, such as annual reports, financial records, and ministerial files. Nevertheless, it is through student sources that we can take the next step in understanding the impact of these innovative training programs by looking at the relation between education and work. The systematic training in skills offered in institutes became the foundation, in whole or in part, of many of the professions taken up by its graduates. As the investigative techniques of science became more complex, it seems reasonable to assume that students became more proficient in some techniques than in others. The increased use of sophisticated instruments and equipment helped to promote a division of labor as students learned to operate with ease the latest tools of investigation. In this way the teaching program of an institute, as well as its research activity, promoted a division of labor in science. Evident first in observatories where rigorous techniques of data analysis led to the separation of "the observer from the calculator and the mathematician,"[52] a division of labor evolved naturally as university institutes gained in strength. The observer at the Munich physiological institute who "likened its operation . . . to a factory, which nevertheless had to function with the precision of a watch," revealed through these metaphors of industry the presence of task-oriented individuals committed to a common goal. A division of labor at Munich must have been necessary for the large-scale physiological investigations executed there, especially the experiments on respiration. Specialization in investigative techniques ultimately promoted the formation of "schools." At Munich, for example, investigative techniques (such as the input-output method) and standards of accuracy shaped a research and training program that constituted a "school" of like-minded individuals whose greatest commonality was that they worked in similar ways. Likewise, Ludwig's attribution to Henle of a "microscopical school" also indicates that schools were identified by investigative techniques rather than exclusively by a problem-oriented research program.

The strength of the relation between scientific training on the one hand and professions, division of labor, and schools on the other can be determined only by a thorough examination of student clienteles and their career patterns which goes beyond superficial statistical analyses. Without a doubt, the professional identity of those who participated in training programs was tied very closely to the disciplinary knowledge they studied. One does not hear of *innere Beruf* but of *Physiker von Beruf* and *Chemiker vom Fach*.[53] Especially in Prussia the connection between professional identity and functional expertise was strengthened by the state examination system and sanctioned by society at large.[54] Without knowledge of the workaday world of institute graduates, however, we cannot know how successful these innovative training programs actually were at democratizing learning.

In replacing talent by training, the gifted by the rank-and-file, and privilege by objective qualifications, the transformation in scientific training should have contributed to the expansion of social, political, economic, and professional opportunities for German university graduates. It also created the possibility of stark disappointment. The hope that training and the possession of an examination certificate would lead to a productive and satisfying professional life often proved false. In our own century, Sir Peter Medawar believed that the democratization of learning led to the possibility that "anyone who combines strong common sense with an ordinary degree of imagination can become a creative scientist, and a happy one besides, insofar as happiness depends upon being able to develop to the limits of one's abilities."[55] But in the past, and perhaps even now, it sometimes proved to be an illusion that individuals with sophisticated scientific training could find personal and professional satisfaction in positions, such as secondary school teaching, that did not provide the material and intellectual conditions for exercising the specialized knowledge and skills of their training. In such cases, according to Charles Rosenberg, one's "professional life becomes then a compromise defined by the sometimes consistent and sometimes conflicting demands of [the] discipline and the condition of [one's] employment."[56] The most tragic consequence, however, was the fact that the German governments offered to their citizens so limited an opportunity to exercise in a political sphere the critical ways of thinking that had been cultivated in university institutes.

In the classroom, however, critical dialogue of various kinds did take place. Perhaps at the lowest levels it did not amount to much. Students no doubt asked for explanations, clarifications, and assistance; instructors taught, guided, and offered advice on matters that were second nature to them. It seems reasonable to expect, though, that the questions asked and the difficulties encountered by students at introductory levels forced instructors to rethink their manner of teaching. Rudimentary skills practiced in exercises may not have led so smoothly to more complicated investigative techniques. Knowledge that seemed straightforward enough at an advanced level may not have lent itself so readily to the simplification necessary at an introductory level. The dialogue between teacher and student at the entry level, then, tested the strength and meaningfulness of the pedagogical form of scientific knowledge and skills. In which direction those skills and knowledge would move in response to those tests depended on more than classroom experiences. Trends in education and pedagogy, the nature of professional qualifications in science, as well as advances in disciplinary knowledge are just some of the factors that, in a tug-of-war, pulled instruction toward either pedagogical simplification or intellectual sophistication. Undoubtedly the immediate and direct pressure of local circumstances most strongly conditioned classroom experiences and dialogues. Introductory students helped to shape in local settings—institutes, seminars, and laboratories—the pedagogical structure of disciplinary knowledge and skills.

At an advanced level, classroom dialogue probably approximated the intellectual exchange that took place in the more sophisticated scientific settings described by Lesch and Frank. Both authors explored circumstances in which the investigative techniques and standards of precision, accuracy, and protocol in experimentation were challenged and debated. There are pedagogical parallels to the situations they addressed. Frank's discussion of the comparison of electrocardiograms and the attempt to "align" graphs reminds one of the practice in astronomy of comparing the conditions under which two or more sets of data were taken and of reducing one set to another. In advanced science instruction that task translated into a comparative analysis of two or more well-known methods designed to achieve the same end (such as the determination of specific heats) and of the data produced by them. Such comparative exercises probably led to the refinement of these methods. The interpretation of graphical results examined by Frank was also troublesome in nineteenth-century science instruction. In Prussia, for example, graphical methods were not introduced into secondary-school mathematical instruction until late in the century, making it difficult for those university science instructors who did wish to analyze data graphically, and whose students were not concurrently taking mathematics courses, to introduce this interpretive technique in the classroom. They did so nonetheless and engaged students in measuring exercises that provided the impetus for discussing issues concerning measurement, quantification, and mathematical expression. Pariset's activity, as described by Lesch, was very much like that of an instructor training a class. He was able to keep matters under control only by cultivating common standards of judgment, rigor, accuracy, and precision, and he saw the need to demand "more order, connection, and coordination" in physiological experiments. Finally, the demands placed on clinical instruments, as described by Frank—that their records be precise and that their data be accessible and unambiguous—are not unlike the requirements that would have to be satisfied by instruments used in a pedagogical setting.[57] In short, many of the decision-making strategies discussed by Lesch and Frank, such as the comparison of experimental methods and the assessment of the reliability of instruments, could probably be found in well-formed classroom exercises in science instruction. So whereas at the introductory level classroom dialogue probably challenged the pedagogical form of scientific knowledge, at the advanced level classroom dialogue probably tested the limits of the techniques and protocol of science.

That any kind of dialogue at all could take place in the classroom, the seminar, or the laboratory was dependent upon the development of the means whereby students could be introduced systematically to the foundations of the discipline they studied. In scientific institutes, as in humanistic seminars, there was a pedagogical imperative to present knowledge and skills in teachable sequences and learnable forms. Accumulated research results did not constitute the corpus of what would be learned or taught; disciplinary knowledge had to be organized and represented in a manner suited to the classroom. Sophisticated research methods could not be learned at once; investigative techniques could be learned best through exercises that broke them down. The survival of a discipline would seem to depend upon pedagogical creations such as these, all of them falling short of research but preparatory to it. It goes without saying that exceptional and dedicated instructors were required for this task. In their hands teaching became a creative enterprise in its own right.

Obviously the demand for pedagogical innovation was not the same at all times. His own teaching methods matured, Ludwig could concentrate on the subtle and more difficult task of guiding research in his Leipzig institute. Frank has surmised that Ludwig's involvement with students, from training them to encouraging their research, was a key factor in Ludwig's success in drawing students to physiology. The "standard array" of courses that Holmes found at the Munich physiological institute was likewise a sign of a mature pedagogical state. At an earlier time that array was undoubtedly not as cohesive or well defined, but intended no less for the task of training students. At both Leipzig and Munich training was essential for the local survival of physiology. The success of instruction at both institutes confirms Ben-David's observation that training "did not discourage innovation" or "[diminish] dissent and independence of thought."[58] Rather, training was one factor that made possible scientific innovation and creativity.

Why these pedagogical changes took place at all is, as several authors in this volume have indicated, a very complicated matter. The introduction into the German universities of innovative means of instruction, including especially participation in the research process and the creation of university institutes, led some authors to search for reasons in the economic and political contexts of the German states. To a greater or lesser extent they have suggested that state efforts at modernization created an environment that was either conducive to or necessary for these innovations. It cannot be denied that the state was a dominating force in Germany's educational systems, as it was in other sectors of German life. Controlling the budgets of institutes and the appointments of professors, the state made its presence known. Its approval of university institutes shifted with each change in the wind of politics. The period from the 1820s through the mid-1830s was especially vexing to ambitious and innovative university professors desirous of change, for the governments of the German states, especially Prussia, uniformly refused most requests for progressive educational institutes, mostly to prevent, it seems, political activism among students. (During this time the Prussian government nonetheless approved three science seminars, two at Königsberg and one at Bonn.) For other reasons they regarded institutes with suspicion until midcentury.[59] Their motives for approving university institutes before and after then were complex.

Tuchman and Lenoir have argued most strongly that the context of economic and political modernization was essential for the educational innovations in physiology that took place at Heidelberg in Baden and Leipzig in Saxony. Though suggestive, the connections that they have drawn between modernization and educational change are also not universal, so dependent are they upon a thorough understanding of sharply defined local contexts. Political modernization of the type described by these two authors was for the most part an unwanted goal in authoritarian Prussia, where even economic modernization was scarcely visible before the 1860s. Instead, at the end of the eighteenth century the Prussian government embarked upon a program of social modernization through the reform of state examinations. Prussia's examinations for medicine, law, theology, and secondary school teaching changed early and radically. By the second decade of the nineteenth century all examinations were based upon the notion of "functional expertise," which stressed skills and the ability to perform with them, thus providing the state with a powerful instrument to modernize its professions.[60] This reform shaped an important part of the environment in which educational innovations eventually flourished. A medical license before 1869 required a doctorate and clinical experience, so a physician's training included both.[61] A license to teach secondary school required intensive disciplinary training and later an original investigation not too different from a doctoral thesis. Trained as scholars, these teachers brought with them to secondary schools the knowledge and the innovative investigative techniques they had learned in the university, now translated for classroom use, thus producing educational changes that could be viewed in turn as products of Prussia's social modernization. At the university level institutes were sometimes approved and educational reforms inaugurated in part to accommodate the needs of the professions treated in Prussia's examination system. Differences such as these between Prussia and other states provide compelling reasons for viewing university and other educational institutes, and to some extent the sciences taught and practiced in them, through regional studies that explore the nuances of political, economic, and social changes.[62]

From Max Weber to Jürgen Habermas to, most recently, Jean-François Lyotard, there has been a way of viewing the role of science in the modern world through the emergence and impact of rational skills, technical execution, or, in Lyotard's language, of "performativity."[63] This view encourages us to consider science not only in terms of its intellectual or technical products but also in terms of its activities: its training, its labor, and its workaday world in general. The largely unwritten history of these activities, all a part of the investigative enterprise of science, poses an intriguing challenge for the future.

NOTES

1. Dominick LaCapra, *History and Criticism* (Ithaca, N.Y.: Cornell University Press, 1985), p. 142.

This commentary is written from the perspective of the history of German scientific education rather than from the perspective of the history of physiology or medicine. In the common problems and styles of instruction shared by members of the philosophical and medical faculties of the German universities, there are compelling reasons, I believe, for taking a closer look at the role of scientific pedagogy in shaping scientific and medical practice.

2. Joseph Ben-David, *The Scientist's Role in Society* (Englewood Cliffs, N.J.: Prentice-Hall, 1971; reprinted with a new introduction, Chicago: University of Chicago Press, 1984); R. Steven Turner, "The Growth of Professorial Research in Prussia, 1818–1848—Causes and Context," *Historical Studies in the Physical Sciences* 3 (1971): 137–182. Also see idem, "The Prussian Universities and the Research Imperative, 1806–1848" (Ph.D. diss., Princeton University, 1973).

3. Theodor Billroth, *The Medical Sciences in the German Universities. A Study in the History of Civilization* (New York: Macmillan, 1924); Wilhelm Lorey, *Das Studium der Mathematik an den deutschen Universitäten seit Anfang des 19. Jahrhunderts* (Leipzig: B. G. Teubner, 1916). Almost all German university histories contain separate essays on institutes; see, e.g., Max Lenz, ed., *Geschichte der Königlichen Friedrich-Wilhelms Universität zu Berlin*, 4 vols. (Halle: Waisenhaus, 1910–1918).

4. For example, the study of Justus Liebig's laboratory by B. H. Gustin, "The Emergence of the German Chemical Profession, 1790–1867" (Ph.D. diss., University of Chicago, 1975); Christoph Meinel, *Die Chemie an der Universität Marburg seit Beginn des 19. Jahrhunderts. Ein Beitrag zu ihrer Entwicklung als Hochschulfach*, Akademia Marburgensis, 3 (Marburg: Elwert, 1978); Gert Schubring, "Die Entwicklung des Mathematischen Seminars der Universität Bonn, 1864–1929," *Jahresberichte der Deutschen Mathematiker-Vereinigung* 87 (1985); 139–163; and Arleen M. Tuchman, "Science, Medicine and the State: The Institutionalization of Scientific Medicine at the University of Heidelberg" (Ph.D. diss., University of Wisconsin, 1985).

5. On the socioinstitutional history of German education, see the exemplary historiographical essay and bibliography by Peter Lundgreen, "Historische Bildungsforschung," in *Historische Sozialwissenschaft. Beiträge zur Einführung in die Forschungspraxis*, ed. Reinhard Rürup (Göttingen: Vandenhoeck & Ruprecht, 1977). Also see idem, *Sozialgeschichte der deutschen Schule im Überblick. Teil I: 1770–1918* (Göttingen: Vandenhoeck & Ruprecht, 1980); Charles E. McClelland, *State, Society and University in Germany 1700–1914* (Cambridge: Cambridge University Press, 1980); Konrad H. Jarausch, *Students, Society, and Politics in Imperial Germany. The Rise of Academic Illiberalism* (Princeton: Princeton University Press, 1982); James Albisetti, *Secondary School Reform in Imperial Germany* (Princeton: Princeton University Press, 1983); Detlef K. Müller, *Sozialstruktur und Schulsystem. Aspekte zum Strukturwandel des Schulwesens im 19. Jahrhundert*, Studien zum Wandel von Gesellschaft und Bildung im Neunzehnten Jahrhundert, vol. 7 (Göttingen: Vandenhoeck & Ruprecht, 1977); Margret Kraul, *Das Deutsche Gymnasium 1780–1980)* (Frankfurt-am-Main: Suhrkamp, 1984); and Fritz K. Ringer, *Education and Society in Modern Europe* (Bloomington: University of Indiana Press, 1979). Past and current trends in this literature are reviewed by Konrad H. Jarausch, "The Old 'New History of Education': A German Reconsideration," *History of Education Quarterly* 26 (1986): 225–241.

On the different route to professionalization in Germany see volume 6 of *Geschichte und Gesellschaft* (1980), esp. Lothar Burchardt, "Professionalisierung oder Berufskonstruktion: Das Beispiel des Chemikers im wilhelminischen Deutschland," pp. 326–348. Also see Charles E. McClelland, "Professionalization and Higher Education in Germany," in *The Transformation of Higher Learning 1860–1930*, ed. Konrad H. Jarausch (Chicago: University of Chicago Press, 1983), pp. 306–320; idem, "Zur Professionalisierung der akademischen Berufe in Deutschland," in *Bildungsbürgertum im 19. Jahrhundert. Teil I. Bildungssystem und Professionalisierung in internationalen Vergleichen*, Industrielle Welt, Bd. 38, ed. Werner Conze und Jürgen Kocka (Stuttgart: Kletta-Cotta, 1985), pp. 233–247. The special nature of the German professions extends to the Nazi period. See, e.g. Konrad H. Jarausch, "The Perils of Professionalism: Lawyers, Teachers and Engineers in Nazi Germany," *German Studies Review* 9 (1986): 107–137.

6. See, e.g., the review essay by David Cassidy, "Recent German Perspectives on German Technical Education," *Historical Studies in the Physical Sciences* 14, pt. 1 (1983): 187–200.

7. Dominick LaCapra, "Rethinking Intellectual History and Reading Texts," in *Modern European Intellectual History. Reappraisals and New Perspectives,* ed. Dominick LaCapra and Steven L. Kaplan (Ithaca, N.Y.: Cornell University Press, 1982), pp. 47–85; on 47–49. Also see the editor's introduction, pp. 7–9.

8. Fritz K. Ringer, *The Decline of the German Mandarins: The German Academic Community, 1890–1933* (Cambridge, Mass.: Harvard University Press, 1969); Kenneth D. Barkin, "Fritz K. Ringer's *The Decline of the Mandarins,*" *Journal of Modern History* 43 (1971): 276–286; on 282.

9. The conventional image of the seminar system is projected by, among others, Friedrich Paulsen, *Geschichte des gelehrten Unterrichts auf den deutschen Schulen und Universitäten vom Ausgang des Mittelalters bis zur Gegenwart,* 3d ed., ed. Rudolf Lehmann, 2 vols. (Berlin and Leipzig: W. de Gruyter & Co., 1921), 2: 25–30, 38–43, 46–47, 80–82, 226–229, 258–267, 271–278. To my knowledge no one, including Paulsen, has commented on the meaning of the notion of *innere Beruf.* On *innere Beruf,* see "Reglement für das philologische Seminar der Universität zu Halle. Vom 18. November 1829," in *Die preußischen Universitäten. Eine Sammlung der Verordnungen,* ed J. F. W. Koch, 2 vols. (Berlin: Mittler, 1839) 2.2: 775–778; on 777. "Reglement für das philologische Seminarium [Bonn Universität]. Vom 16. Februar 1819," in ibid., pp. 621–624; on 623. The transformations in the notion of *Beruf* brought on by curricular and instructional changes in the university deserve further study.

Unless otherwise noted, the discussion of the seminar system that follows is drawn from Prussian examples. Seminars sometimes functioned differently in other German states, especially in Bavaria where they emphasized to a greater extent the pedagogical side of teacher training and thus were less involved in shaping disciplinary knowledge and introducing students to the skills of research. See, e.g., Karl Neuerer, *Das höhere Lehramt in Bayern im 19. Jahrhundert* (Berlin: Duncker & Humblot, 1978).

10. For seminars in the *Geisteswissenschaften,* see Wilhelm Erben, "Die Entstehung der Universitäts–Seminar," *Internationale Monatsschrift für Wissenschaft, Kunst & Technik* 7 (1913): cols. 1247–1264, 1335–1348. Seminar statutes are found in Koch, *Die preußischen Universitäten;* L. M. P. von Rönne, *Das Unterrichtswesen des preußischen Staats in seiner geschichtlichen Entwicklung,* 2 vols. (Berlin: Veit & Co., 1854); L. Wiese, *Das höhere Schulwesen in Preußen. Historisch-statistische Darstellung,* 4 vols. (Berlin: Wiegandt & Grieben, 1864–1902); idem, *Verordnungen und Gesetze für die höhere Schulen in Preußen. Zweite Abteilung. Das Lehramt und die Lehrer* (Berlin: Wiegandt & Grieben, 1875); and *Centralblatt für die gesammte Unterrichtsverwaltung in Preußen,* 1859–1934. For a recent discussion of the seminar system, see McClelland, *State, Society and University,* pp. 174–181. According to Anthony Grafton, the practice of philology changed in part because of the institutional transformation in teaching and learning that occurred in the German universities, especially in research-oriented seminars. See Anthony Grafton, "Polyhistor into *Philolog*: Notes on the Transformation of German Classical Scholarship, 1780–1850," *History of Universities* 3 (1983): 159-192. An earlier version of his essay was presented at a

conference on *"Wissenschaft als Beruf,* The Context and Content of Academic Learning in Germany, 1780–1850," held at Princeton University on 3 April 1982.

11. Hans H. Simmer, "Principles and Problems of Medical Undergraduate Education in Germany during the Nineteenth and Early Twentieth Centuries," in *The History of Medical Education,* ed. C. D. O'Malley (Berkeley and Los Angeles: University of California Press, 1970), pp. 173–200; on 178.

12. Wilhelm von Humboldt, "Der Königsberger Schulplan," in *Quellen zur deutschen Schulgeschichte seit 1800,* ed. Gerhardt Giese (Göttingen: Musterschmidt Verlag, 1961), pp. 64–71.

13. Leo Königsberger, *Carl Gustav Jacob Jacobi* (Leipzig: B. G. Teubner, 1904, pp. 144–145; Walter Langhammer, "Some Aspects of the Development of Mathematics at the University of Halle-Wittenberg in the Early 19th Century," in *Epistemological and Social Problems of the Sciences in the Early Nineteenth Century,* ed. H. N. Jahnke and M. Otte (Dordrecht: Reidel, 1981), pp. 235–254; Lenz, *Universität zu Berlin,* 3: 247–249; Friedrich von Bezold, ed., *Geschichte der Rheinischen Friedrich-Wilhelms-Universität. Zweiter Band. Institute und Seminare, 1818-1933* (Bonn: Friedrich Cohen Verlag, 1933), pp. 252–254.

14. "Reglement für das theologische Seminarium der Königl. Universität zu Halle. Vom 4. Juni 1826," in Koch, *Die preußischen Universitäten,* 2.2: 767–772; on 767–768.

15. See, e.g., "Reglement für das evangelisch-theologische Seminarium [Breslau Universität]. Vom 15. Juni 1812," in ibid., pp. 674–676; "Vorläufige Statuten der mathematisch-physikalischen Seminars an der Königsberger Universität," in ibid., pp. 858–859. The Königsberg statutes were one of the rare ones that stipulated entrance requirements in terms of mastery of a textbook.

16. See, e.g., the statutes for the Greifswald history seminar, for the natural science seminars at Königsberg and Bonn, and for theology seminars at all Prussian universities in ibid.

17. "Reglement für das philologische Seminarium [Berlin Universität]. Vom 8. Mai 1812," in ibid., pp. 560–562; on 562.

18. On the importance of the pedagogical consolidation of knowledge for the definition of a discipline, see Rudolf Stichweh, *Zur Entstehung des modernen Systems wissenschaftlicher Disziplinen. Physik in Deutschland, 1740–1890* (Frankfurt-am-Main: Suhrkamp, 1984), p. 7. That the transition from subject classes to year classes in the Prussian Gymnasium forced a systematization of subject matter, thus contributing to a firmer pedagogical definition of certain fields, has been argued by Brita Rang-Dudzik, "Quantitative Aspects of Curricula in Prussian Grammar Schools during the Late 18th and Early 19th Centuries and Their Relation to the Development of the Sciences," in *Epistemological and Social Problems,* pp. 207–233; on 229.

19. Bezold, *Geschichte der Rheinischen Friedrich-Wilhelms-Universität,* 2: 256; Lenz, *Universität zu Berlin,* 3: 254.

20. Bezold, *Geschichte der Rheinischen Friedrich-Wilhelms-Universität,* 2: 136.

21. Lenz, *Universität zu Berlin*, 3: 203, 206.

22. Charles E. McClelland, "Structural Change and Social Reproduction in German Universities, 1870–1920," *History of Education* 15, no. 3 (1986): 177–193; on 183.

23. Robert S. Leventhal, "The Emergence of Philological Discourse in the German States, 1770–1810," *Isis* 77 (1986): 243–260; on 260.

24. McClelland, "Structural Change," p. 181.

25. Wilhelm Schrader, ed., *Geschichte der Friedrichs-Universität zu Halle*, 2 vols. (Berlin: Dummler, 1894), 2: 455–460; Kathryn M. Olesko, *Physics as a Calling. Discipline and Profession in the Königsberg Seminar for Physics* (in press), pt. IV.

26. "Reglement für das Seminar für Romanische und Englische Philologie an der Universität zu Breslau," *Centralblatt für die gesammte Unterrichtsverwaltung in Preußen* 18 (1876): 359–360; on 359.

27. "Reglement für das historische Seminar an der Königlichen Universität zu Kiel," in ibid., 24 (1882): 533.

28. Lenz, *Universität zu Berlin*, 3: 234.

29. Ibid., 3: 239, 244. On Germany's social imperialism, see Hans-Ulrich Wehler, *Das Deutsche Kaiserreich, 1871–1918*, 3d ed. (Göttingen: Vandenhoeck & Ruprecht, 1977), pp. 172–176.

30. Several of the issues concerning the Prussian seminar system only touched upon here are discussed in greater detail in Olesko, *Physics as a Calling*, Introduction. That the ideal of *Bildung* was not realized in practice and was challenged from several segments of Germany's educational systems has been commented upon by Grafton, "Polyhistor into *Philolog;*" Albisetti, *Secondary School Reform;* Jarausch, *Students, Society, and Politics;* and others.

31. See, e.g., Turner, "The Growth of Professorial Research in Prussia," pp. 148–149. The differences between seminars and institutes are obscured somewhat by a common German archival practice to catalogue seminars as institutes. Although it is true that seminars were one type among many of university institutes, they were nonetheless qualitatively and quantitatively different from laboratory-based natural science institutes.

32. Professor Wilhelm Weber to Colonel Sabine, 20 February 1845, in *Wilhelm Eduard Webers Werke*, ed. Königliche Gesellschaft der Wissenschaften zu Göttingen, 6 vols. (Berlin: Springer, 1892–1894), 2: 274–276; C. F. Gauss, "Die neue Einrichtung des mathematisch-physikalischen Instituts in Marburg," in *C. F. Gauss' Werke*, ed. Königliche Gesellschaft der Wissenschaften zu Göttingen, 6 vols. (Göttingen: Kgl. Gesellschaft der Wissenschaften, 1870–1877), 5: 596–598; Stichweh, *Physik in Deutschland*, pp. 381–382.

33. See, e.g., Paul Forman, John L. Heilbron, and Spencer Weart, "Physics circa 1900. Personnel, Funding, and Productivity of the Academic Establishments," *Historical Studies in the Physical Sciences* 5 (1975): 1–185; David Cahan, "The Institutional Revolution in German Physics, 1865–1914," in ibid. 15, pt. 2 (1985): 1–65; Meinel, *Die Chemie an der Universität Marburg*.

34. See, e.g., Gert Schubring, "The Rise and Decline of the Bonn Natur-

wissenschaften Seminar: Conflicts between Teacher Education and Disciplinary Differentiation"(unpublished manuscript, 1986).

35. Ludwik Fleck, *Genesis and Development of a Scientific Fact*, trans. Fred Bradley and Thaddeus J. Trenn (Chicago: University of Chicago Press, 1979).

36. Joseph Ben-David, "Organization, Social Control, and Cognitive Change in Science," in *Culture and Its Creators. Essays in Honor of Edward Shils*, ed. J. Ben-David and T. N. Clark (Chicago: University of Chicago Press, 1977), pp. 244–265; on 254; cf. Ben-David, *Scientist's Role*, pp. 108, 123–124. The ambiguity in Ben-David's discussion of the function of university institutes is a sign, I believe, of his attempt to reconcile contradictory evidence concerning them. While he did speak of institutes primarily in terms of their research function, and hence in terms of their role in training scientific elites, he also acknowledged that "the development of laboratory research at the universities occurred by default," having evolved from institutes such as "teaching laboratories in chemistry (established mainly for training pharmacists) and physiology (created for training doctors)." According to Ben-David, these "turned into research laboratories" when "a few of the able students conducted original research under the guidance of a professor" (Ben-David, "Organization, Social Control, and Cognitive Change," p. 255). Although several authors in this volume argue that for the case of physiology the training of elites in laboratory methods preceded the training of the "rank-and file," Ben-David's observation suggests that at least some of the rank-and-file were present among the student clientele of laboratory courses from the beginning and that they were trained in the methods of science. A heterogeneous student clientele was also found in at least two other university institutes: Liebig's chemical laboratory at Giessen and Wilhelm Weber's mathematico-physical seminar at Göttingen. The question of the constitution of student clienteles in laboratory instruction may turn out to be less a matter of a transformation from elite to rank-and-file clienteles than of a transition from *elective* (or private) courses to *required* (or public) ones for medical students or for those who, in modern terms, wished to major in a science. That early exercise sessions, seminars, and laboratory courses were electives did not necessarily mean that "non-elite" students did not attend them. The presence of rank-and-file students in early laboratory courses would not diminish the interpretations presented in this volume but would enhance them by reorienting them more directly toward an understanding of the origin of an important part of the modern science curriculum, the laboratory course. Cf. R. Steven Turner, "Justus Liebig versus Prussian Chemistry: Reflections on Early Institute-Building in Germany," *Historical Studies in the Physical Sciences* 13, pt. 1 (1982): 129–162; on 158.

37. Thomas S. Kuhn, *The Structure of Scientific Revolutions*, 2d ed. (Chicago: University of Chicago Press, 1970); Michael Polyani, *Personal Knowledge* (London: Routledge & Kegan Paul, 1958); Jerome Ravetz, *Scientific Knowledge and Its Social Problems* (New York: Oxford University Press, 1971), pp. 75–108.

38. Jarausch, "The Old 'New History of Education,' " p. 235.

39. *Göttingische Gelehrte Anzeigen. Nachrichten von der Georg-Augusts Universität und der Kgl. Gesellschaft zu Wissenschaften zu Göttingen*, no. 6 (11 March 1850), pp. 73–79; on 73. Complementing the curricular development in separate sciences was the rigid curriculum of the Bonn seminar for the natural sciences which in principle required students to take a wide variety of scientific subjects, thus providing a general education in all of the sciences. "Reglement für das Seminarium für die gesammten Naturwissenschaften [Bonn Universität]. Vom 3. Mai 1825," in Koch, *Die preußischen Universitäten*, 2.2: 624–630.

40. Olesko, *Physics as a Calling*, pts. II and III.

41. J. E. Purkyně, "Über den Begriff der Physiologie, ihre Beziehung zu den übrigen Naturwissenschaften, und zu andern wissenschaftlichen und Kunst-Gebieten, die Methoden ihrer Lehre und Praxis, über die Bildung zum Physiologen, über Errichtung physiologischer Institute" (Rede, gehalten bei der Eröffnung des physiologischen Institutes zu Prag am 6. October 1851), in *Opera Omnia/Sebrané Spisy*, ed. V. Kruta and B. Eberhardova, 12 vols. (Prague: Czechoslovakian Academy of Sciences, 1918–1973), 3: 64–79; on 77.

42. Otto Frank, "Das Physiologische Institut und die Physiologische Sammlung," in *Die wissenschaftlichen Anstalten der Ludwig-Maximilians-Universität zu München. Chronik zur Jahrhundertfeier*, ed. Karl Alexander von Müller (München: Oldenbourg, Wolf & Sohn, 1926), pp. 233–237; on 233.

43. Stichweh, *Physik in Deutschland*, pp. 346–351.

44. Lothar Meyer, *Über akademische Lernfreiheit* (Breslau: Schottlaender, n.d.), p. 3.

45. *Vierter Bericht über das naturwissenschaftliche Seminar bei der Universität zu Königsberg [1838–1839]* (Königsberg: Hartung, 1839), p. 33. The needs of medical students were considered in early discussions concerning the establishment of the Bonn seminar in the natural sciences. In addition, the directors of that seminar requested, in their report for 1826–1827, three microscopes, all equipped with micrometric apparatus and all for student use, because they felt that they could not continue to use their own microscopes and because they believed that "many of the most recent physiological discoveries require not only the greatest possible magnification, but also the most accurate microscopic measurements." Acta betreffend die Einrichtung eines Seminars für die naturwissenschaftlichen Studien auf der Universität Bonn, Rep. 76Va Sekt. 3 Tit. X Nr. 4 Bd. I: 1823–1831. Zentrales Staatsarchiv, Merseburg, pp. 96, 138, 168; on 138.

46. Thomas S. Kuhn, "The Function of Measurement in Modern Physical Science," in *The Essential Tension. Selected Studies in Scientific Tradition and Change* (Chicago: University of Chicago Press, 1977), pp. 178–224; on 186. Fleck, *Scientific Fact*, pp. 112, 161.

47. Emil du Bois-Reymond to Carl Ludwig, 17 February 1852, 1 October 1855, in *Two Great Scientists of the Nineteenth Century. Correspondence of Emil du Bois-Reymond and Carl Ludwig*, ed. Paul Cranefield (Baltimore: Johns Hopkins University Press, 1982), pp. 72, 90. Ludwig's textbook appeared as

Lehrbuch der Physiologie des Menschen, 2 vols. (Heidelberg: C. F. Winter, 1852–1856).

48. John Harley Warner, *The Therapeutic Perspective: Medical Practice, Knowledge and Identity in America, 1820–1885* (Cambridge, Mass.: Harvard University Press, 1986), p. 346.

49. Fleck, *Scientific Fact*, p. 35.

50. Justus Liebig, *Anleitung zur Analyse organischer Körper* (Braunschweig: F. Vieweg & Sohn, 1837); Friedrich Kohlrausch, *Leitfaden der praktischen Physik* (Leipzig: B. G. Teubner, 1870).

51. This discussion of "first papers" was based upon a thorough study of the papers published by the graduates of the Königsberg mathematico-physical seminar and, to a lesser extent, upon a general familiarity with student papers issuing from the Bonn and Königsberg natural sciences seminars, Magnus's laboratory at Berlin, and Weber's mathematico-physical seminar at Göttingen. Although papers issuing directly from the more mature and sophisticated scientific institutes that appeared after 1860 displayed these traits to a lesser degree, they nonetheless show some signs of the teaching activity of the institute in question. Cf. *Arbeiten aus der Physiologischen Anstalt zu Leipzig. Dritter Jahrgang [1868]*, mitgetheilt durch Carl Friedrich Wilhelm Ludwig (Leipzig: Hirzel, 1869). Of the seven papers in this volume, two were coauthored by Ludwig.

52. Carl Theodor Anger, "Grundzüge der neueren astronomischen Beobachtungs-Kunst," in *Programm. Städtische Gymnasium, Danzig 1846–1847*, p. 16.

53. The phrase "Physiker von Beruf" was used by Franz Neumann. See his undated essay [1876] on the necessity of a physical laboratory at Königsberg, 61.7 Kampf um das Laboratorium, Franz Neumann Nachlaß, Handschriftenabteilung, Staats- and Universitätsbibliothek Göttingen; reprinted with alterations in Luise Neumann, *Franz Neumann. Erinnerungsblätter von seiner Töchter* (Tübingen and Leipzig: Mohr, 1904), pp. 455–456; on 456. Hermann Kolbe called his more serious laboratory students at Marburg "Chemiker vom Fach" in the 1850s. Turner, "Liebig versus Prussian Chemistry," p. 159.

54. R. Steven Turner, "The *Bildungsbürgertum* and the Learned Professions in Prussia: The Origins of a Class," *Histoire Sociale–Social History* 13 (1980): 105–135.

55. Peter B. Medawar, "Lucky Jim," in *The Double Helix*, Norton Critical Edition (New York: W. W. Norton & Co., 1980), pp. 218–224; on 222.

56. Charles Rosenberg, "Toward an Ecology of Knowledge: On Discipline, Context and History," in *The Organization of Knowledge in America, 1860–1920*, ed. Alexandra Oleson and John Voss (Baltimore: Johns Hopkins University Press, 1979), pp. 440–455; on 444.

57. The requirements that had to be satisfied by clinical instruments, as described by Frank, also parallel those that had to be fulfilled by scientific instruments when used by technicians. See, e.g., Oskar Frölich, "Über Messung starker elektrischer Ströme," *Electrotechnische Zeitschrift* 1 (1880): 197–202; on 198–199.

58. Ben-David, "Organization, Social Control, and Cognitive Change," p. 260.

59. McClelland, "Structural Change," p. 186. In Prussia a period of conservatism emerged on university campuses after the assassination of the political activist Karl Sand in 1819 and the subsequent issuance of the Karlsbad Decrees. Societies dedicated to scholarship were often suppressed or censored by the Prussian government in an effort to control what remained of the *Burschenschaften*.

60. Turner, "The *Bildungsbürgertum* and the Learned Professions," pp. 113, 119, 123; idem, "The Prussian Professoriate and the Research Imperative," in *Epistemological and Social Problems*, pp. 109–121; on 117.

61. Turner, "The *Bildungsbürgertum* and the Learned Professions," pp. 117–120; Simmer, "Medical Undergraduate Education in Germany," p. 192. In Baden, by contrast, physicians could practice without a medical degree provided they passed the state examination.

62. Among recent regional studies of German industrialization are the works of Hubert Kiesewetter, "Erklärungshypothesen zur regionalen Industrialisierung in Deutschland im 19. Jahrhundert," *Vierteljahrschrift für Sozial- und Wirtschaftsgeschichte* 67, no. 3 (1980): 306–333; idem, "Regionale Industrialisierung in Deutschland im 19. Jahrhundert," *Archiv und Wirtschaft* 16, no. 4 (1983): 135–137; idem, "Industrialisierung und Landwirtschaft. Sachsens Stellung im regionalen Industrialisierungsprozeß Deutschlands im 19. Jahrhundert" (Habilitationsschrift, Freie Universität Berlin, 1984). The problematic nature of linking educational curricula and reform to economic change is mentioned by Robert Fox and Anna Guagnini, "Education and Industry. Some Problems and Perspectives," *Lettre d'information/Newsletter* (Education and Industry/Education et industrie), no. 1 (Summer/Fall 1986): 5–8; on 6. It also might be possible to view state interest in the reform of medical instruction and in the certification of physicians in terms of what Michel Foucault called the medicalization of society, which included steps taken by the state to increase its power by monitoring the health of the body politic. Michel Foucault, "The Politics of Health in the Eighteenth Century," in *Power/Knowledge. Selected Interviews and Other Writings, 1972–1977,* ed. Colin Gordon (New York: Pantheon Books, 1972), pp. 166–182.

63. Max Weber, "Science as a Vocation," in *From Max Weber. Essays in Sociology,* ed. H. H. Gerth and C. Wright Mills (New York: Oxford University Press, 1946), pp. 129–156; Jürgen Habermas, "Technology and Science as Ideology," in *Toward a Rational Society. Student Protest, Science and Politics,* trans. Jeremy J. Shapiro (Boston: Beacon Press, 1971), pp. 81–122; Jean–François Lyotard, *The Postmodern Condition: A Report on Knowledge,* Theory and History of Literature, vol. 10 (Minneapolis: University of Minnesota Press, 1984), esp. pp. 41–52.

Index

Designer: U.C. Press Staff
Compositor: Huron Valley Graphics, Inc.
Text: 10/13 Palatino
Display: Palatino
Printer: Braun-Brumfield, Inc.
Binder: Braun-Brumfield, Inc.